KORO
Epidemics in India

KORO
Epidemics in India

Indian Psychiatric Society Publication

Editor

Arabinda N Chowdhury

MBBS MD PhD FAMS FRCPsych PhD (Soc Anthrop) DSc Psychoanalyst

Consultant Psychiatrist

Child and Adolescent Mental Health Services (CAMHS)

Lancashire & South Cumbria NHS Foundation Trust

Preston, UK

Former Professor and Head

Department of Psychiatry

Institute of Postgraduate Medical Education and Research, Kolkata

Superintendent

Institute of Psychiatry

Kolkata, West Bengal, India

Foreword

Kamaldeep Bhui

JAYPEE

JAYPEE BROTHERS MEDICAL PUBLISHERS

The Health Sciences Publisher

New Delhi | London

Jaypee Brothers Medical Publishers (P) Ltd.

Headquarters
Jaypee Brothers Medical Publishers (P) Ltd
EMCA House, 23/23-B
Ansari Road, Daryaganj
New Delhi 110 002, India
Landline: +91-11-23272143, +91-11-23272703
+91-11-23282021, +91-11-23245672
Email: jaypee@jaypeebrothers.com

Corporate Office
Jaypee Brothers Medical Publishers (P) Ltd
4838/24, Ansari Road, Daryaganj
New Delhi 110 002, India
Phone: +91-11-43574357
Fax: +91-11-43574314
Email: jaypee@jaypeebrothers.com

Overseas Office
JP Medical Ltd.
83, Victoria Street, London
SW1H 0HW (UK)
Phone: +44 20 3170 8910
Fax: +44 (0)20 3008 6180
Email: info@jpmedpub.com

Website: www.jaypeebrothers.com
Website: www.jaypeedigital.com

Inquiries for bulk sales may be solicited at: jaypee@jaypeebrothers.com

Koro Epidemics in India

First Edition: **2024**

ISBN: 978-93-5696-221-7

Printed in India

Dedicated to
All the Koro researchers of the world

Contributors

Amitava Dan MD
Associate Professor
Department of Psychiatry
Burdwan Medical College
Bardhaman, West Bengal, India

Arabinda Brahma DNB PhD
Director
GS Bose Clinic
Hon. Lecturer
Indian Psychoanalytical Society
Kolkata, West Bengal, India

Arabinda N Chowdhury MBBS MD PhD FAMS FRCPsych PhD (Soc Anthrop) DSc Psychoanalyst
Consultant Psychiatrist
Child and Adolescent Mental Health Services (CAMHS)
Lancashire & South Cumbria NHS Foundation Trust
Preston, UK
Former Professor and Head
Department of Psychiatry
Institute of Postgraduate Medical Education and Research, Kolkata
Superintendent
Institute of Psychiatry
Kolkata, West Bengal, India

BK Bhowmic MD
Senior Consultant Psychiatrist
Modern Psychiatry Hospital
Singarbil, Tripura, India

Debjit Misra
Post Graduate Trainee
Department of Psychiatry
Burdwan Medical College
Bardhaman, West Bengal, India

Dipayan Sarkar DPM
Senior Consultant Psychiatrist
Modern Psychiatry Hospital
Singarbil, Tripura, India

Hemendraram Phookun MD
Ex-Professor and Head
Department of Psychiatry
Guwahati Medical College
Guwahati, Assam, India

JM Ghosh DPM
Senior Consultant Psychiatrist
Modern Psychiatry Hospital
Singarbil, Tripura, India

Kunjappan Promodu
MA MPhil & SP PhD
Consultant Clinical Psychologist and Sex Therapist
Dr Promodu's Institute of Sexual & Marital Health Pvt Ltd
Kochi, Kerala, India

Monali Chowdhury PhD
Associate Professor
Department of Psychology
Allegheny College
Pennsylvania, USA

Sakal Kumar Gupta MD
Senior Consultant Psychiatrist
Modern Psychiatry Hospital
Singarbil, Tripura, India

Saswati Nath MD
Professor and Head
Department of Psychiatry
Bankura Sammilani Medical College and Hospital
Bankura, West Bengal, India

Sayanti Ghosh MD
Associate Professor
Department of Psychiatry
NRS Medical College and Hospital
Kolkata, West Bengal, India

Indian Psychiatry Society

(Plot 43, Sector 55, Gurugram, Haryana 122003)

Human emotions and their morbidities have been nearly the same since antiquity, but it has been noticed and documented as well that their expressions change with time. These changes are mainly duc to milieu exterior which has two main components—environmental and sociocultural. We appreciate the extensive and deep research in biological psychiatry but cannot ignore the role of sociocultural components which not only are integral to the human mind but also closely and interactively circumvent it. It is heartening to see that the enthusiasm for the study of sociocultural factors has not been dampened in this biological psychiatry era. We congratulate the researchers who identified and documented the epidemic presence of culture-bound syndrome, Koro in India. We especially congratulate Professor Arabinda N Chowdhury for his research, sense of timing and editorial capabilities.

Since 2016, the Indian Psychiatric Society is in publishing field, and it gives us satisfaction that we have refrained from publishing just another book in the market. We have always tried to publish something which is not only unique but also needed. "Koro Epidemics in India" is also unique because it is first of its kind and has enough material to update us on this culture-bound conundrum.

The Indian Psychiatric Society is thankful to Professor Arabinda N Chowdhury and all the contributors for their hard work. We thank the publication committee led by Professor Anil Kakunje for pubishing one more unique book. We thank Shri Jitendar P Vij (Group Chairman), Mr Ankit Vij (Managing Director), Mr MS Mani (Group President), Ms Chetna Malhotra (Senior Director—Professional Publishing, Marketing, and Business Development), and Ms Manpreet Kaur (Development Editor) of M/s Jaypee Brothers Medical Publishers (P) Ltd, New Delhi, India, for beautiful production.

Long Live IPS!

Vinay Kumar
President, IPS

Lakshmikanth Rathi
Vice President

Arabinda Brahma
Hony Secretary, IPS

Message from the Publication Committee

It is a matter of great pleasure to write a message for a unique book on Koro which is a culture-bound/related disorder.

It is heartening to see IPS coming up with a lot of books in Psychiatry; it is not just textbooks but books on many specialty topics and niche areas. There is a need to get in-depth knowledge of each illness with special emphasis to Indian context; not only for students but also for all mental health professionals and researchers.

Psychiatry is now not limited to treating mainly severe mental illness in mental hospitals. Psychiatrists now handle varied illness and many are related to culture, region, beliefs and so on. I feel glad to highlight that this unique book on Koro covers every aspect of this disorder in great detail covering history to current scenario.

The author Arabinda N Chowdhury has put in real hard work to make this book a reality. The cover page photo was personally designed by him and it was his idea to have a photo related to the illness itself. The publication committee congratulates him for editing this book.

I on behalf of the publication committee thank the IPS office bearers for their continued support and cooperation. I also thank M/s Jaypee Brothers Medical Publishers (P) Ltd, New Delhi, India for their efforts. I am sure this book will be a hugely popular and will be 'the' book to read on Koro.

Long Live IPS!

Anil Kakunje DPM MD
Professor and Head
Department of Psychiatry
Yenepoya Medical College
Yenepoya Deemed to be University
Mangaluru, Karnataka, India
Chairman, IPS Publication Committee
anilpsychiatry@yahoo.co.in

Mrugesh Vaishnav
Advisor

Sai Krishna Tikka
Co-Chairperson

Shahul Ameen
EC Representative

Snehil Gupta
Convener

Foreword

Professor Arabinda N Chowdhury is the world expert on Koro syndromes, a collection of expressions of distress including a fear of penile shrinking, accompanied by anxiety, a fear of dying, and taking measures to prevent such occurrences. The syndrome is often presented in textbooks as a culture-bound syndrome, as if restricted to specific cultural groups and as if the presentations were bizarre and beyond comprehension, exotic even. This impressive volume dispels those myths and presents important reflections in a humane and thoughtful manner, enabling readers to appreciate the cultural contexts within which the syndrome manifests, and the distress of those afflicted. The authors show a range of presentations with case studies from India, alongside a historical and wider geographical syntheses of where and how Koro presents. For example, there is comparison with syndromes in China, Malaysia, and Indonesia to those in India. Detailed case studies and research studies are provided by a number of scholars from India, including drawings and schematics and photographs to illustrate cultural and cognitive elaborations of physiological processes to form the syndrome in diverse ways across the continent. The authors present explanations for how epidemics of fear and cognitions recognizable as Koro spread as infectious ideas and fears in rural and urban settings. There are also examples of female correlates of Koro, and tracing of expressions of distress to reflect common folk beliefs of health and illness, including humoral theories of hot and cold influences on health status. We must thank Professor Arabinda N Chowdhury for this Herculean effort. He has dedicated his life to the study of this syndrome, in all its manifestations, with and without co-occurring mental illnesses, and shows how to approach classification and therapeutic efforts. There are nostalgic pictures of scholars at scientific gatherings, through which one can sense the intense debate around complex presentations. The Indian Psychiatric Society does a great service publishing and preserving these intriguing collection of studies as the foundation for future research and education. A delightful read and thought provoking with lessons for clinicians, those training to become health professionals, for social and cultural scientists, and Indian scholars.

Kamaldeep Bhui
CBE MD FRCPsych FRCP(E) FRSA PFHEA
Professor of Psychiatry
Department of Psychiatry and Nuffield
Department of Primary Care Health Sciences Medical Sciences Division
University of Oxford
Editor in Chief, British Journal of Psychiatry
Director, Synergi Collaborative Centre
Director, World Psychiatric Association Collaborating Centre, UK
Hon. Professor of Psychiatry, QMUL
Hon. Consultant Psychiatrist, East London NHS Trust

Preface

India is now becoming a Koro-prone country like Guangdong of South China. Since 1982, India has experienced at least 12 Koro epidemics involving states like West Bengal, Assam, Tripura, Kerala, Karnataka, and the city of Mumbai. A handful of sporadic Koro cases reporting appeared from different parts of India as well. Psychiatric epidemics are comparatively rare, and Koro epidemics occupy a unique position because of their genital focus and unusual clinical presentations. Koro is usually referred to as a culture-bound syndrome. So, the study of Koro epidemics not only help to develop insight into its phenomenology, but also sheds important light on the sociocultural and ethnic specificity of the concerned regions. Global comparison of Koro epidemics also enriches our transcultural understanding of the phenomenon. This book will serve as a reference document in the global Koro literature.

Moreover, Koro is not a research issue only for mental health professionals. It is also a widely clinical topic of interest to cultural psychiatry, anthropology, medical sociology, and psychosexual medicine. With this aim in view, this book was intended to accumulate different Indian Koro epidemic studies done by eminent academicians and researchers. Their intense study unfolded many new avenues of phenomenological thoughts on Koro in particular and mental epidemics and details of sociocultural dimensions and mechanisms of spread, in general.

This book contains the reports of major Koro epidemics from West Bengal (four accounts), Assam (three accounts), Mumbai, Tripura (one account) and Kerala (one account). It is known that there was an epidemic in Orissa, but there is no published literature yet. Some published reports on the contemporary Koro epidemics (Assam, West Bengal, Mumbai, Tripura, and Bengaluru) are also abstracted by me. I also added a short state description of West Bengal, Assam, Tripura and South India at the beginning of respective state Koro epidemic reports. I am deeply indebted to all the contributors for their excellent presentation of their Koro epidemic research. All the reports meticulously highlighted the sociocultural aspects and modes of the spread of epidemic waves. This research document also helps draw transcultural comparisons with other global Koro epidemics. I hope all researchers in this field will be immensely benefited from these very intensive studies of the Koro epidemics.

I am expressing my sincere thanks to my Indian colleagues, Professor Prakash B Behere, Emeritus Professor of Psychiatry, Jawaharlal Nehru Medical College, Wardha, and Professor Purna Dhar Das, former Head, Department of Psychiatry, Guwahati Medical College, Assam, for their help in this endeavor.

I am deeply indebted to all the contributors for their excellent efforts to make this publication a landmark in the arena of cultural psychiatry.

I am also highly thankful to Dr Kamaldeep Bhui, Professor of Psychiatry, University of Oxford and Editor-in-Chief, British Journal of Psychiatry, for writing the Foreword and to Dr Fabida Aria, Consultant Psychiatrist, and Medical Director, Birmingham and Solihull Mental Health Foundation NHS Trust; and Chair, Transcultural Psychiatry Group, and Specialist Advisor for Medical Trainee Initiative Scheme, Royal College of Psychiatrists, London, for introducing the book.

My sincere gratitude and thanks to Dr Arabinda Brahma, Hon. Secretary, Indian Psychiatric Society and Dr Anil Kakunje, Chairperson of the IPS Publication Committee for accepting this manuscript and enriching the global Koro literature with the first book on Koro epidemic.

30 April, 2023

Arabinda N Chowdhury
Kettering, United Kingdom

Contents

Introduction

It is an honor to introduce this book that has provided an extensive report of Koro epidemics in India in such a detailed and informative way, which will help those reading about Koro for the first time, and also experienced researchers and clinicians. As we know psychiatric epidemics are quite rare, and though there are reports in the literature on mass psychogenic illness and hysterical epidemics in schools and/or in closed communities; to have an extensive compilation for Koro epidemics across several decades across India with excellent detail is a commendable achievement by Professor Arabinda N Chowdhury.

In a hugely populated country like India, Professor Arabinda N Chowdhury has described Koro epidemics effectivity among rural, urban, and cosmopolitan population groups. The book is rich in both the length of time between the first and last epidemic, and covers reports from various parts of India including the West (Mumbai) to East (Assam) of India and also from North (Darjeeling) to South (Kerala) of India. This book documents different aspect of Koro epidemics and a model of spread along with demography of Koro-affected people. This book provides a strong and valuable base for transcultural comparison among Indian, Chinese, Indonesian, Thai, and Singapore Koro epidemics.

It is really interesting to read all the clinical materials provided by different Indian researchers and will provide as extremely valuable data to all those involved in cross-cultural and psychosexual research projects. In addition to his first published book on clinical and historical developments of Koro, this is the first book on Koro epidemics in India. As a world expert on this topic, Professor Arabinda N Chowdhury has done an excellent contribution to psychiatry. The Indian Psychiatric Society has done a very praiseworthy job by publishing this book for the mental health and psychosocial academia of the world. The readers will get a deep insight with this fascinating account of Koro epidemics in India.

Fabida Aria
MBBS FRCPsych MSc
Consultant Psychiatrist and Medical Director
Birmingham and Solihull Mental Health Foundation NHS Trust, UK
Chair, Transcultural Psychiatry Group
Specialist Advisor, Medical Trainee Initiative Scheme
Royal College of Psychiatrists, London, UK

Chapter 1

Introduction: The Universe of Koro

Arabinda N Chowdhury

INTRODUCTION

Koro is a Malay term, and in Chinese, it is called *Shook yang* or *Suo yang*. Historically, Koro is a culture-bound syndrome (CBS), mainly found in southern China.[1] It is also reported from other Southeast Asian countries where the south Chinese people have migrated, viz., Malaysia, Indonesia, Thailand, and Singapore.[2,3] A Dutch physician, Dr JC Blonk, in 1895, first introduced the term "Koro" and its clinical features to the Western medical press from Nederlandsch-Indie (now Indonesia).[4] It was reported that the disease was indigenous to the southern Sulawesi people. Koro illness has a long historical track record in China from 476 to 221 BC.[5,6] Most recent Chinese reference is Pao Sian-Ow, a traditional Chinese physician. His treatise "New Collection of Remedies of Value", published in 1834, described the genital retraction disorder during intercourse.[7] Koro was known as a CBS in the literature from the 1960s.[8] Then two radical changes have taken place in its nosology. The first one was the renaming of Koro as Genital Retraction Syndrome (GRS) in 1984.[9] There was a shift in the conceptual framework of CBSs from culture-bound to culture-related disorders in 2006.[10] So the DSM-5 (Diagnostic and Statistical Manual of Mental Disorders, Fifth Edition) in 2013 pruned Koro's long association with "culture-boundness" and Koro was placed under the category of "Other specified Obsessive-Compulsive and Related Disorders" (ORCD) with a diagnostic code-300.3.[11]

Koro epidemic is reported in recent history from China in 1908 among teenage school students in Szechwan.[12] Later in the 19th Century, China and India were marked as "Koro-prone" countries.[13,14] Guangdong, a coastal province in South China, has evidenced a series of Koro epidemics almost every year since 1984.[15,16] Similarly, in India **(Fig. 1)**, at least 12 epidemics have involved many states since 1982. From 1981, Koro started appearing by name in the Indian medical press with increasing frequency, especially after the 1982 Koro epidemic in India's North-Eastern states. Since 1982, there have been at least four epidemics in West Bengal, two in Assam, three in Tripura, one in Mumbai, and two in South India. In India, the first Koro case was reported from Jhansi (Uttar Pradesh state), in 1981[17] and the second case

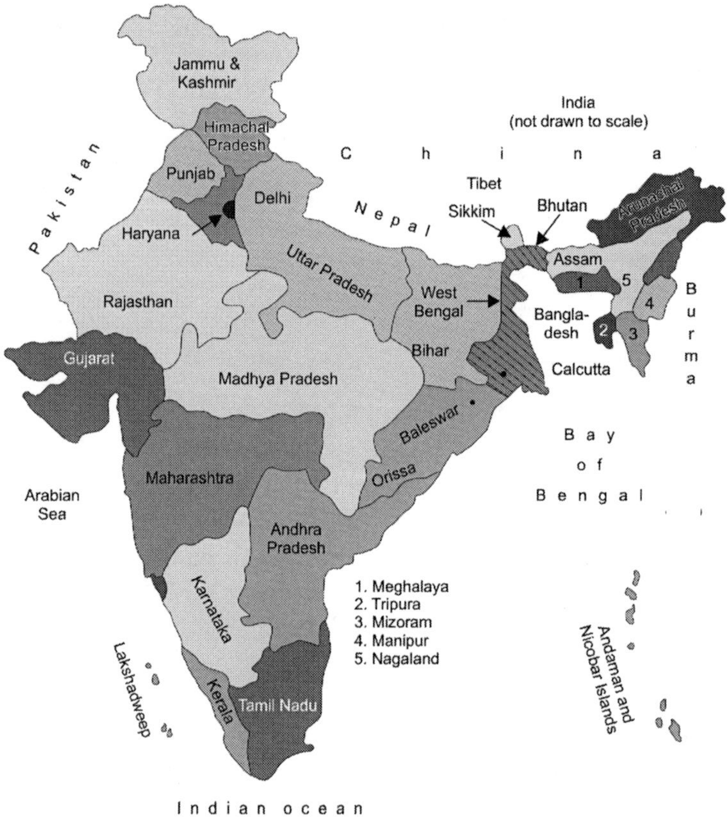

Fig. 1: Map of India (in 1982), not to scale.

was from Ahmedabad (Gujarat State), 1982.[18] It is interesting to note that in Mumbai and South India epidemic, the index cases were (migrant workers) from Northeastern Indian states such as West Bengal, Assam, and Orissa. Interestingly, none of these researchers found any Chinese or Indonesian contact or context in these Indian epidemics. How this disease landed on the Indian soil in the North-Eastern region is still a mystery!

Following is a brief discussion that will address the clinical picture of Koro along with a short note on its different local names used in India and the global distribution of Koro epidemics, including India.

CLINICAL FEATURES

Koro is a culturally related psychogenic syndrome, clinically characterized by acute panic reaction concerning the perception of genital shrinkage or retraction and fear of impending death. In the male, the cardinal feature is shrinking or retracting of the penis and testes into the abdomen. In the female, shrinkage of vulval labia into the belly and/or nipple or breast into the chest cavity is the predominant presentation.[19]

The symptom manifestations have four distinct features: (1) *Cognitive (Perceptual):* perception of shrinkage and, or retraction of the penis/testes (or nipple and or labia) due to an intra-abdominal (or intrathoracic) pull; (2) *Psychological:* fear of impending death (or sexual disability) out of this penile (or breast and or labial) involution or dissolution; (3) *Emotional:* there are accompanying symptoms of an intense panic reaction with feelings of collapse, palpitations, sweating, nausea, breathlessness, visual blurring, body spasms, pain and paresthesia, and (4) *Behavioral:* patients' (or others') idiosyncratic remedial measures or maneuvers to prevent the apparent disappearance of the penis or vulva into the abdominal cavity or the breast into the chest. This last component may be prone to penile or nipple injury or other health hazards as a complication.

DIFFERENT CLINICAL PRESENTATION OF KORO

Over the years, the various clinical presentations of Koro have been reported. The typical clinical presentation described above is usually referred to in the literature as *Classical Koro*. A partial clinical presentation (only perception of penile pull with or without fear of death but with other fears, is often described as *Koro-like symptoms (KLS)*.[20,21] Some authors preferred to label these presentations as complete or incomplete Koro.[22,23] When Koro is the only clinical presentation, it is often referred to as *Primary Koro*. When Koro is associated with other medical, psychiatric, neurological, or urological diseases or drug abuse, they are called *Secondary Koro*.[19] Perception of penile retraction in the background with paranoid ideas or schizophrenic illness is often referred to as "Koro delusion."[24] It is also important to note that the conceptual component of accompanied panic or Koro anxiety is the "fear of death." But many reports also identified other ideational contents such as fear of infertility, fear of sexual disability or impotence, fear of sex change, fear of insanity, fear of loss of penis, or fear of loss of childbearing capacity (in females). It is also a point of concern in the differential diagnosis of Koro (both in sporadic or epidemic cases) to review carefully the genitally focused obsessive-compulsive disorder (OCD)—preoccupation or hypochondriacal genital health concern of the subject. Association of drug abuse (especially cannabis, amphetamine, and heroin) with Koro perception should constantly be screened.[6] Recurrent Koro, though usually rare, may be encountered in sporadic or epidemic settings.[25]

CULTURAL BACKGROUND OR ETHNOMEDICAL PERCEPTION

Koro always occurs against the backdrop of sociocultural beliefs and myths. There are ample examples in the literature where a particular traditional idea or social or folk construct acts as a triggering factor and helps the spread of Koro. Historical records in Chinese medical classics stressed that improper sex or intercourse during physical illness might precipitate a solitary Koro attack.[26] In epidemic cases, the myth of the female fox-spirit cult (*Huli Jing*) is implicated, who in a desperate attempt to steal male penises.[27] In India, "excessive body heat" is involved in the retraction of the penis.[28] Supernatural cause or black magic is also implicated in some Indian Koro epidemic patients.[29] Cultural vulnerability enhances the number of people affected in a particular community and accelerates its spread in the locality.[30]

Koro and tortoise: Gwee[31] traced several Malay lexical terms as a possible origins for the disease name, e.g., *Kuru, Kerukul, Keroh,* and *Keruk.* In Malay and Indonesian dialects, the tortoise is known by *Kura* or *Kura-Kura.*[32] and in Macassarese by *Koero.*[33] Both the Malay and Chinese use the tortoise head symbolically for the glans penis, and coitus reservatus is linked in ancient Chinese writings to retracting a tortoise's head.[34,35] The similarity between the tortoise withdrawing head under its wrinkled neck and ultimately within the body **(Fig. 2)** with that done by the shrinking penis may have given rise to the term's folk-etymological expression *Kuro* or *Kura* and eventually by corruption to Koro.[36] Slot[33] reported many rituals regarding tortoise and Koro from his study of Macassares people of South Celebes of Dutch-Indies and noted that the illness might affect many people simultaneously. In China, belief in the fox spirit cult is associated with genital stealing in Koro epidemics.[37,38]

- **The different *ethnolinguistic* terms used to designate Koro illness in India**
  - *Jha-Jha:* Lower Assam
  - Jhinjhini Bemar in Guwahati, Assam, and Tripura
  - *Jhin-Jhinia:* Assam, and Jalpaiguri of North Bengal
  - *Beriberi:* Darjeeling district (Kharibari block) of West Bengal
  - *Kattaow (small tortoise/"cut off"):* Cooch-Bihar district of West Bengal

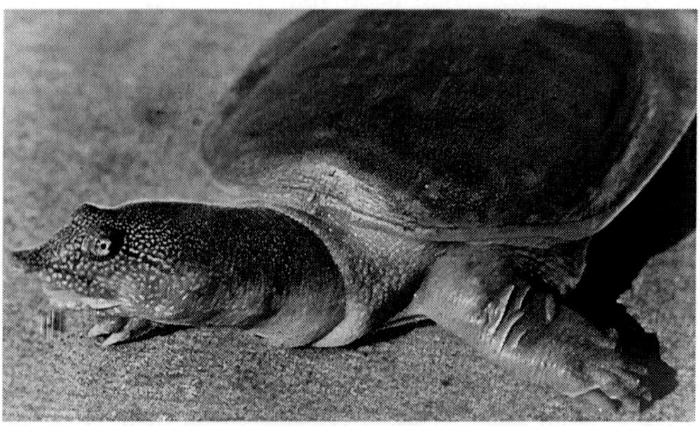

Fig. 2: Retracting head-neck of the tortoise.

- *Disco, Disco-fever:* South Bengal and Calcutta of West Bengal and Baleswar district of Orissa
- *Viral (Flu) disease:* West Bengal (South 24 Parganas district)

GLOBAL DISTRIBUTION OF KORO OR GENITAL RETRACTION EPIDEMICS

In an excellent historical review, Mo et al. (1995)[27] traced the Koro epidemic in different years since the 19th century in China's Guangdong region. That were from as early as 1862, 1864, and then in 1920, 1952, 1962, 1966, 1976, 1984, 1987, and 1988. All available references and cross-references show the following years as a reasonable chronology of global Koro epidemics.

1908: Koro epidemic in Szechwan, China[12]
1952: Suoyang epidemic in Guangdong, China
1955: Koro epidemic in Guangdong[3]
1962: Suoyang epidemic in Guangdong, China
1966: Suoyang epidemic in Guangdong, China[3]
1967: Singapore Koro epidemic[39,40]
1972: Koro epidemic in Thailand[41,42]
1974: Koro epidemic in Guangdong, China[3]
1975: Koro epidemic in Palembang, Indonesia[43]
1976: Koro epidemic in Thailand[44]
1979: Koro-like epidemic in Lagos, Nigeria, Africa[45]
1982: Koro epidemic in Thailand
1982: Koro epidemic in North-East India (Assam and West Bengal state)
1984–1985: Koro epidemic in Guangdong, China
1987: Koro epidemic in Guangdong, China
1988: Koro epidemic in Tripura, India
1988: Suoyang epidemic in Warring County, Hainan, Guangdong[46]
1992: A "magical penis loss" epidemic in Nigeria[47]*993*: A mini Koro epidemic in South 24 Parganas district of West Bengal, India.
1999: Koro epidemic in Ende city of Flores, Indonesia[48]
2010: Koro epidemic in India (West Bengal, Assam, Tripura, Mumbai, Kerala states).
2015: Koro epidemic in Tripura, India.

A NOTE OF CAUTION

Since the mid-1990s, some epidemics concerning "penis vanishing or genital theft" (breast/vagina vanishing also) were reported in West African nations: Ghana (in 1997), Senegal (1997), Benin (2001), Gambia (2003), Sudan (2003), Nigeria (2001–2010), Cameroon (2008), and Congo (2008). It is variously described in the literature as Koro-like or magical penis-loss[47] or "Vanishing Sexual/genital Organ Syndrome" (VSOS)[49] or as "Genital Shrinking Panic" (GSP) or Mass Psychogenic Illness[50] or "penis snatching phenomena."[51] In the strict nosological sense, they are not Koro but may be considered as a Koro variant or a form of genital neurosis (the core symptom being the penis).

REFERENCES

1. Yap PM. Koro or Suk-yeong: An atypical culture-bound psychiatric disorder found in Southern Chinese. Transcul Psychiatric Res Rev. 1994;1:36-8.
2. Rin H. A study of the aetiology of Koro in respect to the Chinese concept of illness. Int J Soc Psychiat. 1965;11:7-13.
3. Jilek WG. Epidemic of "Genital Shrinking" (Koro): Historical review and report of a recent outbreak in South China. Curare. 1986;9:269-82.
4. Blonk JC. Koro. Geneeskunding Tijaschrift voor. Nederlandsch-Indie. 1895;35:562-3.
5. Ng BY, Kua EEH. Koro in ancient Chinese history. Hist of Psychiat. 1996;7:563-70.
6. Chowdhury AN. Koro: Clinical and Historical Developments of the Culturally Defined Genital Retraction Disorder. Palgrave Macmillian. Switzerland: Springer Nature; 2021.
7. Gwee AL. Koro—A Cultural Disease. Singapore Medical J. 1963;4:119-22.
8. Chowdhury AN. Hundred years of Koro. Int J Soc Psychiat. 1998;44:182-9.
9. Edwards JW. Indigenous Koro: A genital retraction syndrome of insular Southeast Asia: A critical review. Cul Med Psychiat. 1984;8:1-24.
10. Tseng W-S. From peculiar psychiatric disorders through culture-bound syndromes to culture-related specific syndromes. Transcul Psychiat. 2006;43(4):554-76.
11. Diagnostic and Statistical Manual of Mental Disorders. 5th Edition. Arlington, USA: American Psychiatric Association; 2013.
12. Legendre J. Une curieuse epidemie. Annales de Med Coloniale. 1908;11(2):280-1.
13. Guangdong Transcultural Psychiatric Research Group. The koro epidemic in Hainan island (A preliminary report). Paper read at the Regional Conference of the World Psychiatric Association's Transcultural Psychiatry Section, Beijing, August 17-31, 1985.
14. Chowdhury AN. Koro and the Indian Psychiatrists. Ind J Soc Psychiat. 1995;11:78-80.
15. Tseng WS, Mo KM, Hsu J, Shuen LL, Wah OL, Qian CG, et al. A socio-cultural study of Koro epidemics in Guangdong China. Am J Psychiat. 1988;145:1538-43
16. Tseng WS, Mo KM, Li LS, Chen GQ, Qu LW, et al. Koro epidemics in Guangdong, China, A questionnaire survey. J Nerv Ment Dise. 1992;180:117-23.
17. Shukla GD, Mishra DN. Koro-like syndrome: A case report. Ind J Psychiat. 1981;23:96-7.
18. Chakrabarty PK. Koro: A peculiar anxiety neurosis (A Case Report). Ind J Psychiat. 1982;24:192-3.
19. Chowdhury AN. Definition and classification of Koro. Cul Med Psychiat. 1996;20:41-65.
20. Garlipp P. Koro—A culture-bound phenomenon: Intercultural psychiatric implications. Germ J Psychiat. 2008;11(1):21-8.

21. Chowdhury AN. Cultural Koro and Koro-like symptom (KLS). Germ J Psychiat. 2008;11:81-2.
22. Damodaran SS, Nizamie SH. "Incomplete Koro"—A forerunner for mood disorders: two case reports. Ind J Psychiat. 1993;35:60-2.
23. Panigrahi M, Padhy SK, Behere PB. Understanding and managing complete from sporadic koro syndrome associated with depression. J Postgrad Med Ed Res. 2012;46(2)104-5.
24. Kendell EM, Jenkins PL. Koro in an American man. American J Psychiatry. 1987;144;12:1621.
25. Chowdhury AN, Brahma A. Update on Koro research methodology. Ind J Psychiat. 2020;62(1):102-4.
26. Wong KC. An inquiry into some Chinese sexual diseases. Nat Medical J China. 1918;4:26-31.
27. Mo GM, Chen GQ, Li LX, Tseng WS. Koro epidemic in Southern China. In: Lin TY, Tseng WS, Yeh EK, (Eds). Chinese societies and mental health Hong Kong: Oxford University Press; 1995. pp. 231-43.
28. Chowdhury A. Ethnomedical concept of heat and cold in Koro: Study from Indian patients. World Cul Psychiat Res Rev. 2008;3:146-158.
29. Ghosh S, Nath S, Brahma A, Chowdhury AN. Fifth Koro epidemic in India: A review report. World Cul Psychiat Res Rev. 2013;8(1):8-20.
30. Chowdhury AN. Psychic infectivity: The role of positive illness cognition in psychiatric epidemic. J Personality Clin Stud. 1992;8:125-8.
31. Gwee AL. Koro—Its origin and nature as a disease entity. Singapore Medical J. 1968;9:3-6.
32. Wilkinson RL. A Malay-English Dictionary. Greece, Mytilene: Salavopoulos & Kinderlis; 1932.
33. Slot JA. Koro in Central Celebes. Geneeskundig Tijdschrift voor. Nederlandsch-Indie. 1935;75:811-20.
34. Rubin RT. Koro (Shook Yang): A Culture-bound Psychogenic Syndrome. In, Extraordinary Disorders of Human Behavior. In: C. T. H. Friedmann and R. A. Faguet (Eds.) New York: Plenum Press. 1982; pp. 155-172.
35. Chowdhury AN. Tortoise: A psycho-anthropological perspective. East Anthropol. 2003;56:51-9.
36. van GRH. Sexual Life in Ancient China. The Netherlands, Leiden: E. J. Brill; 1961.
37. Prince RH. Koro and the Fox Spirit on Hainan Island (China). Transcul Psychiatric Res Rev. 1992;29:119-32.
38. Chowdhury AN. Psychiatric morbidity and the fox connection. Transcul Psychiatric Res Rev. 1993;30(4):399-401.
39. Ngui PW. The Koro epidemic in Singapore. Aus N Z J Psychiat. 1969;3:263-6.
40. Gwee AL; Koro Study Team. The Koro epidemic in Singapore. Singapore Med J. 1969;10:234-42.
41. Suwanlert S. Koro epidemic in northeast Thailand. J Psychiatric Assoc Thailand. 1978;23(1):1-38.
42. Jilek W, Jilek-Aall LA. Koro epidemic in Thailand. Transcul Psychiatric Res Rev. 1977;14:57-9.
43. Moekti S, Denin SK. A non-rational dissemination of castration anxiety in Palembang, 1975. Paper presented at the First Asian Teaching Workshop on Mental Health and Culture, Jakarta, 1978. Personal Communication.

44. Suwanlert S, Coates D. Epidemic Koro in Thailand—Clinical and Social aspects. Transcul Psychiatric Res Rev. 1979;16:64-6.
45. Murphy HBM. Comparative Psychiatry: The International and Intercultural Distribution of Mental Illness. Heidelberg: Springer-Verlag;1982. pp. 269-77.
46. Mo KM, Li LS, Ou LW. Report of koro epidemic in Leizhou Peninsula, Hainan Islands. Chinese J Neuropsychiat. 1987;20:232-4.
47. Illechukwu STC. Magical penis loss in Nigeria: Report of a recent epidemic. Transcul Psychiatric Res Rev. 1992;29:91-108.
48. Mitchell D. Is shrinking penis syndrome a delusion or real thing? Paper presented at the 'History of Medicine in Southeast Asia Symposium' at the Indonesian Academy of Sciences, 27-30 June, 2018. [online] Available from https://theconversation.com/is-shrinking-penis-syndrome-a-delusion-or-a-real-thing- 99631. [Last accessed March, 2023].
49. Sackey BM. The vanishing organ phenomenon in the context of Ghanaian religious beliefs. African Anthropol. 1997;4(2):110-25.
50. Adams G, Dzokoto VA. Genital-shrinking in Ghana: A cultural-psychological analysis. Cul Psychol. 2007;13:83-104.
51. Mather C. Accusations of genital theft: a case from northern Ghana. Cul Med Psychiat. 2005;29(1):33-52.

Chapter 2

Koro Epidemics in West Bengal

INTRODUCTION

West Bengal[1] is a state in the eastern Indian region along the Bay of Bengal, with over 91 million inhabitants. It is the fourth most populous state and the 14th largest state by area. It covers 88,752 km^2. Bangladesh bounds the state in the east, and Nepal and Bhutan in the north. It also borders the Indian states of Odisha, Jharkhand, Bihar, Sikkim, and Assam.

According to the 2011 national census, West Bengal is 4th most populated state in India.

West Bengal[1] is a state in the eastern Indian region along the Bay of Bengal, with over 91 million inhabitants. It is the fourth most populous state and the 14th largest state by area. It covers 88,752 km^2. Bangladesh bounds the state in the east, and Nepal and Bhutan in the north. It also borders the Indian states of Odisha, Jharkhand, Bihar, Sikkim, and Assam.

According to the 2011 national census, West Bengal is the fourth-most-populous state in India, with a population of 91,347,736 (7.55% of India's population). It is also the eighth most populous country subdivision of the world.[2] As of 2017, scheduled castes and tribes form 28.6% and 5.8% of the population, respectively, in rural areas and 19.9% and 1.5% in urban areas. As of 2011, West Bengal had a population density of 1,029 inhabitants per square kilometer (2,670/m^2), making it the second most densely populated state in India, after Bihar. West Bengal has 23 districts.

As of 2011, Hinduism is the most common religion, representing 70.54% of the total population. Muslims, the second-largest community, comprise 27.01% of the total population; Sikhism, Christianity, Buddhism, and other religions make up the rest. The state's official languages are Bengali and English. Nepali has another official status in the three subdivisions of the Darjeeling district. As of the 2011 census, 86.22% of the population spoke Bengali, 5.00% Hindi, 2.66% Santali, 1.82% Urdu, and 1.26% Nepali as their first language. The literacy rate is 77.08%, higher than the national rate of 74.04%.

The main river in West Bengal is the Ganges, which divides into two branches. One branch enters Bangladesh as the Padma, while the other flows through West Bengal as the Bhagirathi and later Hooghly River. The northern part above the river Ganges is the North Bengal region, while the southern part is known as South Bengal. Roads and railways well connect the state in both interstate and intrastate places. It has two international and one domestic airport. Kolkata is a major river port in eastern India.

The capital and largest city of the state is Kolkata—the third largest urban agglomeration and seventh largest city in India. The city has a long cultural, social, and political history. Kolkata was the workplace of several renowned social reformers, including Raja Ram Mohan Roy, Iswar Chandra Vidyasagar, and Swami Vivekananda. This city is also associated with the works of four Nobel laureates (Rabindranath Tagore, CV Raman, Amartya Sen, and Abhijit Banerjee) and is often called the "Cultural Capital" of India.[3] Satyajit Ray is widely regarded as one of the greatest filmmakers of the 20th century.[4]

Interestingly, Koro first appeared in West Bengal state in epidemic form, in 1982 and then again in 2010. Both the epidemics were massive and affected all the districts of West Bengal. In between there are some reports of mini epidemic and few sporadic Koro case reportings are evident.

REFERENCES

1. West Bengal. [online] Available from https://en.wikipedia.org/wiki/West_Bengal. [Last accessed April, 2023].
2. Provisional population totals paper 1 of 2011: West Bengal. [online] Available from https://www.censusindia.gov.in/2011-prov-results/prov_data_products_wb.html. [Last accessed April, 2023].
3. Chaudhuri S. Calcutta, the Living City: The past. New Delhi: Oxford University Press; 1990.
4. Tmh General Knowledge Manual. Noida: Tata McGraw-Hill Education; 2007.

1982 NORTH BENGAL KORO EPIDEMIC: DEMOGRAPHICS, CLINICAL, AND SOCIAL RESPONSE STUDY

Arabinda N Chowdhury

PREAMBLE

A massive Koro epidemic took place in the entire North Bengal region of West Bengal State of India **(Fig. 1)** in July 1982. The northern region includes five districts. They are Cooch Behar, Darjeeling, Jalpaiguri, Malda, and West Dinajpur. The River Ganges separates these from the southern part of the

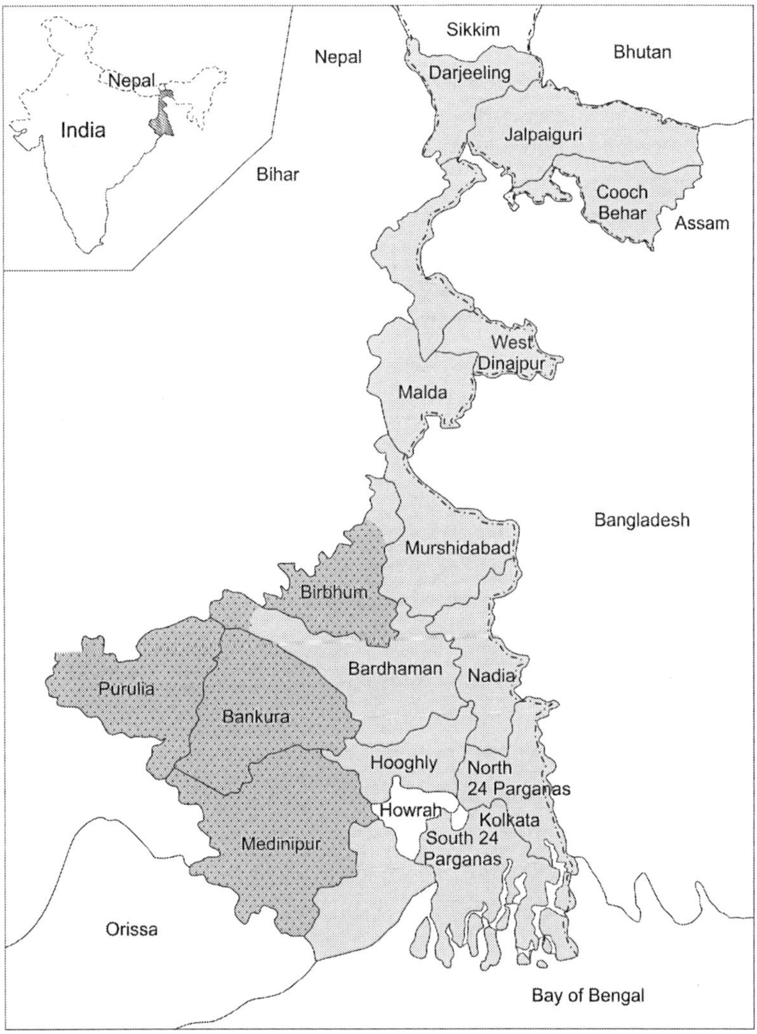

Fig. 1: West Bengal state with North Bengal region in 1982 (not to scale).

State. The epidemic started on the first week of July from a village in Jalpaiguri districts and then gradually spread throughout the North Bengal region and eventually coursed to the different districts of South Bengal, including the State capital Calcutta and probably stopped at Baleswar, a town of the adjoining state of Orissa. All the 16 districts of the state have been affected. The estimated number of cases of this Koro epidemic may be well over 3,000. At the same time, the present author has personally tracked and confirmed the affectivity figure of 631:405 from the North Bengal region.[1] 186 from the South Bengal region (Murshidabad, Nadia, Burdwan, Hoogly, and South 24-Parganas) and 40 from Baleswar town, Orissa.[2]

During this time, the author organized two symposia in the Department of Medicine, North Bengal Medical College, and Hospital. The first one, "Social Psychiatry Symposium," was held from 20 to 21 February, 1985 It was inaugurated by Professor DB Dutta, Vice Chancellor, North Bengal University, and was attended by Dr Mitchell Weiss, Department of Psychiatry, The Cambridge Hospital, and Harvard Medical School, Massachusetts, USA. The second one was a "Koro Symposium," which held from 20 to 21 December, 1986 and was inaugurated by Professor DB Dutta, Vice Chancellor, North Bengal University. It was attended by Dr Alain Bottero, Chief de Clinique, Assistant, Hospital De La Salpetriere, Paris, France. Professor NC Chowdhury, then Head, Department of Sociology and Social Anthropology, North Bengal University, graced both the symposia as Guest of Honor and resource person. The symposia themes were on different sociocultural aspects of Koro illness, case presentation, and field visits to Koro-affected families and local healers of the tea gardens. The symposia generated good academic interactions and transcultural views between Indian and foreign experts. Field visits helped us understand the sociocultural landscape of the region, especially in the tea gardens. The Koro Symposium Monograph is attached in **Appendix II**, containing the symposia theme, lecture abstracts, and photographs. Other authors' published studies of the 1982 Koro epidemic are abstracted in **Appendix III**.

Organization of the Chapter: The following discussion is grouped under the following parts:

- *Part One:* The Land and the People
- *Part Two:* General Epidemic Character
- *Part Three:* Clinical Profile: Male Cases; Female cases, Koro and Psychiatric Morbidity
- *Part Four:* Koro Social Response Study
- *Part Five:* Medical and Social Treatment of Koro

PART ONE: THE LAND AND THE PEOPLE

DARJEELING DISTRICT

Darjeeling, the northernmost district of Jalpaiguri division, is located between 27° 13′ 05″ and 27′ 10″ north latitudes and 88° 53′ 00″ and 87° 59′ 30″ east longitudes. International frontiers hem in its boundary. Nepal to the west, Sikkim—a state of India to the north, and Bhutan and Bangladesh to the east **(Fig. 2)**.

District Name

The district is named after *Darje-ling,* a Buddhist monastery that once stood on Observatory Hill near the Mall. The name Darjeeling appears to be a corruption of Dorjeeling—*ling* means place and *dorje* standing for the ecclesiastical scepter or the double-headed thunderbolt which the Lama holds in their hand during service.[3]

Topography

The district consists of a portion of the outlying hills of the lower Himalayas and a stretch of territory lying along their base known as Tarai. The mean height of the Tarai is 300 ft above sea level, while some of the hills rise to more than 10,000 ft. The perpetual snow line is approximately 16,000 ft. Sandakphu (altitude 11,923 ft) is at its base. Ghum is the highest point of

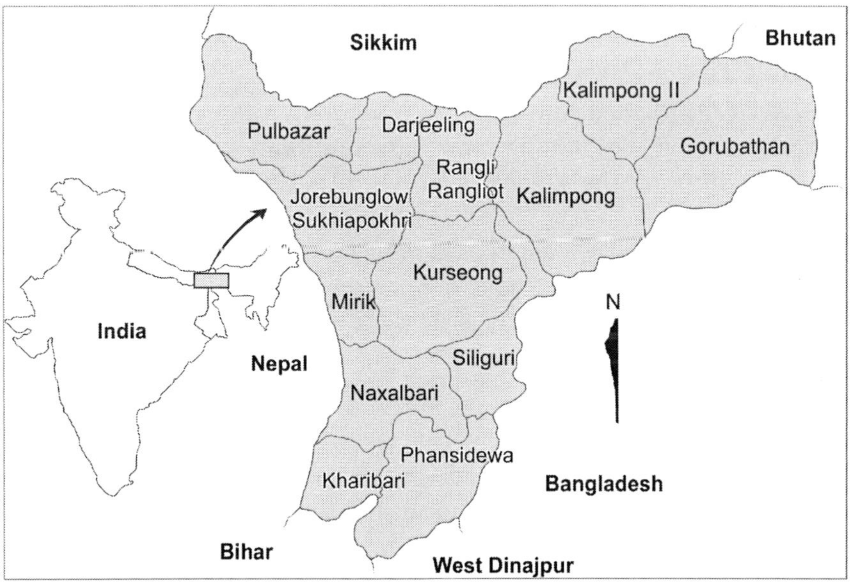

Fig. 2: Darjeeling District.
Source: https://www.researchgate.net/figure/Location-map-of-the-study-area-not-to-the-scale_fig1_254861440.

human habitation (8,163 ft). Tiger Hill (8,482 ft) is a famous tourist spot. Kalimpong subdivision falls within the hill portion, the highest point is Sonchonglu (6,255 ft).

Tea Plantation

The tea plantation in this district was introduced by Dr Arthur D Campbell, superintendent of the district, in 1839. The first commercial tea plantation was started in 1856 at Aloobari and Lebong. The expansion of the tea plantation is the primary cause of the development of this entire area in terms of new settlements, commerce, trade, and industry. In 1966, 144 gardens covered 28,121 hectares of land with a yearly yield of 1,73,98,000 kg tea involving a workforce of >3,00,000 people, 31.5% of the total district population.

Forest

The vast forest region with varieties of plants and trees and several tea plantations add scenic beauty to the district and provide a livelihood to its people. More than 1,46,112 acres of the district are covered with forest, having two main groups—the plain forest and the hill forest. Timber and different medical plants (both of medical and traditional folk value) are essential forest products. The variations in altitude and climate offer a rich and diverse animal life, especially avifauna. There is no record of crocodiles and testidunes from the mountainous parts, although at least one tortoise species is found in the Terai region.

Administrative Division and Population

The district is divided into the hills (comprising three subdivisions—Darjeeling Sadar, Kalimpong, and Kurseong) and the plains and the Terai (constituting the Siliguri subdivision). Terai is a Persian word meaning "dampness." The Terai lies between the mountains and the plains and is traversed by numerous hill streams. The total area of the district is 3,005 sq. km. The district's total population numbered 7,81,777 persons (males: 4,15,442 and females: 3,66,335) as per the 1981 census.[4]

Religion and Language

The Census of 1971 shows that 81.4% of the district population were Hindus, 11.7% Buddhist, 3.7% Christians, and 3% Muslims. Among the Indo-Aryan language family, Nepali speakers form the largest single group (59.1%), followed by Bengali (18.4%), Hindi (7.7%), and Oria (1.4%). Oraon (2.8%) is the primary dialect of the Dravidian language family. Of the Austric group of languages, Santali accounts for 1.2% of the population, followed by Munda (0.9%).

Koro cases were reported from the following places:

- *Darjeeling Sadar:* This is the district headquarters, situated at the height of 5,970 ft. It is a municipal town with 13 wards spread over 4.08 sq miles. It is well connected by road with different hill communities and by rail to Siliguri town. It is a tourist spot and has a more or less cosmopolitan character. It is 87 km by rail from New Jalpaiguri railway station and about 79 km by road from Siliguri town.
- *Ghum:* A small township in Jorebungalow Police Station, 6.4 km South of Darjeeling town, situated at an elevation of 7,400 ft. It is an important trade center and has a good road connection with Darjeeling, Kalimpong, and Sukhiapokhri at the Nepal border. It has a railway connection to the New Jalpaiguri-Darjeeling section of the North-East Frontier Railway (NEFR), standing at the height of 7,407 ft, is supposed to be the highest railway station in India.
- *Kurseong:* This is the headquarter of a subdivision of the same name, situated at an elevation of 4,860 ft above sea level and 32 km from Darjeeling.
- *Sonada:* This is situated 6,552 ft above sea level in Jorebungalow Police Station and is 14 km from Darjeeling town. The name, "Sonada" originated from the Lepcha word *Sona* (bear) and *dah* (abode).
- *Mirik:* This is situated at an elevation of 5,000 ft from sea level. It is well connected with other parts of the district by a motorable road and is 45 km from Darjeeling Sadar and 51 km from Siliguri town. Mirik Bazaar, on the northern edge of a lake, is one of the biggest orange markets of the district.
- *Tista Bazar:* Situated 710 ft above sea level in Kalimpong subdivision, is 16 km from Kalimpong and 35 km from Darjeeling along the Pashok road. It is on the west bank of river Tista. There is a weekly hat (market) and a primary health center.
- *Siliguri* is the headquarter of the plain subdivision by the same name and is situated at 26° 43′ north latitude and 88° 26′ east longitude. It is the most essential cosmopolitan, commercial town in the Darjeeling district and the entire northeastern part of the country. It is the gateway to the whole of northeastern India. It is a municipal town having 12 wards, spread over 15.54 km^2. It has a road National Highway (NH31) and rail connection to Calcutta (584 km), Assam, and Bihar. This town has the North Bengal University, the North Bengal Medical College and Hospital, Siliguri subdivisional hospital, and the Airport (Bagdogra).
- *Matigara:* It is a prominent marketplace, 6 km northwest of Siliguri town along the NH 31. It is one of the most important trading centers for different commodities, jute, and domestic animals. The milk-producing government organization Himul is situated 4 km away on the road to Mirik.

- *Bagdogra:* A small developing town on the NH 31 is in the northwest direction of Siliguri. The airport is situated here.
- *Nakshalbari:* The headquarter of the police station of the same name on the Nepal border is 24 km from Siliguri town. It has a large village market (hat) and some rice and sawmills.
- *Phansidewa:* A big village situated near the Bangladesh border, is 24 km north-east of Siliguri town. The North Bengal Medical College is 4 km away from this place.
- *Kharibari:* A big village situated near the Bihar border, is 29 km south of Siliguri town. A weekly hat is vital for the trading of jute and domestic animals.
- *Bidhan Nagar:* A small town by NH 31 before the Bagdogra area.

JALPAIGURI DISTRICT

Jalpaiguri district **(Fig. 3)** lies between 26° 16′ and 27° 0′ north latitude and 88° 53′ east longitude. It comprises an area of 6,245 sq. km and total population 2,789, 827 (males: 1,447,106 and females: 1,342,721) as on 1991. The district has derived its name from the Olive trees (*Jalpai* in Bengal), which grew in large numbers around early 1900. The suffix *guri* means place. The name could also be associated with "Jalpes," the presiding deity (Lord Shiva) of the entire region.

The district has two subdivisions: Jalpaiguri or Sadar and Alipurduar. The district has many rivers and streams intersecting the area with extensive forests, reed jungles, and tea gardens. Tista is the largest river in North Bengal. It originates from the glaciers of north Sikkim at an altitude of 6,400 meters. A Vedic and mythological connection regarding this river is a vital cultural and folk belief in the region.[5]

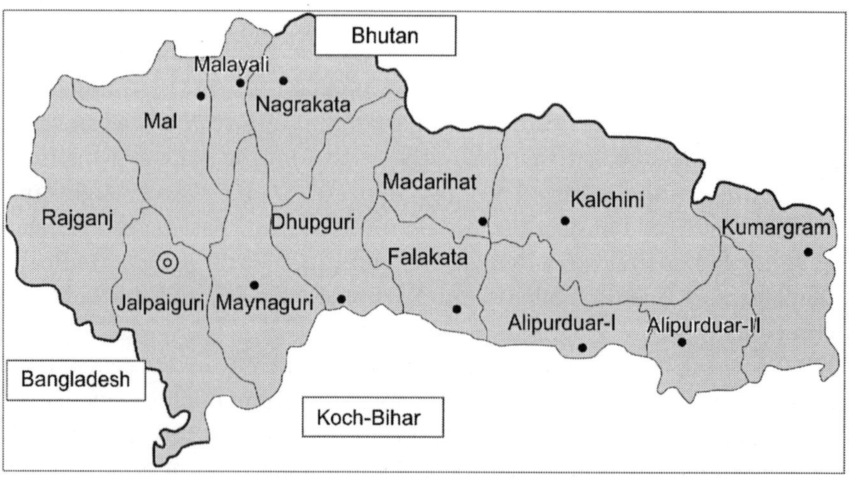

Fig. 3: Jalpaiguri district (not to scale).

Rural-urban Division

There are 744 inhabited villages (402 in Sadar division and 342 in Alipurduar subdivision). The rural area aggregates to 61,653 sq. km, containing 90.39% of the total district population.[6] The two towns, Jalpaiguri and Alipurduar, have municipal bodies.

Language

54.5% of the total population speak Bengali; 11.9% Kurukh-Oraon; 8.3% languages of Nepali origin; 7.1% Hindi; 5.6% Sadri; 3.2% Munda; 2% Santali, and 5.9% Rajbansi.[6] Rajbansi can hardly be regarded as a language, being a dialect of Bengali, spoken by Rajbansi. Totopara is a small village on the hill, inhabited by only 376 ethnic Totos, an autochthonous tribe that speaks nonpronominalized Himalayan group Tibeto-Burman family languages.

Religion

Hindus are numerically the most prominent religious groups. Worship of Siva in different forms is widespread. The *Puranic* (mythological) link of Lord Siva in his dynamic and malevolent form (Mahakal), being worshiped by the Koches, Meches, and Rahabas of this region. The most famous Siva temple of Jalpaiguri is Jalpeswar. The most famous Mahakal deity of the district is honored in an enormous lingam or phallic symbol at Jayanti of Alipurduar subdivision.

Islam (8.9% of the total population) and Christianity (3.2%) have their people, though of smaller dimension. The first mosque of Jalpaiguri town was built in 1875, and the first Church was founded in 1882. Protestants predominate among the Christens and are found mainly among the Orans, Mundas, Hos, Bhutias, Mechs, and Santal in descending order. Most of the Himalayan group of Tibeto-Burman language-speaking Bhutias and Sherpas from Nepal and Sikkim follow Buddhism (0.9% of the population).

Past Evidence of Koro

A young priest of a temple of *Siva* at Jattaswar village (Mainaguri) told the author that he had heard from his father that some 40 years ago, there were a few cases of a penis shrinking illness in this locality. This author, however, failed to trace any proof of this record.

Places from where Koro cases were reported:

- *Alipurduar:* A subdivisional town, about 110 km from Jalpaiguri town. It is a trading center and has a big railway colony.
- *Ambari-Falakata:* A village in Rajgang police station, on the bank of river Karatoya.
- *Bagrakot:* A station on the Katihar (Bihar)—Lumding (Assam) section of the NEFR. There are four tea gardens.

- *Banarhat* is a village under Dhupguri Police Station, surrounded by many tea gardens. It has a railway station on the Katihar-Lumding section of NEFR.
- *Bhelakoba:* A jute-growing area under the Jalpaiguri Police Station. It has a big jute market.
- *Falakata:* It is 88 km away from Jalpaiguri town, on the east bank of the river Mujnai close to the boundary of Koch Bihar district.
- *Chalsa:* A place under Malati Police Station. Matiali Hat (Market) is one of the largest markets in the tea garden area.
- *Dhupguri:* The station has the Police Station of the same name on the Chamargram—New Bongaigaon section of NEFR. It has a big jute market.
- *Jaipaiguri:* The district town and headquarter of the Jalpaiguri Civil Division. It is situated on the right bank of the Tista river, and the river Karala divides the city into two parts. It is the commercial center of the district—tea is the essential item of trade, though tobacco, jute, and timber are also important.
- *Lataguri:* A village in Mal Police Station, famous for timber.
- *Madarihat:* It is a marketplace on the right bank of river Torsa.
- *Maynaguri:* It is about 12 km from Jalpaiguri town and is on the bank of the Jhorda river.
- *Mal:* A prominent marketplace with junction station of the New Mal-Changrabandha section of NEFR.
- *Nagrakata:* Mainly a tea garden area with a railway station on the Katihar-Lumding section.
- *Oldabari:* It is a village in Mal Police Station, surrounded by four tea gardens.
- *Rajgang:* A prominent marketplace for jute, situated between Jalpaiguri and Siliguri town.
- *Sannyasir Hat:* A village in Rajgang Police Station by the side of the Sikarpur tea garden area. It is named after a *Sannyasi* (sage)—probably the legendary sage Bhavani Pathak, a character in novelist Bankim Chandra Chatterjee's "Devi Chuddhurani."
- *Chakchaka:* A small village at the southeastern corner of the district, close to the Koch-Bihar border.

KOCH-BIHAR DISTRICT

Cooch Behar or Koch-Bihar district is the northeastern frontier of India with Bangladesh **(Fig. 4)**. A feudatory prince, Maharaja of Koch-Bihar, ruled Koch-Bihar on 28th August, 1949. It was annexed with the territory to the Dominion Government of India on the 12th of September, 1949. It was merged with the Province of West Bengal on 1st January, 1950.[7]

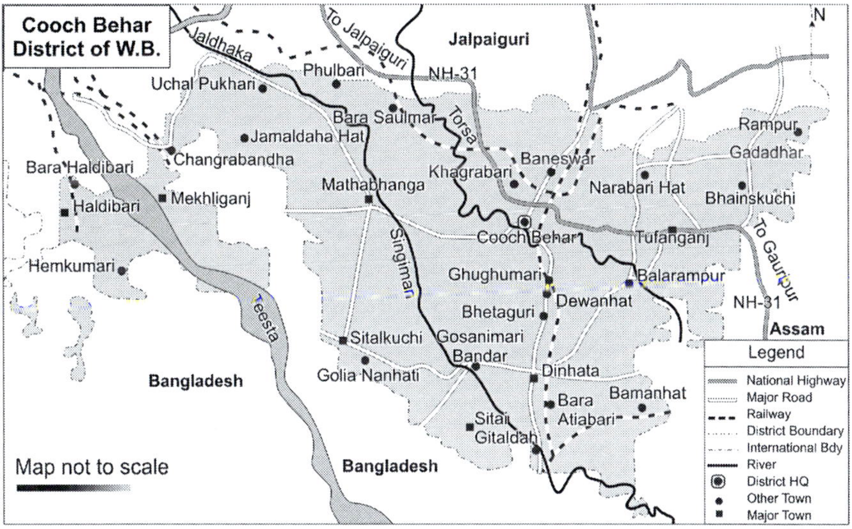

Fig. 4: Cooch Behar District (http://coochbehar.nic.in/htmfiles/CoB_map.htm).

Location and Boundary

Koch-Bihar lies between 26° 32′ 46″ and 25° 57′ 56″ north latitudes. The longitudes of the easternmost and the westernmost point are 89° 52′ 00″ east and 88° 45′ 02″ east, respectively. The northern and most of the western boundaries are formed by the district of Jalpaiguri. The district of Rangpur of Bangladesh has many indents on the southern border. The eastern edge consists of the district of Goalpara of Assam. The district's total area is 3,386 sq. km, with a population of 1,414,183.[8]

Origin of the Name of the District

The present name Koch-Bihar is of comparatively recent origin. The name Koch-Bihar was probably first used in *Sha Jahan Nama* about the middle of the 17th century. In the treaty between East India Company and King of Koch-Bihar in 1763, the Kingdom was referred to as Koch Behar and its capital as Behar Fort. Hamilton (1838),[9] in his record, mentioned only "Behar." There is a possibility of a link of "Behar" with an early Buddhist monastery in the region. Etymologically, "Bihar" means "a place or abode or sport." Koch-Bihar thus is an abode of the Koch tribe. There is a mythological story linked with this orthography. Lord Mahadeva (Siva) had engaged in dalliance with Koch maidens at once, and the word "Vihara" also means dalliance. The name has finally become Koch-Bihar or Cooch-Behar, and both forms are in use currently.

Administrative Division

The district have five divisions, viz., Koch-Bihar Sadar (Police Station Kotowali), Dinhata (Dinhata and Sitai), Tufangang (Tufangang), Mathabhanga (Mathabhanga and Sitalkuchi), and Mekhligang (Mekhligang and Haldibari).

River System

Almost all the rivers in Koch-Bihar originate in the Himalayas. There are six major river systems in the district. Kura: Due to the weighty rainfall in the district, these remain full of rain and local drainage water. These *bils* (ponds) and marshes are used to grow fish and small tortoises and help the cultivations by providing water for the steeping of jute. Locally, these water collections or bills are known as *chhara, dara, doba* or *kura.*[7]

Literacy, Immigration, Language, and Religion

The 1971 census found that 21.9% of the population was literate. Of the five districts of North Bengal, Koch-Bihar is in the third position according to literacy percentage. Bengali is the principal language spoken (96%), followed by Hindi (3.1%). Hindus (78.4%) and Muslims (21.1%) are the predominant religious communities. The Rajbanshis is the district's largest schedule caste class comprises 54% of the total Hindu population. There are a considerable number of immigrants from Bangladesh and other Indian states.

Rajbanshi

The Rajbanshi is a Hinduized tribe. The origin of the tribe is not precisely known. Generally, they are a mixed people from Dravidian stock with a considerable admixture of Mongoloid blood. They follow the Hindu custom of marriage and worshipping of Gods. Wild animals such as tigers, crocodiles, and some minor village deities are also worshipped. Though they follow the Hindu custom and ritual, they have unique health and healing methods and different world views with more significant stress on the magicoreligious principle.

The places from where Koro cases were reported:

- *Changrabandha:* It is under Mekligang police station, an export center for jute and tobacco.
- *Deewan* Hat*:* It is a marketplace, 8 km south of Koch-Bihar town.
- *Dinhata:* It is the headquarter of the subdivision of the same name and is located 16 km to the south of Koch-Bihar town.
- *Fulbari:* A small marketplace under the Mathabhanga police station.
- *Haldibari:* A small town separated by river Tista from the mainland of the district.

- *Koch-Bihar Sadar:* It is the district headquarter. It is also the North Bengal State Transport Corporation headquarter, which maintains passenger services to Calcutta, Assam, and Bhutan. The NH31 passes through the town, and there is an airport.
- *Mathabhanga:* It is a small town and the headquarter of the subdivision.
- *Pundibari:* It stands on either side of NH31.
- *Sitalkuchi:* It is the headquarter of the police station of the same name. It is 13 km from Mathabhanga town.
- *Tufangang:* The subdivisional headquarter of the same name is situated to the east of Koch-Bihar town.

The geographical descriptions above of all the districts are well illustrative that there are extensive communication networks by rail or road inside and outside of each district, and there is a weekly hat (market) in each town. This easy socializing and communicability is one of the factors probably that facilitated the spread of Koro illness during the epidemic.

PART TWO: GENERAL EPIDEMIC CHARACTER

EPIDEMIC CASE FREQUENCIES AND DEMOGRAPHIC PROFILE

Methodology

Koro Study Team collected a total of 405 Koro cases (357 males and 48 females) from different sub-divisional hospitals, General Practitioners (GP) clinic, and by the local community survey by key informants of the four districts of North Bengal (Darjeeling, Jalpaiguri, and Cooch-Behar mainly and some part of the adjoining West Dinajpur) during the epidemic in the region. The epidemic started from the first week of July 1982 and persisted until the end of December 1982, though with decreasing incidence of the cases later. This entire period is regarded as the epidemic period. 395 Koro cases (347 males and 48 females) were collected from this epidemic period **(Table 1)**. In the following 3 years, i.e., 1983, 1984, and 1985, 10 more male Koro cases were reported.

TABLE 1: Gender distribution of Koro cases (1982–1985) of North Bengal.

	Male		*Female*		*Total*	
District	*No.*	*%*	*No.*	*%*	*No.*	*%*
Darjeeling	154	43.1	12	25.0	166	41.0
Cooch-Behar	129	36.1	28	58.3	157	38.8
Jalpaiguri	69	19.3	7	14.6	76	18.8
West-Dinajpur	5	1.4	1	2.1	6	1.5
Total	357	88.15	48	11.85	405	

Of the data, 78% of the case interview were obtained directly within 1–2 weeks of the onset. The remaining case reports were obtained through different professional and community informers like subdivisional, primary, and subsidiary health center medical officers, medical officers of the tea gardens, pharmacists and paramedical staffs of clinics and laboratories, general and private medical practitioners, health workers (malaria and filarial prevention program), managers and other staffs of the tea gardens, Panchayat members, village leaders, schoolmasters, medicine shopowners, quacks, and faith healers (Jikri) of the region. A Koro study team was formed for the ease of data collection from the various areas of the districts. The group consisted of Dr A Chatterjee, Medical Specialist, and Dr M Roy, Child Specialist of the Siliguri Subdivisional Hospital, Dr P Pal, Psychiatrist, and Dr AN Chowdhury (Team Lead), Lecturer, Psychiatry Department of North Bengal Medical College and Hospital and Dr BB Das Chowhury, General Physician of Siliguri and Mirik Town.

These are not actual representations of the total caseloads in each district, as only a portion attended hospitals and clinics. The number of cases varies at different data analysis steps because only those data were analyzed, authentic, and cross checked. This is, of course, not an all-inclusive information gathering network for such a vast region, so the incidence of Koro cases of the districts is not comparable to their respective population composition. This is an unavoidable limitation in studying psychiatric epidemics and is also evident in the investigations of Koro epidemics of Singapore[10,11] and Thailand.[12] Therefore, a careful note regarding the interpretation of the result of this study is not to consider the result as a generalized representation of the whole epidemic but be taken obviously as a judicious prospective data of maximum available/reported Koro cases of the epidemic.

Instrument

"Demography Schedule" is a brief format that includes identification data such as age, marital status, education, occupation, ethnicity, economic class, family type, and family size.

"Economic class" was divided into five categories according to a monthly family earning viz., Class V: up to ₹ 1000/-; Class IV: between ₹ 1,001 and 2,000/-; Class III: between ₹ 2,001 and 3,000/-; Class II: between ₹ 3,001 and 4,000/- and Class I: ₹ 4,001 and above.

"Single family" refers to the husband, wife, and unmarried children. "Joint family" consists of other relatives (e.g., parents of the spouse, other in-laws, married children) who generally live under one roof. They eat food cooked at one hearth, hold property in common, participate in common worship, and are related to one another.

Results

Table 1 shows that out of 405 Koro cases, males constituted 88% and females 12%. The highest number of cases was from the Darjeeling district (40.9%). Male affectivity was also highest in this district (43.1%). Female patients were highest in the Cooch-Behar district (58.3%).

Table 2 and Figure 5 depict the calendar-month distribution of cases with a week-wise breakup of July. The highest total percentage (41.3%) and highest male affectivity (43.5%) was from the Darjeeling district. Cooch-Behar was in the second-highest position (38.9%) with the highest female affectivity (58.3%). 18.5% cases of the total were from Jalpaiguri and 1.3% from the West-Darjeeling district.

The highest toll of the epidemic was noted throughout July, 82% of the total cases. Especially the third week of July showed the maximum number of cases, both sex-wise (males 42.9%, females 41.7%) and in total number (42.8%). The month of August revealed a precipitous decrement of this number to 4.6% only, followed by a small peak (9.6%) in September, followed by an abrupt fall.

The first case was reported at the Siliguri sub-division hospital in the *Darjeeling district* at 2 AM on 9th July, 1982. The third-week toll was the highest (37.4%), and by the fourth week, 83.4% of the total cases occurred and was followed by an abrupt decline to 4.9% in August, while in September there was a slight rise (7.9%), succeeded by a fall of incidence to 1.2% in November **(Fig. 6)**.

The first case in the *Jalpaiguri district* was supposed to be from the village Bagaribari under Dhupguri police station on 2nd July. The next ones rapidly spread to the close-by district from Jalpaiguri and reached the highest toll (50.7%) during this week. By the fourth week of July, the case reporting dropped to 2.7% **(Fig. 7)**.

Identification of the first case in the *Koch-Bihar district* was uncertain. The outbreak probably started from the village Mohischaru under the Mathabhanga police station on the second week of July. The third-week toll was the highest in total (62.3%). By the end of July, 77.9% of cases were reported, followed by a sharp fall of new-onset to 3.9% in August. In September, a new epidemic wave with a peak (14.3) was observed **(Fig. 8)**.

The ease of transport system in the West Dinajpur district prompted the cases to attend the Malda subdivision hospital. Therefore, very few cases were collected from this district. Only five cases attended the North Bengal Medical College Hospital from West Dinajpur adjoining the Darjeeling district. The first case was reported on 6 September from a semiindustrial colony (of Oil India Corporation) at Dhumdangi.

TABLE 2: Sex-wise calendar-month distribution of Koro epidemic cases.

Year 1982	*Darjeeling*			*Jalpaiguri*			*Koch-Bihar*			*West-Dinajpur*			*Total*		
	M	*F*	*T*	*M*	*F*	*T*	*M*	*F*	*T*	*M*	*F*	*T*	*M*	*F*	*T*
July 1st week	–	–	–	36 54.5	1 14.3	37 50.7	–	–	–	–	–	–	36 10.4	1 2.1	37 9.4
2nd week	32 21.2	–	32 19.6	15 22.7	2 28.6	17 23.3	6 4.8	2 7.1	8 5.2	–	–	–	53 15.3	4 8.3	57 14.4
3rd week	58 38.4	3 25.0	61 37.4	9 13.6	3 42.9	12 16.4	82 65.1	14 50.0	96 62.3	–	–	–	149 42.9	20 41.7	169 42.8
4th week	38 25.2	5 41.7	43 26.4	2 3.03	–	2 2.7	11 8.7	5 17.9	16 10.4	–	–	–	51 14.7	10 20.8	61 15.4
Total	128 84.8	8 66.7	136 83.4	62 93.9	6 85.7	68 93.2	99 78.6	21 75.0	120 77.9	–	–	–	289 83.3	35 72.9	324 82.0
August	6 3.97	2 16.7	8 4.9	3 4.55	1 14.3	4 5.5	4 3.2	2 7.1	6 3.9	–	–	–	13 3.75	5 10.4	18 4.6
September	11 7.3	2 16.7	13 8.0	–	–	–	19 15.1	3 10.7	22 14.3	2 50.0	1 100	3 60.0	32 9.22	6 12.5	38 9.6
October	4 2.6	–	4 2.5	1 1.52	–	1 1.4	2 1.6	2 7.1	4 2.6	2 50.0		2 40.0	9 2.59	2 4.2	11 2.8
November	2 1.3	–	2 1.2	–	–	–	–	–	–	–	–	–	2 0.58	–	2 0.5
December	–	–	–	–	–	–	2 1.6	–	2 1.3	–	–	–	2 0.58	–	2 0.5
Total	151 92.6	12 7.4	163	66 90.4	7 9.6	73	126 81.8	28 18.2	154	4 80.0	1 20.0	5	347 87.8	48 12.2	395

M = Male, F = Female, T = Total

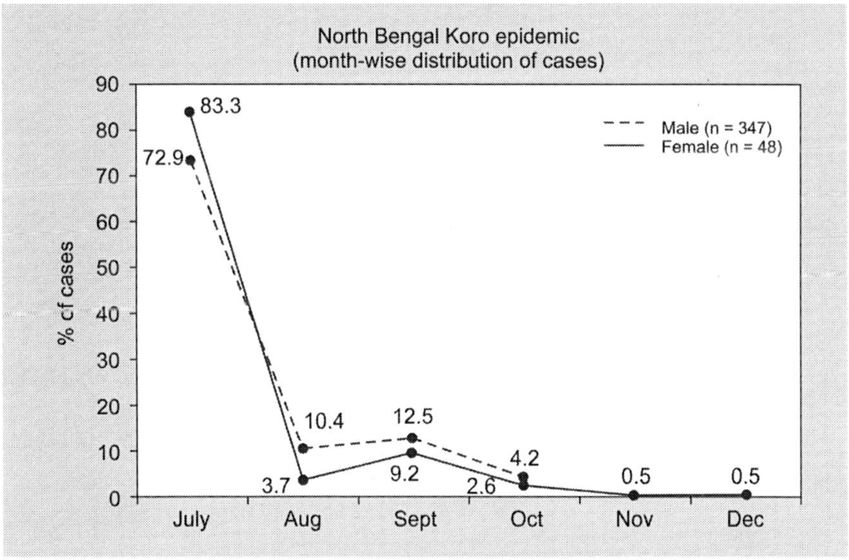

Fig. 5: Calendar-month distribution of cases.

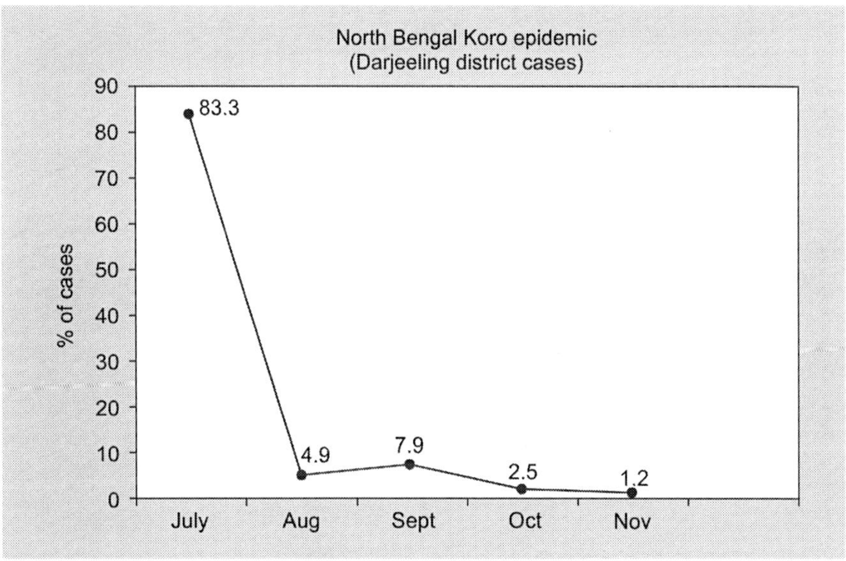

Fig. 6: Darjeeling district cases.

A total of 10 patients (all males) were reported. In 1983, 6 cases; in 1984, 3, and in 1985, one case. **Table 3** shows the district-wise distribution of patients during the postepidemic years (1983–1985).

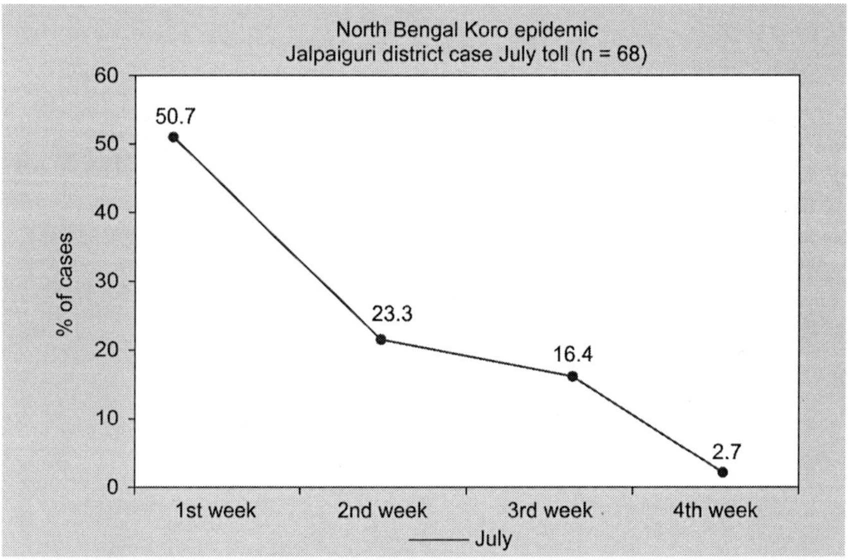

Fig. 7: Case reporting in July.

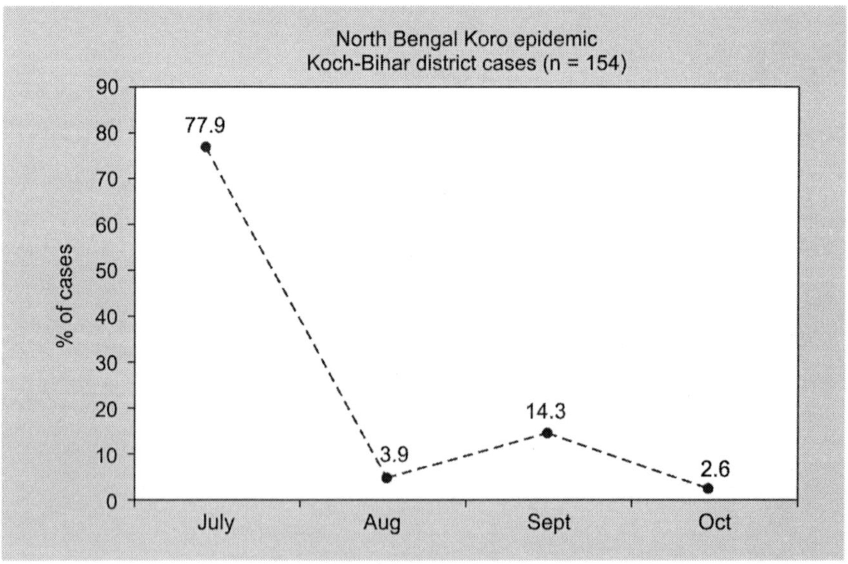

Fig. 8: Koch-Bihar district cases.

DEMOGRAPHIC PROFILE OF CASES OF DARJEELING DISTRICT

Table 4 shows the demographic profile of the Koro cases of Darjeeling district. The mean ages for the males were 14.3 ± 7.6 years and for females 21.4 ± 8

TABLE 3: Calendar-month distribution of Koro cases* in postepidemic years (1983–1985) in North Bengal.

	1983					1984			1985	
District	*Feb*	*July*	*Aug*	*Sept*	*Oct*	*May*	*July*	*Oct*	*Mar*	*Total*
Darjeeling			1		1		1			3
Koch-Bihar		2				1				3
Jalpaiguri	1			1			1			3
West-Dinajpur									1	1
Total			6				3		1	10

*All cases were males.

years. The highest and lowest ages recorded for the males were 8 and 47 years and for females 8 and 41 years respectively. Single marital status was standard in males (62.9%) and females (58%). In both sexes, "No formal schooling" was maximum (male 44.8%, female 50%) as "no occupation" (males 36.4%; females 58%). The highest number of cases came from the economic class IV (males 33.1%; females 33.3%). In the male, joint family was more common (53.8%), while in the females, this was the single-family (58.3%). Maximum cases were from 6–10 members (males 49.2%, females 50%). Hinduism was the commonest religion of both the sexes (males 32.3%, females 33.3%).

DEMOGRAPHIC PROFILE OF CASES OF JALPAIGURI DISTRICT

Table 5 shows the mean age of the male cases to be 25.3 ± 7.4 and females 28.6 ± 7.5 years. The lowest and highest ages of patients reported were 11 and 44 years in males and 18 and 40 in females, respectively. The highest frequencies are the single marital status in males (68.1%) and females (71.4%). Primary education was the commonest (in males 37.5% and in females 42.8%). No occupation was maximum in both sexes (males 33.3%, females 42.8%). The economic class status of IV was leading in males (31.2%) while that of class V was in females (42.8%). The joint family was more in males (56.3%) while in females it was single-family (57.2%). Maximum cases of both the groups were from families having 6–10 members (males 45.8%, females 57.2%). Maximum males were Behari Hindus (41.7%), while females showed equal distribution (28.6) among Bengali, Behari Hindus, and Rajbansis.

DEMOGRAPHIC PROFILE OF CASES OF KOCH-BIHAR DISTRICT

The age mean for the males were 23.2 ± 8.4 years and for females 22.1 ± 9.9 years **(Table 6)**. The lowest and highest ages reported were 8 and 54 years

TABLE 4: Demographic profile of Koro cases of Darjeeling district.

Demography	*Male (n = 154)*		*Female (n = 12)*	
I. Age in years: mean ± sd	24.3 ± 7.62		21.4 ± 8.05	
II. Marital Status	*No*	*%*	*No*	*%*
Single	97	63.0	7	58.3
Married	49	31.8	4	33.3
Once	42	27.3		
Twice	4	2.6		
Thrice	3	1.9		
Separated	6	3.9	1	8.3
Widow/Widower	2	1.3		
III. Education				
No schooling	69	44.8	6	50.0
Primary education	47	30.5	4	33.3
Secondary education	31	20.1	2	16.7
College education	7	4.5		
IV. Occupation				
Nil	56	36.4	7	58.3
Student	27	17.5	1	8.3
Agriculture	23	14.9		
Unskilled laborer	18	11.7		
Skilled laborer	9	5.8		
Business/Trade	15	9.7		
Regular Service	6	3.9		
Housewife			4	33.3
V. Economic Class	*n = 130*	*%*	*n = 12*	*%*
Class I	3	2.3		
Class II	14	10.8	2	16.7
Class III	31	23.8	3	25.0
Class IV	43	33.1	4	33.3
Class V	39	30.0	3	25.0
VI. Family Type				
Single	60	46.2	7	58.3
Joint	70	53.8	5	41.7
VII. Family Size				
1–5	29	22.3	3	25.0
6–10 members	64	49.2	6	50.0
11 and above members	37	28.5	3	25.0

Contd...

Contd...

Demography	*Male (n = 154)*		*Female (n = 12)*	
VIII. Religion				
Bengali Hindu	42	32.3	4	33.3
Behari Hindu	18	13.8	3	25.0
Nepali Hindu	13	10.0	2	16.7
Rajbansi	24	18.5	2	16.7
Islam	6	4.6		
Christian	11	8.5		
Jain	9	6.9		
Schedule Tribe	7	5.4	1	8.3

TABLE 5: Demographic profile of Koro cases of Jalpaiguri district.

Demography	*Male (n = 69)*		*Female (n = 7)*	
I. Age in years: mean ± sd	25.3 ± 7.42		28.6 ± 7.46	
II. Marital Status	*No.*	*%*	*No.*	*%*
Single	47	68.1	5	71.4
Married	16	23.2	1	14.3
Once	14	20.3		
Twice	2	2.9		
Separated	2	2.9	1	14.3
Widow/Widower	4	5.8		
III. Education	*n = 48*	*%*	*n = 7*	*%*
No schooling	17	35.4	3	42.9
Primary education	18	37.5	3	42.9
Secondary education	10	20.8	1	14.3
College education	3	6.3		
IV. Occupation				
Nil	16	33.3	3	42.9
Student	14	29.2	1	14.3
Agriculture	7	14.6		
Unskilled laborer	2	4.2	1	14.3
Skilled laborer	2	4.2		
Business/Trade	4	8.3	1*	14.3
Regular service	3	6.3		
Housewife			1	14.3

Contd...

Contd…

Demography	*Male (n = 69)*		*Female (n = 7)*	
V. Economic Class				
Class I	3	6.3		
Class II	7	14.6	1	14.3
Class III	10	20.8	2	28.6
Class IV	15	31.3	1	14.3
Class V	13	27.1	3	42.8
VI. Family Type				
Single	21	43.8	4	57.1
Joint	27	56.3	3	42.9
VII. Family Size				*0.0*
1–5	23	47.9	3	42.9
6–10 members	22	45.8	4	57.1
11 and above members	14	29.2		
VIII. Religion				
Bengali Hindu	11	22.9	2	28.6
Behari Hindu	20	41.7	2	28.6
Nepali Hindu	2	4.2		0.0
Rajbansi	6	12.5	2	28.6
Islam	1	2.1	1	14.3
Christian	1	2.1		
Jain	4	8.3		
Scheduled Tribe	4	8.3		

*Prostitute

in males and 12 and 54 years in females. The maximum cases in both sexes were single (males 58.9%, females 71.4%) and without formal schooling (males 68.8%, females 39.3%). Agriculture was the most typical occupation in males (21.5%) while the female for unskilled work was maximum (42.9%). Most of the male cases were from economic class V (35.4%), while that for females was class IV (35.7%). The single-family type was more common in males (54.8%) but the joint family in females (67.9%). The maximum cases of both sexes were from families having 6–10 members (males 55.9%, females 60.7%). Leading cases were Bengali Hindus (males 29%, females 35.7%).

TABLE 6: Demographic profile of Koro cases of Koch-Bihar district.

Demography	*Male (n = 129)*		*Female (n = 28)*	
I. Age in years: mean ± sd	23.2 ± 8.4		22.07 ± 9.96	
II. Marital Status	No.	%	No.	%
Single	76	58.9	20	71.4
Married	38	29.5	6	21.4
Once	30	23.3	5	17.9
Twice	8	6.2	1	3.6
Separated	11	8.5	2	7.1
Widower	4	3.1		
III. Education	*n = 93*	%	*n = 28*	%
No schooling	64	68.8	11	39.3
Primary education	20	21.5	9	32.1
Secondary education	8	8.6	8	28.6
College education	1	1.1		
IV. Occupation				
Nil	14	15.1	8	28.6
Student	14	15.1	2	7.1
Agriculture	20	21.5		
Unskilled laborer	12	12.9	12	42.9
Skilled laborer	9	9.7		
Business/Trade	14	15.1		
Regular service	7	7.5		
Housewife			6	21.4
Professional	3	3.2		
V. Economic Class				
Class I	4	4.3	1	3.6
Class II	14	15.1	4	14.3
Class III	20	21.5	5	17.9
Class IV	22	23.7	10	35.7
Class V	33	35.5	8	28.6
VI. Family Type				
Single	51	54.8	9	32.1
Joint	42	45.2	19	67.9
VII. Family Size				
1–5 members	18	19.4	5	17.9
6–10 members	52	55.9	17	60.7
11 and above members	23	24.7	6	21.4

Contd…

Contd...

Demography	*Male (n = 129)*		*Female (n = 28)*	
VIII. Religion				
Bengali Hindu	27	29.0	10	35.7
Behari Hindu	24	25.8	4	14.3
Nepali Hindu	2	2.2		
Rajbansi	23	24.7	7	25.0
Islam	3	3.2	5	17.9
Christian	4	4.3		
Jain	2	2.2		
Tribe	8	8.6	2	7.1

DEMOGRAPHIC PROFILE OF CASES OF WEST-DINAJPUR DISTRICT

Table 7 shows that the male cases age means 23.8 ± 12.9 years, the lowest and highest ages recorded being 14 and 46 years, respectively. Following were the maximum frequencies in male cases: single marital status (60%), no schooling (60%), agriculture occupation (60%), joint family (60%), and Rajbansi by religion (60%). Economic classes IV and V were equally noted (40% each), as also family sizes of 1–5 and 6–10 members (40% each).

DEMOGRAPHIC PROFILE OF TOTAL KORO CASES (N = 405) OF NORTH BENGAL

Tables 8 and 9 show the overall demographic characteristics of the total Koro cases of this study cohort. The age mean of the male cases was 24 ± 8 years and that of female cases 23.6 ± 10.8 years. The lowest and highest ages recorded for both sexes were 8 and 54 years. The maximum cases were from 16–20 years (males 31.9%, females 27.1%). Single marital status was the most typical finding in both sexes (males 62.5%, females 66.7%). In the males, 13.3% and 2.9% cases were twice and thrice-married, respectively. 8.3% of females were separated in contrast to 5.3% of males. About half of the cases in both sexes had no formal school education (males 51%, females 41.7%). 3.6% of the males had college-level education. The highest educational standards recorded were: a case with double MA in English and Economics; one was a Medical (MBBS) student, one a BA student, and one a Pharmacy (B. Pharm.) student. "No occupation" status was highest in both the sexes (males 29%, females 37.5%) following by student status (18.3%) and agricultural work (17.6%) in males and unskilled labor (27%) and housewife status (25%) in females. 11% of males were occupied in private,

TABLE 7: Demographic profile of Koro cases of West Dinajpur district.

Demography	*Male (n = 5)*		*Female (n = 1)*	
I. Age in years: mean ± sd	23.8 ± 12.9		51	
II. Marital Status	No	%	No	%
Single	3	60.0		
Married	2	40.0	1	100.0
III. Education				
No schooling	3	60.0		
Primary education	1	20.0		
Secondary education	1	20.0		
IV. Occupation				
Nil	1	20.0		
Student	3	60.0		
Regular service	1	20.0		
Housewife			1	100.0
V. Economic Class				
Class III	1	20.0		
Class IV	2	40.0	1	100.0
Class V	1	20.0		
VI. Family Type				
Single	2	40.0	1	100.0
Joint	3	60.0		
VII. Family Size				
1–5	2	40.0	1	100.0
6–10 members	2	40.0		
11 and above members	1	20.0		
VIII. Religion				
Bengali Hindu	1	20.0		
Rajbansi	3	60.0	1	100.0
Jain	1	20.0		

semigovernment, and government jobs. There were two policemen, one home guard, one fire-brigade employee, one engine operator of Oil India Company, one mechanic of North Bengal State Transport Corporation, and four school teachers. One homeopathic doctor, one pharmacist, and one lawyer were professionals. 61.2% males and 62.5% females were from economic class IV, and V combined. The lower the economic class, the higher

TABLE 8: Age group distribution of Koro cases of North Bengal.

	Male		*Female*	
Age group in years	*n = 357*	*%*	*n = 48*	*%*
8–10	5	1.4	1	2.1
11–15	30	8.4	11	22.9
16–20	114	31.9	13	27.1
21–25	70	19.6	6	12.5
26–30	68	19.0	4	8.3
31–35	35	9.8	5	10.4
36–40	22	6.2	5	10.4
41–45	10	2.8	2	4.2
46–50	2	0.6	–	–
51–54	1	0.3	1	2.1

TABLE 9: Demographic profile of the total Koro cases (n = 405) of North Bengal.

Demography	*Male (n = 357)*		*Female (n = 48)*	
I. Age in years: mean ± sd	24.1 ± 7.97		23.6 ± 10.8	
II. Marital Status	*No.*	*%*	*No.*	*%*
Single	223	62.5	32	66.7
Married	105	29.4	12	25.0
Once	88	24.6		0.0
Twice	14	3.9	1	2.1
Thrice	3	0.8		
Separated	19	5.3	4	8.3
Widower	10	2.8		
III. Education	*n = 300*	*%*	*n = 48*	*%*
No schooling	153	51.0	20	41.7
Primary education	86	28.7	17	35.4
Secondary education	50	16.7	11	22.9
College education	11	3.7		
IV. Occupation				
Nil	87	29.0	18	37.5
Student	55	18.3	4	8.3
Agriculture	53	17.7		
Unskilled laborer	32	10.7	13	27.1
Skilled laborer	20	6.7		

Contd...

Contd...

Demography	*Male (n = 357)*		*Female (n = 48)*	
Business/Trade	33	11.0	1 (Prostitute)	2.1
Regular service	17	5.7		
Housewife			12	25.0
Professional	3	1.0		
V. Economic Class				
Class I	10	3.3	1	2.1
Class II	35	11.7	7	14.6
Class III	62	20.7	10	20.8
Class IV	82	27.3	16	33.3
Class V	87	29.0	14	29.2
VI. Family Type				
Single	134	44.7	21	43.8
Joint	142	47.3	27	56.3
VII. Family Size				
1–5 members	61	20.3	12	25.0
6–10 members	140	46.7	27	56.3
11 and above members	75	25.0	9	18.8
VIII. Religion				
Bengali Hindu	81	27.0	16	33.3
Behari Hindu	52	17.3	9	18.8
Nepali Hindu	17	5.7	2	4.2
Rajbansi	56	18.7	12	25.0
Islam	10	3.3	6	12.5
Christian	16	5.3		
Jain	16	5.3		
Schedule Tribe	18	6.0	3	6.3

the Koro affectivity in both the sexes. The joint family type was more common in both the sexes (males 51.5%, females 56.3%), as also the maximum number of cases came from families with 6–10 members (males 50.7%, females 56.3%). Leading cases were Hindu (males 58%, females 56%). There were no female cases from Christian or Jain religions. Christians were tribal plantation workers, mostly Oran, Santals, and Mech.

SUMMARY OF SALIENT FINDINGS

Analysis of total Koro cases (n = 405) of North Bengal, irrespective of their sexes reveals the following demographic characteristics:

- *Age:* The most common age group was 16–20 years (31.4%).
- *Marital status:* Maximum Koro cases were single (63%).
- *Education:* No formal school education was maximum (49.7%).
- *Occupation:* No occupation was maximum (30.2%).
- *Economic group:* Maximum Koro cases were lower economic classes (IV + V = 61.4%).
- *Family type:* Maximum patients (52.2%) were from joint families.
- *Family size:* Maximum patients (51.5%) were from 6–10 member strength families.
- *Religion:* Hinduism was the most typical (57.7%) religion, and 21% of cases were Rajbansis.

PART THREE: CLINICAL PROFILE OF KORO

MALE KORO CASES (n = 276)

Materials and Method

A total of 276 male Koro cases (130 from Darjeeling; 48 from Jalpaiguri, 93 from Koch-Bihar, and 5 from West Dinajpur District) were interviewed in hospitals, private clinics, and on community visits during the epidemic. Detailed analysis of Koro's clinical characteristics was done for 101 cases, of which 64 (63.4%) were examined during their Koro attack and 37 (36.6%) within 24–72 hours of the episode.[13]

Result and Discussion

Habit and addiction (n = 262): Tobacco chewing was the highest (30.4%), followed by betel leaf chewing (23.2%) and tobacco smoking (21.4%). Alcohol addiction (16.7%) and ganja (Cannabis) smoking (6.5%) was also reported. Gambling with cards or number books was also recorded in 3.9% of cases, all urban slum dwellers.

Past illness and operation (n = 276): Disease affecting the genital area or organs were quite prevalent, viz. phimosis (8.7%); venereal diseases (14.9%); scrotal filarial (13.8%); hydrocele (11.2%); vasectomy (10.9%) and phimosis operation (3.9%) **(Table 10)**. The diagnosis of pulmonary tuberculosis (3.3%) and malaria fever (10.1%) was reported, and such patients received treatment from medical specialists. Psychiatrists made psychiatric diagnoses, and the patients received psychotropic medicines. Two cases of epilepsy were on antiepileptic medications in the past—one of these attempted suicide by hanging and was admitted to the hospital.

CLINICAL PICTURE (n = 101)

- *Onset type:* Acute onset was the most typical presentation mode (86%). A few cases also showed sub-acute onset with a short premonitory period.

TABLE 10: Past history of illness and operations of male Koro cases.

Past history	*n = 276*	*%*
Phimosis present	24	8.7
Phimosis operated	11	3.9
Venereal diseases	41	14.9
Epilepsy (G-M type)	4	1.5
Filariasis		
Scrotum	38	13.8
Legs	6	2.2
Total	44	15.9
Hydrocele	31	11.2
Pulmonary tuberculosis	9	3.3
Malaria fever	28	10.1
Lepromatous patch	2	0.7
Schizophrenia	6	2.2
Manic depressive disorder	2	0.7
Depression	1	0.4
Vasectomy is done	30	10.9
Appendicectomy	8	2.9
Attempted suicide	1	0.4

- *Onset time:* The most familiar onset time was a mid or late night **(Table 11)**. This night-prone Koro attack ($p > .01$) is interesting and may have psychoanalytical significance.
- *Place and situation of Koro attack:* Though the majority (60.4%) of attacks occurred in a sheltered environment of patient's residence, varieties of situations and places were recorded, e.g., in the agricultural field while working (5.9%); in the tea garden while plucking leaves (5.9%); in the market (4.9%); during attempted sexual intercourse either with wife at home (3.9%) or with a prostitute in her hut (3.9%) or with an extra-marital partner in a jungle (0.9%); in the pond or river while fishing or bathing (1.9%); in the playground, while playing (1.9%); in the cinema hall (0.9%); in the cowshed during milking (0.9%) and in a ceremonial get together (5.9%).
- *Duration of attack:* Koro is a short-lived acute attack similar to a panic attack. A careful analysis of duration of Koro attack, i.e., the time interval from the point of perception of penile retraction/shrinkage up to the feeling of normal reposition of the penis, in 64 cases has shown it to be 30 ± 10 minutes, with a range from 5 minutes to 3 hours. The Assam

TABLE 11: Distribution of Koro onset time.

Time	*n = 101*	*%*
6 AM to 12 noon	15	14.9
12 noon to 6 PM	12	11.9
6 PM to12 midnight	33	32.7
12 midnight to 6 AM	41	40.6

Koro epidemic Study[14] also found a similar range of 5 minutes to 5 hours, an average of 25 minutes.

- *Clinical symptoms:* This is divided into four categories as follows:
  1. *Premonitory symptoms:* **Table 12** shows eight types of distress before the Koro attack, felt by 66.3% of the cases. "Heaviness" or "burning inside the head" was the most typical symptom (77.6%), followed by "breathlessness" (64.2%) and "lower abdominal pain" (55.2%). The cases were grouped into two sets based on premonitory symptoms: Those who did (66%) and did not (34%) exhibited symptoms. A comparison of main symptoms—physical, mental, and genital was made by Z-score analysis to see whether there is any difference in these symptoms between the groups.
  2. *Physical symptoms:* **Table 13** shows the distribution and comparison of ten physical symptoms associated with the Koro attack between the groups. Cases with a history of premonitory symptoms showed significant ($p > .05$) excess of four symptoms, viz, choked throat sensation, increased body heat, breathlessness, and abdominal pain compared to those without such histories.

     The maximum frequency percentage distribution of symptoms was palpitation (83.2%) followed by choked throat sensation (75.2%), increased body heat (67.3%), and breathlessness (63.4%).
  3. *Mental symptoms:* **Table 14** shows the distribution of six types of reported mental symptoms. No significant variation concerning the presence of premonitory symptoms was found. "Fear of impending death" (from the hyperinvoluted penis) was the most typical association (87%), followed by "fear of damage of sex organ" (loss of sexual power) in 65%. Fear of nonspecific danger, e.g., heart trouble or "something bursting inside the abdomen" was also reported in 23% of cases. An altered perception of the environment (19%) was mainly informed by those patients who had attacks outside home-setting (e.g., in a field, during finishing, while urinating on the roadside, or way to school). This was described as a sudden experience of strange feelings of changed surroundings. This

TABLE 12: Distribution of Koro premonitory symptoms.

*Symptoms**	*n* = 67	%
1. Heaviness/Burning inside the head	52	77.6
2. Breathlessness	43	64.2
3. Lower abdominal pain	37	55.2
4. Difficulty in micturition	36	53.7
5. Uneasy/uncanny feeling	31	46.3
6. Apprehension/fearfulness	29	43.3
7. Loss of sensation in the penis	17	25.4
8. Sleeplessness	6	8.9

*More than one symptom is present in some cases.

TABLE 13: Physical symptoms with Koro.

	With premonitory symptoms		*Without premonitory symptoms*		*Z score*	*Total*
Symptoms#	*n* = 67	%	*n* = 34	%		%
1. Palpitation	59	88.1	25	73.5	1.71	83.2
2. Choked-throat sensation	61	91.0	15	44.1	5.10*	75.2
3. Increased body heat (feeling hot inside head or body)	38	56.7	30	88.2	3.858*	67.3
4. Breathlessness	51	76.1	13	38.2	3.85*	63.4
5. Lower abdo-minal pain	48	71.6	9	26.5	4.83*	56.4
6. Difficulty in articulation (stammering)	37	55.2	14	41.2	1.35	50.5
7. Muscular weakness	23	34.3	9	26.5	0.82	31.7
8. Restlessness	18	26.9	8	23.5	0.37	26.7
9. Nausea/vomiting	11	16.4	4	11.8	0.65	14.9
10. Feeling of fainting	9	13.4	5	14.7	0.17	13.9

*$p > 0.05$
#More than one symptom in some cases.

TABLE 14: Distribution of mental symptoms.

*Symptoms**	*n = 101*	*%*
1. Fears of impending death	88	87.1
2. Fears of damage to the sex organ	66	65.3
3. Fears of nonspecific physical danger	23	22.8
4. Feeling of an altered perception of the world around	19	18.8
5. Hearing odd sounds	17	16.8
6. Feeling of being chased or talked about	6	5.9

*More than one symptom is present in the cases.

TABLE 15: Distribution of genital symptoms.

Symptoms	*n = 101*	*%*
1. Penile retraction only	79	78.2
2. Alteration of penile shape with retraction	9	8.9
3. Loss of penile muscular tone with retraction	6	5.9
4. Complete loss of penile sensation only	4	4.0
5. Shortening of penile length/shaft girth without retraction	3	3.0

phenomenon was mainly associated with the experience of hearing an odd or unclear monosyllabic sound (17%) just before their attack. Many patients (mainly from the Koch-Bihar district) articulated this fear-rousing sound by the syntax of "Kottash." Interestingly, the "Kattow" is the local syntax for small tortoise of river beds. Koro illness was locally called by the term "Kattaw" in Koch-Bihar district, which also means "cut off."[15,16] Among the patients who complained of "being chased or talked about (6%), one had a concurrent diagnosis of schizophrenia."

4. *Genital symptoms* **(Table 15)**: Though the retracting penis was the cardinal presentation (78%), in the present series, two other Koro-equivalent features without penile retraction was also noted, viz., feelings of complete loss of penile sensation (3.9%) and shortening of the penis without retraction (2.9%). Two associated symptoms were also noted: these are alterations of penis morphology (8.9%) (reduced glans size, reduced penis-shaft girth) and loss of penile muscular tone (5.9%).

- *Attack frequency:* Customarily, Koro is characterized by a solitary attack. An analysis of 357 male Koro cases here revealed that quite a large number of cases did have more than one attack within a single day, usually interspersed 30–40-minute intervals. **Table 16** shows the attack frequencies.

TABLE 16: Koro attack frequency in males.

Frequency	*n = 357*	*%*
Single attack	226	63.3
Two attacks	78	21.9
Three attacks	44	12.3
Four or more attacks (within 1–4 days)	9	2.5

A clinical severity gradation of Koro intensity based on attack frequencies may be helpful in research methodology. The rating of clinical severity may be done as: mild (solitary attack), moderate (two spells), and marked (three or more episodes).

- *Relapse:* Koro is a benign disease so far as the recurrence is concerned. All Koro researchers also noted that the relapse frequency in Koro is virtually negligible. 1-year follow-up of 101 cases of this series revealed relapse in two patients only, one after a gap of 4 weeks from the first attack and the other after 19 days.

CONCLUSION

This analysis reveals that the hallmark of Koro symptoms, i.e., the penile retraction with fear of death, is also associated with different types of symptoms, many of which have not been reported earlier. The presence of premonitory symptoms, mainly reflecting the anxiety spectrum, significantly contributes to developing some of Koro's associated physical symptoms. Shortening of the penis without intra-abdominal retraction may also be found in an epidemic setting and needs careful clinical notice for its proper diagnostic labeling.

FEMALE KORO CASES (n = 48)

This is a comprehensive study of female Koro cases[17] in the literature.

- *Demographic features:*
  - *Age mean: 23.6 ± 10.8 years.*

  The highest and lowest ages were 8 and 54 years, respectively.
  - *Education:* Maximum cases were illiterate (41.7%)
  - *Occupation:* No occupation was maximum (37.5%).
  - *Economic class:* Maximum cases were from the lower economic classes, viz., Class IV and V (combined 62.5%).
  - *Family type:* Maximum cases were from joint families (56%).
  - *Family size:* Maximum cases were from families having 1–5 members strength (56%). Religion—Hinduism was the most familiar religion (including Rajbansi's)—81%.

- *Clinical features:*
  - *Onset type:* 64% acute onset.
  - *Onset time:* 51% during the morning (6 AM to 12 noon).
  - *Place of attack:* 56% at home.
  - *Clinical symptoms:*
    - Premonitory symptoms were present in 43% of cases. The most frequently noted symptoms were: chest pain (64.7%), headache (52.9%), unusual feeling in the abdomen (41%), lethargy (35%), and tremor of hands and legs (17.7%).
    - *Physical symptoms:* Most frequently noted symptoms were: Lethargy—51%; Inability to speak—46%; Chest pain—46.6%
    - *Mental symptoms:* Most frequently noted symptoms were:
      Fear of breast damage: 64%; Fear of death: 38.5%; Bewitched feeling: 25.6%; Fear of heart damage: 15%; Fear of turning into a eunuch: 2.6%
    - *Breast and genital symptoms:* Retraction of the Nipple/Breast: 64%; Labial Retraction: 7.7%; Vaginal/or Breast Pain:12.8%
    - *Associated morbidity:* 17 cases fulfilled the criteria for a secondary diagnosis as follows: hysterical fainting: 9 (23%); neurotic depression: 2 (5.1%); psychotic depression: 1 (2.6%); hypochondriasis: 1 (2.6%); viral fever: 2 (5.1%); migraine: 1 (2.6%); arthritis: 1 (2.6)

Breast image perception: Some Koro patients complained of a feeling of reduced breast mass after their attack. They showed a reduced breast area perception on DABT (Draw-a-Breast Test) compared to their perception of a normal breast (unpublished). This area needs further research.

KORO AND PSYCHIATRIC MORBIDITY

- Koro, in association with 4 schizophrenia and 7 with paranoid schizophrenia (all-male cases), is reported.[18]
- Seven cases of Koro (4 males, 3 females) in association with affective disorder (depression) is reported.[19]
- Twenty-one cases (17 males, 4 females) are reported from 9 families with different kinships, e.g., brother-brother, brother-sister, father-son, father-daughter, and husband-wife.[20]

PART FOUR: KORO SOCIAL RESPONSE STUDY

PREAMBLE

Social support and cultural reference are the two most critical sociomedical variables for any episode of "mental contagion."[21] Mechanic,[22] therefore, stresses the due importance of a sociocultural perspective and states that the concept of illness refers to objective symptoms. In contrast, illness behavior ascribes the personal and social meaning of the symptom. Illness perception and response are socially learned phenomena because the magnitude of symptoms and the resultant disability are products of subjective experience, social expectations, and social definitions of distress. How people in a community respond to a sick person is immensely important because social sanction is one of the most crucial prerequisites for any maladaptive behavior labeled "illness."[23] Social support systems play a decisive role here since the network of friends and primary relationships provide a role model for one's behavior, leading to social credibility and positive sanctions to the individual's behavior.[24] Social labeling requires a positive illness paradigm of a given symptom for its acceptance in the family and community. This individual-social interaction and reciprocal cognitive exchange is a well-established sociopsychological mechanism in the genesis and spread of mental contagion.[25,26] in the community **(Flowchart 1)**. The cultural atmosphere is vital in the labeling process. The content of beliefs about the aberrant behavior held by the family and treatment people and the hypothetical risk and danger of the behavior assessed are essential determinants of the condition under which a behavioral abnormality earns the illness character.[27] Once the symptom patterns are received and confirmed as *illness*; one may expect a very high prevalence rate by transmitting the "illness model" through different sociometric channels.[28]

The social response theory suggests that the labeling of deviation and its messages to the patient about the sick role is consistently strengthened and reinforced by the opinion and the help-providing system of treating

Flowchart 1: Conceptual framework of "Positive Illness Paradigm."

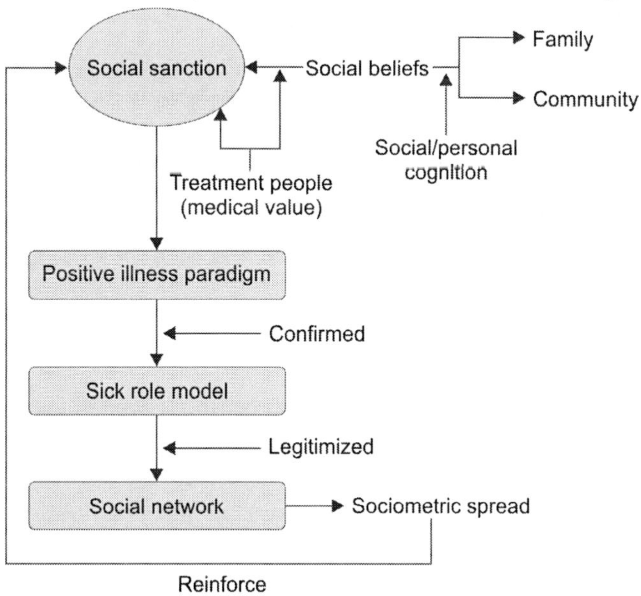

people in the community.[29] Denitz et al.[30] state that sickness may be modeled by the bureaucratic influence of the caregiver system, including the records of diagnosis and prognosis made by the treatment people of a community, which "may circulate through many hands and may become the sole basis for a treatment person's message; to him." Mechanic[22] saw that illnesses and their associated behavior are not static but rather a dynamic response to changing personal and social cognitive interactions. A clinician should guide the process by providing a constructive explanation but not reinforcing maladaptive behavior. The doctor is highly influential because his/her scientific opinion assigns medical value to the illness in question. A doctor should be an essential helper in the patient's adaptive response; otherwise, people accommodate illness perception through social cognitive constructions, search for meaning, sociocultural attribution, and social comparison.[31-33]

Once an illness serves as a model of a set of social relationships, it provides a referential basis for defining the model, and the contagion enters into the social network. It will disperse with increasing rapidity in a chain reaction. Turner and Killian[34] stress the "emergent norm" concept, which may explain the spread of the illness or contagious behavior. In any collective behavior, milling behavior must precede any collective action. Milling behavior is such that persons circulate and share their perceptions of occurring events in their environment. From these shared perceptions, definitions of the situation arise, communicated to others in the background. These shared and communicated perceptions reflect the cultural resources and ethnomedical concepts, then emerge as the basis for norms regarding the deviant behavior model and the coping strategy of the situation after that. The acceleration of the massage of illness or the illness "acting-out" itself is a part of the fact that, as more cases appear, the behavior becomes increasingly legitimized in the community.[35] Since such a contagion is at the very root of psychiatric epidemics, it soon forms, with its accelerated and greater legitimacy in society, a phenomenon of such a proportion that it is an illness. The credibility of such claims can no longer be denied. Thus increasingly reinforcing the "illness paradigm" and vice versa among the affected and the nonaffected segment of the population.[36] The credibility of a case is the initial determining factor in the community perception of contagiousness as the psychiatric epidemic is concerned. Kerckhoff[37] puts this contention nicely as follows:

"There is also a reciprocal reinforcement process involved in the validation of the threat. One or two cases of illness might not impress many of those present. However, as the number of cases increases, it is difficult to avoid believing that *something* must be making those people sick and the more an individual believes in the reality of the threat, the greater the tension(s) he is likely to experience, and the more likely (s)he is to experience symptoms associated with tension. Such symptoms are then very likely to be associated with the suggested threat, and the individual may well become a "case" (p. 204)."

Scheff's[27] classical work on the contagiousness of mental illness is noteworthy here. He provides a series of propositions in this regard: (1) The repeated signs of disease are noted in such outbreaks that follow a stereotypic snowballing pattern. (2) Every victim learns the typical clinical signs; thus, the cases express the same learned phenomenon. (3) The immediate peer group reaction is critical in determining both the duration and the outcome of the disability. (4) There may be a reward for playing out stereotypical behavior in some situations. The victim shares the experience with others, thus making the behavior a collective one and reinforcing the actor's perception of the reality of the event.

The Psychiatric Epidemic Process: Sirois[38] described the different perspectives of epidemic hysterical manifestations elegantly. He very aptly points out that any episode of a mental epidemic is a conjoint agendum for psychiatrists, psychologists, sociologists, and anthropologists. The interactions of all the aspects are crucial for understanding a psychiatric epidemic. These are: the psychological attributes like personality, anxiety profile, suggestibility of the individual; his spectrum of coping strategies and strength of defense mechanism, conflicts areas and morbidities (signs/symptoms), the social support system and the sociometric communicative network and their environment—the cultural beliefs and attitudes, folklore, and mythological references. The expert analysis of Sioris of the last hundred and ten years (1870–1980) world literature consisting of 88 reports of epidemic hysteria is valuable in this context.[39]

The Metaphoric Model of Psychic Infectivity: The element of *contagiousness* in the psychiatric epidemic is an issue of much debate. The word "contagion" of an infectious medical model dictates that some psychic stuff is transmitted from one individual to another. Sioris[28] asserts that an epidemic mental contagion is an acute group syndrome that resolves a conflicting situation. In many episodes, the conflict stems from a fantasized[40,41] or a real threat.[42] The response of pathological defense to the conflictive issues rather than the usual coping is dependent on at least four psychodynamic attributes of the individual, viz., (1) the identification of the people in the group with the wish of the index cases; (2) the regression fostered by the group situation; (3) the unconscious or preconscious nature of the conflict or the underlying fantasy; and (4) the neurotic or suggestible personality disposition of the persons involved. They are intrinsic or personal vulnerability factors. There are three extrinsic vulnerabilities: the existing myth regarding the justification of stress of the conflictive/fantasized situation, the affected population's conducive social behavior, and the geopolitical situation. Both the factors,

Flowchart 2: Mental contagiousness in a psychiatric epidemic.

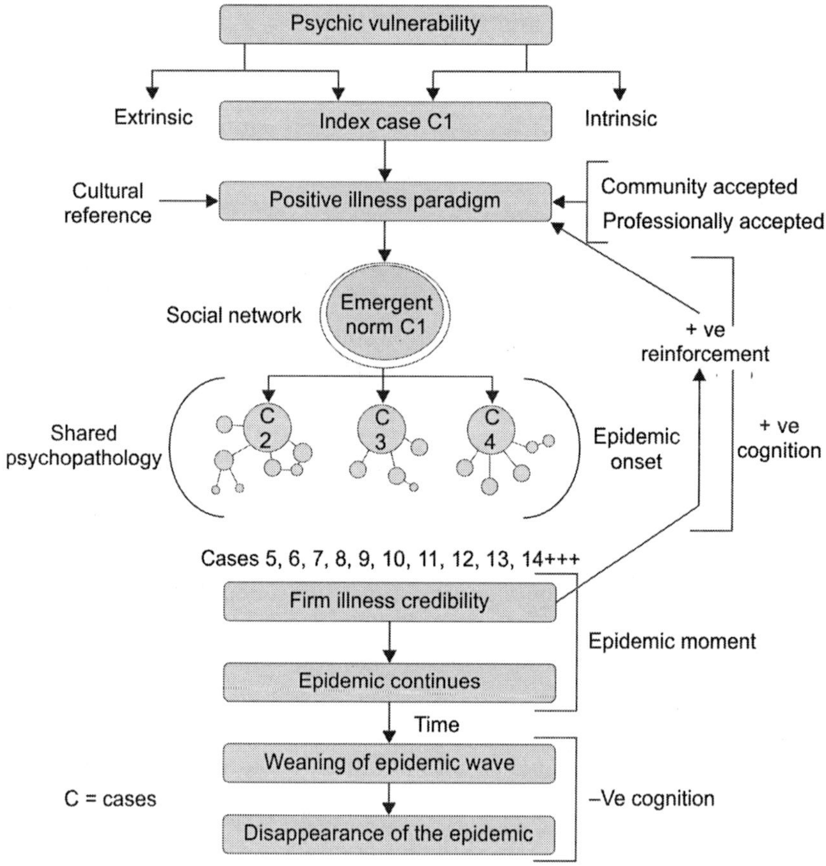

i.e., intrinsic and extrinsic, guide the manifestation of the conflict through displaced or symbolic maladaptive behavior. **Flowchart 2** shows the schematic chart of mental contagiousness, the process of an epidemic wave, and its weaning in a simplified manner.

This investigation was aimed to explore the different social responses to the epidemic of Koro in the Darjeeling district. This study examines some extrinsic or sociocultural factors intimately related to Koro's social acceptance and the acceleration of the Koro-contagion in the community. Some social aspects were assessed longitudinally and others cross-sectionally to understand the mass psychological dynamics.

The following is the summary heading of this Koro Social Response study design.

- Positive Illness Paradigm of Koro as perceived by:
    - *Community:* (1) Rural group/ (2) Urban group > Longitudinal study

- Professional Group
- Intra- and intercomparison of both the groups.

- *Koro Cause Perception* by: (1) Community: (a) Rural group/(b) Urban group. (2) Treatment people and (3) Koro patients (Ethnomedical study)
- *Treatment Opinion for Koro* by: (1) Community: (a) Rural group, (b) Urban group. (2) Treatment people.
- *Account of Social Treatment* used in North Bengal epidemic Koro cases.
- *Profile of Koro Acquaintance Source* of the total samples studied.

MATERIALS AND METHODS

Study Sample

Koro Study Population

Rural sample: Koro social responses were taken from 70 heads (or elders) of families (all males) of two villages (Naxalbari and Kharibari) of Darjeeling districts. These families had no Koro-affected members. 45 responses were taken by random sampling without replacement for this study. Similarly, reactions of 43 family heads were taken by random sample from a total of 63 who had at least one Koro-affected member in their family from the Dabgram village of the same district. Thus a total of 88 responses were studied and are referred to here as the *rural group.*

Urban sample: Koro Social Responses of 60 family heads (or elder, male persons) of non-Koro affected families were taken by random sampling from a total of 98 responses from three municipal wards (Nos. 3, 6, 11) of Siliguri town of Darjeeling district. 58 heads out of 72 responses from Koro-affected families from the same localities were taken by random sampling. Thus a total of 118 responses was taken for this study under the *urban group.*

Professional sample: Koro Social Responses were elicited from four groups of treatment people and health providers working in modern medicine of the Darjeeling district. They are Physicians (having diploma or degree in any branch of medicine); General Practitioners (medical graduates); Surgeons (having a diploma or degree in any branch of Surgery), and Paramedical Staff (Working in medical laboratories and physiotherapy or optometry clinics). 40 responses were taken randomly from each of the four groups, viz. 61 Physicians (P); 87 General Practitioners (GP); 51 Surgeons (S) and 47 Paramedical Staff (PMS). Thus a total of 160 persons were taken here as constituting the *professional group.* Two-point inclusion criteria was followed: (1) They must be willing to take part in the study, and (2) Respondent has seen or here about Koro's illness in the community.

The Koro Study Team collected all the responses through field visits.

Instrument

Social Response Pattern Schedule: It is a simple 12-item forced-choice questionnaire **(Appendix I)** for recording the social responses to Koro illness, made in consultation with the Department of Sociology and Social Anthropology of North Bengal University, Darjeeling. It has five sections: (1) *Brief Demography,* (2) *Illness Paradigm of Koro,* (3) *Koro etiology,* (4) *Koro Treatment option,* and (5) *Koro Acquaintance Source.*

Illness Paradigm of Koro: This section includes the following items:

- Identification of Koro Illness type as either *physical/mental or nil.*
- Grades of Koro Seriousness, viz., *nil/mild/moderate or severe.*
- Infective Potential of Koro illness, viz., *nil/mild/moderate/severe or highly infectious.*
- Risk imposition by Koro illness, viz.. *nil/life threatening/risk of sexual power loss/risk of general health problems or a combination of the last two.*

Each respondent was asked to express their best estimate of the items of their choice in each category. Koro Positive illness Paradigm study was also done longitudinally over time in the same rural and urban samples.

Koro Etiology or Cause Perception: This part includes the enlistment of nine items. Eight of them, except "mischievousness" (unknown, high fever, physical strain, excessive body heat, sexual reason, supernatural cause, fear, and mental), were selected based on the finding of most frequently expressed (57%) perception related to illness causation in this region, elicited in a previous pilot study on the "Social Cognition of Mental Illness" at the Psychiatry Unit of North Bengal Medical College and Hospital, Darjeeling and also based on participant observations during the epidemic. The item "mischievousness" was added while working with the Koro social cognition study because many respondents attributed this concept, including professional people.

Koro Treatment Option: This section includes four response options or categories, viz.:

1. *Treatment Option,* i.e., medical (allopathic)/natural (folk treatment) or no treatment
2. *Medicine Option,* i.e., nil/Allopathic/Kabiraji or Ayurvedic
3. *Natural (folk) Treatment Option,* Water pouring/penile pull, either manual or mechanical/saltwater feeding
4. *Mental Treatment Option,* i.e., whether the respondent would consider any scope of (yes/no) mental treatment in Koro cases.

Koro Acquaintance Source: This section deals with the source of Koro's acquaintance of the respondent, viz., *direct viewing of a case of Koro or hearsay.*

Time of Social Response Ratings

The responses (all cross-sectional studies) were collected at the height of the Koro epidemic in the district. The mean time intervals from the onset of the outbreak in the district (9th July—first case reporting at the Subdivisional hospital, Siliguri) were 2.4 ± 1.7 weeks for the urban group; 3.5 ± 2.1 weeks for the rural group, and 2.2 ± 1.2 weeks for the professional group.

A longitudinal study of the "Positive Illness Paradigm" of the Koro on the rural and urban groups was also done. The same respondents, twice in the rural group and thrice in the urban group, were rated. The details of the time intervals of these longitudinal responses are given in the respective sections.

Statistical analysis of the response-data was done using the "t", Chi square, "z", and Tau tests of significance.

STUDY OF ILLNESS PARADIGM OF KORO

Introduction: The cultural impact on the perception of health and illness has been documented in many studies.[43,44] Culture also shapes the cognitive and behavioral options for help-seeking attitudes of an individual and society. In organic illness, the fundamental nature of symptoms, the host-pathogen immunological reaction, and the therapeutic responses to specific antidotes are not usually directly related to the individual or society's cultural dimension and psychological disposition. The concept of "infectivity" is associated with the disease progression by microbes. In Preventive and Social Medicine, this context of infectivity is categorized by a different mechanism, which is primarily independent of the individual's cognitive status (about the illness).

A series of research in biological psychiatry has failed to pinpoint any substantial evidence favoring direct biological causative organisms in mental illness. Cultural aspects of the cognitive disposition of an individual or a group, on the other hand, claim to play an essential role in the labeling and help-seeking attitudes for abnormal behaviors.[45,46] When an illness shifts from an individual to a group, then it follows a sociometric patterns of hysterical cognition,[47] as seen in the mass psychogenic illness (MPI) in industries.[48] The cognitive process concerning the sick-role model is the basis that fosters a cognitive differentiation between categories of normal and abnormal behaviors[49] and generates an element of psychic infectivity that accelerates the spread of mental epidemics among vulnerable individuals in the community.

Study design: Home visits elicited a koro Social Response rating from 88 respondents (45 from non-Koro and 43 from Koro affected families). *The First rating* was done during the height of the epidemic (3rd/4th week of July and 1st week of August). *The Second rating* from the same respondents was done at an interval (from the first) of 36.8 ± 5 days.

RESULTS

ILLNESS PARADIGM: STUDY OF RURAL GROUP

- Pattern and comparison of responses between first and second social ratings.

Table 17 and Figure 9 show a comparison between the two ratings.

On "Illness Perception," 100% of the respondents identified Koro as a form of physical illness in the first rating. In contrast, in the second rating, 13.6% identified it as a form of mental illness. This change in "Illness Perception" between the ratings is significant ($p < .01$).

Comparison of the perceived "seriousness" of Koro responses: In the first rating, there was no "nil" response; all the reactions varied from mild (6.8%), moderate (19.3%), and severe (73.9%). In the second rating, not only 19.3% of the responses referred to the "nil" category, but the distribution of responses in different severity intensities also changed significantly ($p < .01$): i.e., 25% mild, 28.4% moderate, and only 27.3% were severe.

Comparison of "Risk" perception between the ratings: Everyone perceived that Koro entailed a substantial risk in the first rating; so the "no danger" response was virtually unendorsed. However, 12.5% of the respondents thought Koro carried no danger to the sufferer in the second rating. The response to the "life-threatening" item also demonstrated a changed perception from 48.9% to 18.2% in the second rating. "Weakness and general health problem" though perceived by only 10.2% of the respondents in the first rating, more respondents (28.4%) positively endorsed this item in the second rating. This difference in the pattern of risk perception between the two ratings is significant ($p < .01$).

Comparison of Koro "Infectivity" perception between the ratings: In the first rating, the highest endorsement was to "highly infectious" (56.8%), and the lowest was "nil" response (2.3%). In the second rating, the picture was quite contrary, i.e., the "highly infectious" answer scored the lowest percentage (9.1%), and the "nil" response was increased to 18.2%. These changes in cognitive appraisals over time, are significant ($p < .01$).

Observation: The first social response of illness cognition about Koro was elicited at the height of the epidemic. It is evident from the result that Koro's cognitive construct as a form of "physical illness" of "serious" nature, with "high risk" (life-threatening) and "highly infectious" was the predominant social understanding construct about Koro illness. This positive illness paradigm **(Fig. 9)** was instrumental in Koro's spread through these social cognitive appraisals. Over time (gaining more experience), a negative shift occurred in this cognition, which eventually restricted its occurrence and spread. The disease cognition waned gradually **(Fig. 10)**, as manifested in the second rating.

TABLE 17: Comparison of cognitive assessments between two ratings (n = 88).

	First rating		*Second rating*		
	No.	**%**	**No.**	**%**	X^2
Rural illness cognition					
Nil	–	–	–	–	*(df = 1)* 12.88*
Physical	88	100	76	86.4	
Mental	–	–	22	13.6	
Rural seriousness cognition					
NIl	–	–	17	19.3	*(df = 1)* 46.55*
Mild	6	6.8	22	25	
Moderate	17	19.3	25	28.4	
Severe	65	73.9	24	27.3	
Rural risk cognition					
No danger			11	12.5	*(df = 4)* 32.21*
Life-threatening	43	48.9	16	18.2	
Sexual power (S)	29	32.9	27	30.7	
General health (H)	9	10.2	25	28.4	
S + H	7	8.0	9	10.2	
Rural infectivity cognition					
Nil	2	2.3	16	18.2	*(df = 4)* 54.29*
Mild	4	4.6	19	21.6	
Moderate	14	15.9	25	28.4	
Severe	18	20.4	20	22.7	
Highly infectious	50	56.8	8	9.09	

$^*p < .01$

- Pattern and comparison of responses between members of non-Koro (NKF) and Koro families (KF) in the First Social Response rating

Table 18 exhibits a comparison of "Illness perception" between the non-Koro (NKF) and Koro families (KF) in the first social response rating, which shows virtually identical responses, viz. Koro is a physical illness between the two groups.

Table 19 compares perceived "Seriousness" "between the two groups in the first rating. The NKF group also perceived that Koro entailed mild (13.3%), moderate (22.2%), and severe (64.4%) seriousness, and these differences from Koro families" responses were significant ($p < .05$).

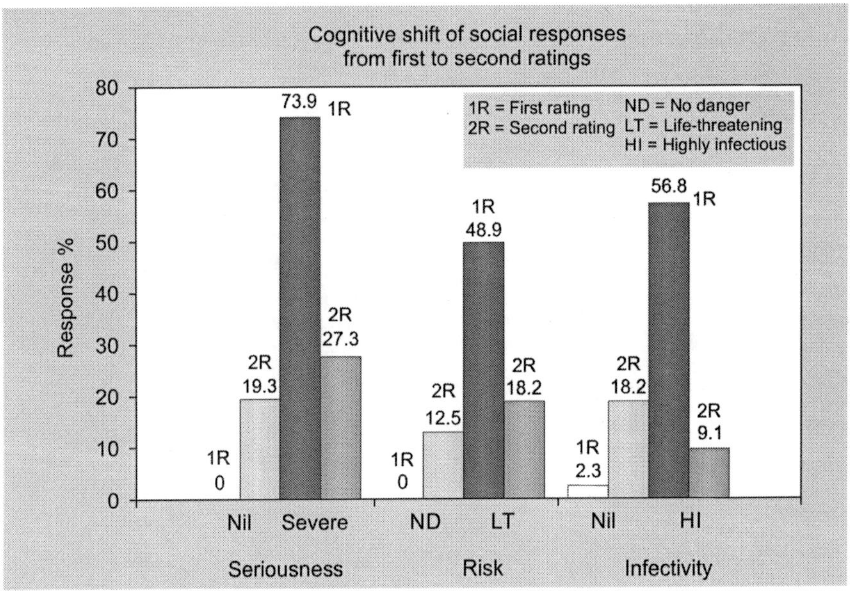

Fig. 9: Comparison of responses between the two ratings.

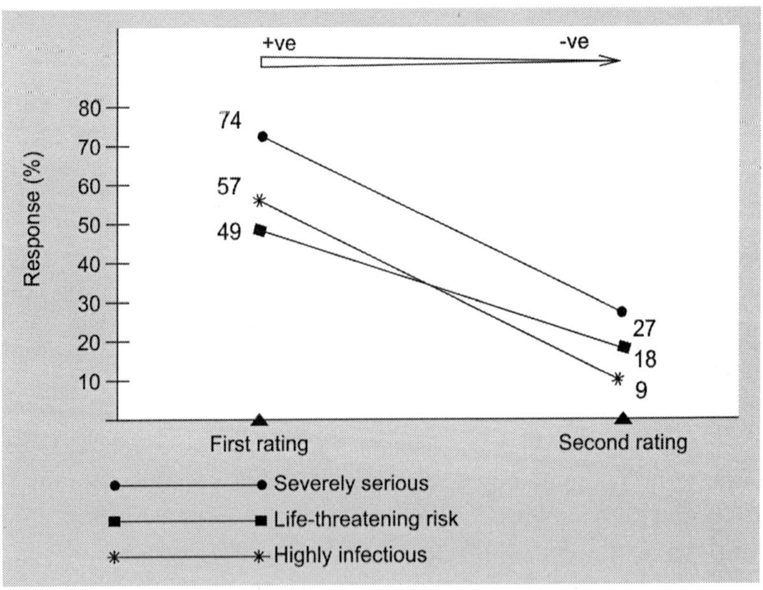

Fig. 10: The cognitive shift from positive to negative illness paradigm over time.

Comparison of "Risk" perception between NKF and KF groups in the first rating showed that the NKF group showed higher endorsement in all the items except "life-threatening" than the KF group. This difference was significant ($p < .01$).

TABLE 18: "Illness perception" of non-Koro families (NKF) and Koro families (KF) members in the first rating.

	NKF (n = 45)		*KF (n = 43)*	
	No.	*%*	*No.*	*%*
Nil	–	–	–	–
Physical	45	100	43	100
Mental	–	–	–	–

TABLE 19: Comparison of opinions on seriousness, risk estimation, and infectivity between non-Koro families (NKF) and Koro families (KF) groups in the first rating.

	NKF (n = 45)		*KF (n = 43)*		
	No	*%*	*No*	*%*	X^2
Seriousness					
Nil	–	–	–	–	*(df = 2)*
Mild	6	13.3		100	*7.24**
Moderate	10	22.2	7	16.3	
Severe	29	64.4	36	83.7	
Risk estimation					
No danger	–	–	–	–	*(df = 3)*
Life-threatening	14	31	29	67.4	*14.88***
Sexual power (S)	18	40	11	25.6	
General health (H)	6	13	3	6.9	
(S + H)	7	16	–	–	
Infectivity					
Nil	2	4.4	–	–	*(df = 4)*
Mild	4	8.9	–	–	*7.40 (NS)*
Moderate	5	11	9	20.9	
Severe	10	22	8	18.6	
Highly Infectious	24	53	23	60.5	

**p*< .05; ***p*< .01/NS = Nonsignificant

Comparison of opinions on "Infectivity" between NKF and KF groups showed that though few NKF members endorsed nil (4.4%) and mild (8.9%) infectivity potential of Koro, the responses of both the groups showed no significant difference.

Observation: The KF members showed more favorable responses regarding the seriousness (severe) and the risk (life-threatening) from Koro illness than NKF members. So far as infectivity opinion is concerned, both groups evinced almost identical understanding, which played a role in the epidemic spread of Koro in the region **(Fig. 11)**.

- Pattern and comparison of responses between NKF and KF in the second social response rating **(Table 20)**.

Opinion on "illness" type between the NKF and KF groups in the second rating showed no differences.

Comparison of opinion on "Seriousness" between the two groups in the second rating: NKF members endorsed more the nil (37.8%) and mild (26.7) categories, whereas KF members did so in the moderate (37.2%) and severe (39.5%) items. These differences between the groups were significant ($p < .01$).

Comparison of "Risk" perception between the NKF and KF groups in the second rating showed no differences.

In the second rating, the comparison of opinion on "Infectivity" between NKF and KF groups showed no significant differences.

Observation: The most exciting finding in this second social response rating is that members of both non-Koro and Koro-affected families showed almost identical perceptions in the positive illness paradigm, like severely serious, sexual power loss, and severe infectivity. This positivity was due to the distress family members underwent during the Koro episodes in their family members. Even well after the epidemic, this cognitive endorsement

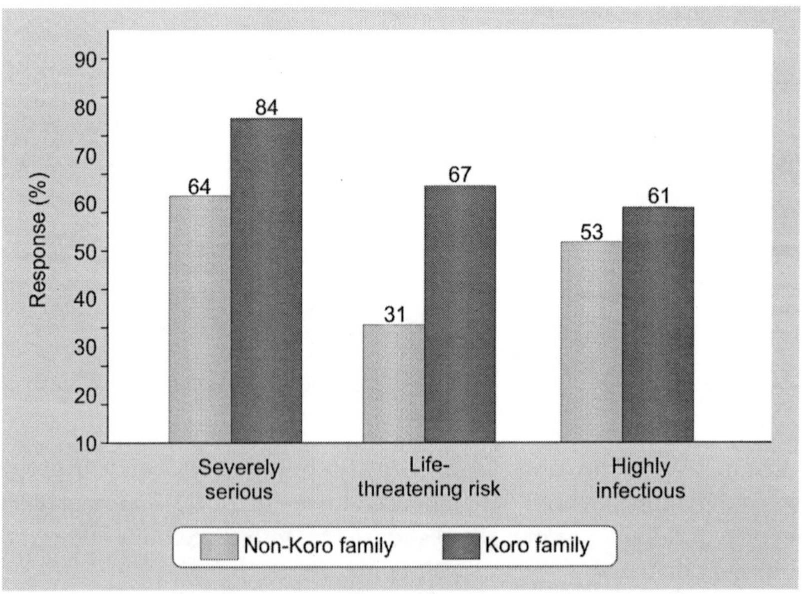

Fig. 11: Comparison of non-Koro (NKF) and Koro family (KF) members responses in the first social response rating.

TABLE 20: Comparison of opinions between non-Koro families (NKF) and Koro families (KF) groups in the second rating.

	NKF (n = 45)		*KF (n = 43)*		
	No	*%*	*No*	*%*	X^2
Illness					
Physical	40	88.9	36	83.7	*(df = 1)* *0.49 (NS)*
Mental	5	11.1	7	16.3	
Seriousness					
Nil	17	37.8			*(df = 3)* 23.28*
Mild	12	26.7	10	23.3	
Moderate	9	20	16	37.2	
Severe	7	15.6	17	39.5	
Risk					
No danger	4	8.9	7	16.3	*(df = 4)* 5.36 (NS)
Life-threatening	5	11.1	11	25.6	
Sexual power (S)	15	33.3	12	27.9	
General health (H)	15	33.3	10	23.3	
S + H	6	13.3	3	6.9	
Infectivity					
Nil	8	17.8	8	18.6	*(df = 4)* 0.75 (NS)
Mild	10	22.2	9	20.9	
Moderate	13	28.9	12	27.9	
Severe	9	20	11	25.6	
Highly infectious	5	11.1	3	6.9	

$^*p < .01$/NS = nonsignificant.

will help maintain Koro's illness paradigm in the community for a considerable length of time.

- Pattern and comparison of illness paradigm of Koro perception of Koro-affected family members between the First and Second Social Response ratings.

Table 21 shows the changing pattern of opinion about Koro illness between first and second ratings among the Koro-affected families (n = 43).

Illness opinion: In the second rating, they endorsed Koro as a mental illness (16.3%). In the first rating, there was no such endorsement. This difference was significant ($p < .05$).

TABLE 21: Changing pattern of opinions of Koro families between the two ratings.

	Koro family members (n = 43)				
	First rating		*Second rating*		
	No	*%*	*No*	*%*	X^2
Illness opinion					
Physical	43	100	36	83.7	*(df = 1)* 7.62*
Mental	–	–	7	16.3	
Seriousness opinion					
Mild	–	–	10	23.3	*(df = 2)* 20.33**
Moderate	7	16.3	16	37.2	
Severe	36	83.7	17	39.5	
Risk assessment					
No danger	–	–	7	16.3	*(df = 4)* 21.91**
Life-threatening	29	67.4	11	25.6	
Sexual power (S)	11	25.6	12	27.9	
General health (H)	3	6.9	10	23.3	
S + H			3	6.9	
Infectivity potential					
Nil	–	–	8	18.6	*(df = 4)* 36.15**
Mild	–	–	9	20.9	
Moderate	9	20.9	12	27.9	
Severe	8	18.6	11	25.6	
Highly infectious	26	60.5	3	6.9	

*$p < .05$; **$p < .01$

Seriousness opinion: There were endorsements to the "mild" (23.3%) item in the second rating and less percentage loading on the severe category (from 83.7 to 39.5%). These differences were significant ($p < .01$).

Risk assessment: The most remarkable change in the second rating is the endorsement of the "no danger" (16.3%) category with a reduced response in the "life-threatening" opinion from the first rating (67.4 to 25.6%). These differences were significant ($p < .01$).

Opinion on infectivity: The significant ($p < .01$) change observed here was the endorsement of "nil" (18.6%) and "mild" (20.9%) categories with remarkably reduced responses in the "highly infectious" category (from 60.5 to 6.9%) in the second rating.

Observation: The most notable change from the first to second responses of Koro family members is the diminishing perception of Koro's positive illness paradigm over time. This perceptual change reflects the reality inherent in Koro illness itself. It heavily influences the threat perception (from Koro) in all the essential dimensions, viz. seriousness, risk, and infectivity, of illness cognition of the population.

- Pattern and comparison of illness paradigm of Koro perception of non-Koro affected family members (NKF) between the first and second social response ratings.

Table 22 presents the changing pattern of Cognitive appraisal of Koro illness among non-Koro families (NKF, $n = 45$) between the two ratings.

TABLE 22: Changing pattern of cognitive appraisal of Koro illness among non-Koro families (NKF) between the two ratings.

	Non-Koro family members (n = 45)				
	First rating		*Second rating*		
	No	*%*	*No*	*%*	X^2
Illness perception					
Physical	45	100	40	88.9	*(df = 1)* 5.29**
Mental	–	–	5	11.1	
Seriousness perception					
Nil	–	–	17	37.8	*(df = 3)* 32.49**
Mild	6	13.3	12	26.7	
Moderate	10	22.2	9	20	
Severe	29	64.4	7	15.5	
Risk perception					
No danger	–	–	4	8.9	*(df = 4)* 12.47*
Life-threatening	14	31.1	5	11.1	
Sexual power (S)	18	40	15	33.3	
General health (H)	6	13.3	15	33.3	
S + H	7	15.6	6	13.3	
Infectivity perception					
Nil	2	4.4	8	17.8	*(df = 4)* 22.23**
Mild	4	8.9	10	22.2	
Moderate	5	11.1	13	28.9	
Severe	10	22.2	9	20	
Highly infectious	24	53.3	5	11.1	

*$p < .05$; **$p < .01$

Illness perception: 11.1% of the respondents endorsed Koro as a form of mental illness in the second rating. This difference in perception was significant ($p < .01$).

Seriousness opinion: In the second rating, a significant ($p < .01$) shift from "more serious" to "less serious" estimates has been noted and was reflected in 37.8% endorsement in the "nil" item and increase in the "mild" item from the first rating (from 13.3 to 26.7%) and decrease in the "severe" item (from 64.4 to 15.5%).

"Risk" perception: In the second rating, a significant ($p < .05$) positive endorsement was noted in "no danger" (8.9%) and "general health" (from 13.3 to 33.3%) items and more reduced response (negative appraisal) in the "life-threatening" item (from 31.1 to 11.1%).

Infectivity opinion: The significant ($p < .01$) change observed was the shift from the positive towards the negative perception as reflected in the endorsement of "nil" (from 4.4 to 17.8%), "mild" (from 8.9 to 22.2%) and marked reduction in "highly infectious" (from 53.3 to 11.1%) estimations.

Conclusion

It is evident from this study that, during the epidemic days, people from both Koro-affected and nonaffected families endorsed Koro as a severe disease with significant risk to life and sexual disability and with a highly infective potential. This is the social model of Koro illness-construct in the rural communities of North Bengal.

Social evaluative-cognitive dimensions of an illness mainly involve the assessment of seriousness, risk, cause, and prognosis, of which "seriousness" is the most critical variable.[50] Atypical symptoms are usually viewed as severe.[51] The unknown nature of this rare "sexual" disease in this region had no prior social or community cognitive reference. Besides, the very sexual nature of the illness (under its cultural and moral overtone) resulted in its assessment being of a severe nature. The simultaneous occurrences of similar community cases reinforce its "infective" character with the strong endorsement for community cognitive support of Koro-affected and nonaffected family members, which in reality generated a snowballing influence on vulnerable individuals.

The message from the affected families that "Koro is an illness" with "high infectivity" percolated through the interfamilial communicative pathways. It enriched the nonaffected population with Koro information. A positive social environment primed with the cognition of vulnerability of Koro was then generated, and the behavioral dysfunction of Koro follows a "facilitative norm" pathway without any social resistance. Credibility increases the likelihood of more new cases, and the construct of "infectivity" becomes

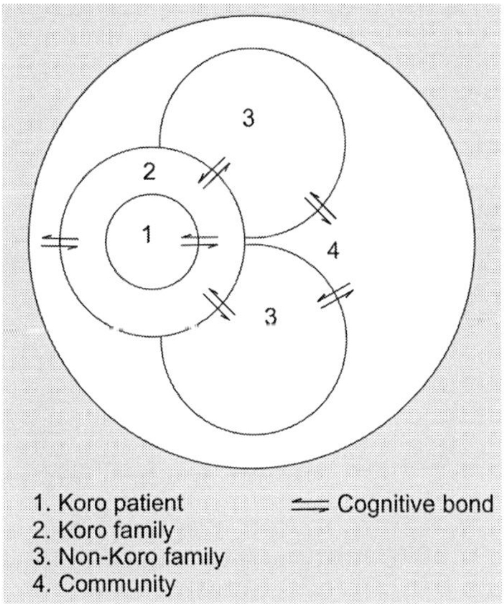

Fig. 12: The dynamic force of psychic infectivity in Koro.

even more strengthened by the various cognitive bonds of the community **(Fig. 12)**.

These positive beliefs' strength and intensity was reflected in the peak incidence of cases during the early part of the epidemic. Koro's benign nature is conceived only with the passing of time when both the positive illness cognitive appraisal and the incidence rate of cases gradually fall and ultimately disappear. Some positive social beliefs remain in the community that serves a dual purpose, viz., as a token of prior societal acknowledgment of the illness and as a cognitive resource or background information for potential future use in a similar context. The latter ultimately helps form a cultural construct or model of a particular dysfunction or disability in a specific community.

ILLNESS PARADIGM: STUDY OF URBAN GROUP

Study design: Koro's social response rating was done by home visits. The first rating (IR) was done during the height of the epidemic (in the third week of the outbreak). The second rating (IIR) was done at an interval from the first of 29.5 ± 3 days, and the third rating (IIIR) from the second at 30.7 ± 4 days. In the third rating, due to absence or unwillingness, the number of respondents was dropped to 38 in non-Koro families and 30 in Koro-affected families. So for comparison between IIR and IIIR, a sub-sample (of the same persons who also responded in IIR) of the IIR was drawn.

Epidemic situation and cases: Social responses were elicited at the following background of Koro epidemic in the Darjeeling district. Out of a total of 151 male cases of this epidemic, 84.8% were reported in July, 3.9% in

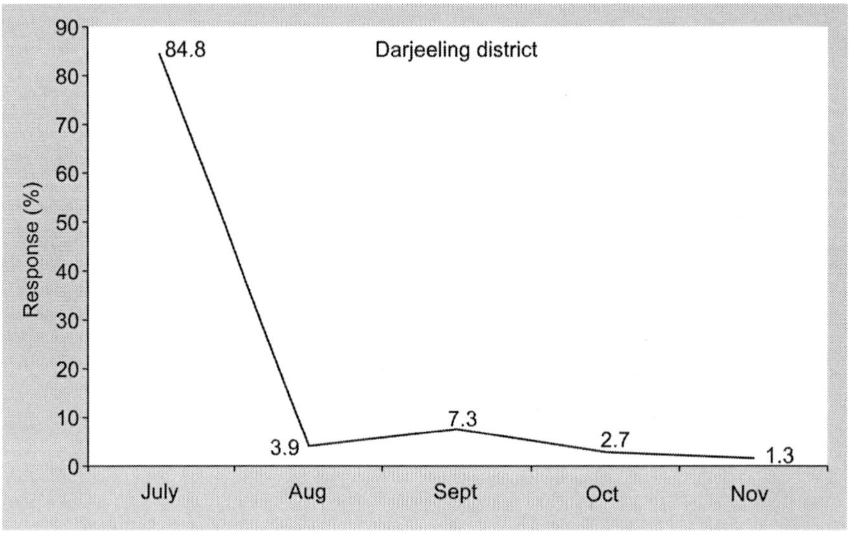

Fig. 13: Male Koro incidence of 1982 epidemic.

August, 7.3% in September, 2.7% in October, and 1.3% in November 1982 **(Fig. 13)**.

Results

Table 23 shows the responses percentage distribution and comparison between the first (IR) and second ratings (IIR).

In the IR most of the respondents from both Koro and non-Koro families perceived Koro as a physical illness with little emphasis on its mental causation. That showed no difference in their perception of illness types. However, in the IIR, this "illness type" perception differed significantly ($p < .01$), where physical-mental typology was endorsed with greater frequency. The previous "physical-type" perception showed decreased response with a slight increase in "mental-type" response. This cognitive shift of illness-type from IR to IIR was significant ($p < .01$) in the non-Koro families. In the cognition about Koro seriousness, both the groups differed significantly ($p < .01$) in the IR perception, where non-Koro families stressed more on the less serious nature of Koro than the Koro family respondents. In the IIR, this trend was noted in higher frequency in the non-Koro families. In the Koro-families, this cognition shift towards "nil" or "mild" serious nature of Koro was evident. These differences from more severe to less severe nature perception were significant ($p <.01$) from IR to IIR in all the groups.

Perception about the assessment of the infective potential of Koro showed no difference between the groups in both the ratings. However, there

TABLE 23: Comparison between first and second response percentages (n = NKF 60 + KF 58 = Total 118).

	First rating (%)			*Second rating (%)*		
	(A)	*(B)*	*(C)*	*(a)*	*(b)*	*(c)*
Perception	*NKF*	*KF*	*Total*	*NKF*	*KF*	*Total*
I. Illness type						
Physical (P)	90.0	91.4	90.7	35.0	75.0	55.10
Mental (M)	6.7	1.7	4.2	16.7	10.3	13.60
P + M	3.3	6.9	5.1	48.3	13.8	31.30
X_2^2: A vs. B = 2.4; a vs. b = 21.03*; C vs c = 38.4*; A vs. a = 40.6*						
II. Seriousness						
Nil	13.3	–	6.8	40	10.3	25.4
Mild	15	–	7.6	28.3	22.4	25.4
Moderate	21.7	19	20.3	16.7	36.2	26.3
Severe	50	81	65.3	15	31.1	22.9
X_3^2: A vs. B = 20.9*; a vs. b = 18.2*; C vs. c = 49*; A vs. a = 22.2*; B vs. b = 30.04*.						
III. Infectivity						
Nil	23.3	17.2	20.3	65	48.3	56.8
Mild	6.7	1.7	4.2	15	17.2	16.1
Moderate	21.7	17.2	19.5	6.7	15.5	11
Marked	10	19	14.4	3.3	5.2	4.2
Highly infectious	38.3	44.8	41.5	10	13.8	11.9
X_4^2: A vs. B = 4.5; a vs. b = 4.2; C vs. c = 57.3*; A vs. a = 30.5*; B vs. b = 30.04.						
IV. Risk						
Nil	10	–	5.1	26.7	5.2	16.1
Life threatening	31.7	55.1	43.2	–	18.9	9.3
Sexual power (S)	35	20.7	27.9	45	13.8	29.7
General health (H)	16.7	12.1	14.4	20	41.4	30.7
S + H	6.6	12.1	9.3	8.3	20.7	14.4
X_4^2: A vs. B = 13.1**; a vs. b = 37.1*; C vs. c = 40.7*; A vs. a = 24.6*; B vs. b = 24.7.						

*$p < .01$; **$p < .05$

was a cognition shift from IR to IIR so far as the "nil" and "highly" infections' endorsement is concerned. The shift from IR to IIR concerning the more or less infective nature of Koro is significant (p <.01) in both the groups and in the total response.

Interesting perceptual differences (p < .05) were evident in the risk perception between the groups in the IR, where non-Koro families perceived more about the "sexual power loss" from Koro. In contrast, Koro families perceived more about the "life-threatening" risk. This trend was also observed in greater frequency in IIR and the non-Koro families" endorsement of "no-life threat" from Koro. Similarly, the Koro families perceived for the first time in IIR that Koro posed no risk and emphasized the general health problem" as a risk of Koro. These perceptual differences between the groups were significant ($p < .01$). Differences in the risk perception from IR to IIR in all the groups were significant ($p < .01$).

Table 24 shows a comparison between II and IIIR percentage responses. In the IIR, mental or mental-physical nature of Koro illness-type was perceived in greater frequency in both the groups. Also, non-Koro families perceived for the first time in IIIR that Koro as not an illness at all. These differences in perception were significant ($p < .05$). A significant shift from IIR to IIIR was observed in non-Koro families ($p < .01$) and the total responses ($p < .05$).

In the "Seriousness" response, though some shift of perception was observed in IIR to IIIR, there were not significant. Similarly, in the reaction of "infectivity," this type of perceptual shift from "highly infections" to "nil" or "mild" was noted though they showed no significance.

The "Risk" response: The total responses from IIR to IIIR showed more significant endorsement on thc "nil" item ($p < .01$). There was a significant difference ($p < .05$) between the two groups in both the ratings.

Discussion: Social response theory suggests that deviance labeling in the form of messages to the patient about how to confirm the sick role is consistently strengthened and reinforced by the community's significant others.[29] As far as illness cognition is concerned, positive cognitive strength is one of the most crucial factors in this reinforcing process. Time is an important variable to influence this cognitive paradigm's strength and direction because it offers the basis of facilitative observational clues and sociometric feedback as to the rational outcome of the initial hypothetical mental construct of the illness in question. Mechanic[22] viewed this process as a dynamic response to changing personal and social comparison, in the process of cognitive shift that accommodates illness perception through the construction of social cognition. In his elegant analysis of Epidemic Hysteria, Sirois[39] stressed the importance of this aspect of mass-cognition in seven psychiatric epidemics, two of which were of Koro.

The present investigation displayed this social cognition pattern about the Koro epidemic in this region. With Koro's outbreak, the Koro as a positive illness paradigm was initially accepted through emergent norm theory.[52] With time, this positive (regarding the illness validity of Koro) perception shifted towards a negative paradigm, both in Koro-affected and non-Koro populations of this region. So gradually, the incidence of new cases falls

TABLE 24: Comparison between second and third response percentages (n = NKF 38 + KF 30 = Total 68).

	Second rating (%)			*Third rating (%)*		
	(A)	*(B)*	*(C)*	*(a)*	*(b)*	*(c)*
Perception	*NKF*	*KF*	*Total*	*NKF*	*KF*	*Total*
Illness type						
Physical (P)	47.4	80	61.8	36.8	60	47.1
Mental (M)	10.5	6.7	8.8	15.8	16.7	16.2
P+M	42.1	13.3	29.4	26.3	23.3	25
Nil	–	–	–	21.1		11.7
X_2^2: A vs. B = 7.78**; a vs. b = 2.96; X_3^2: a vs. b = 8.3**; C vs. c = 11.1**; A vs. a = 10.3*						
Seriousness						
Nil	39.5	16.7	29.4	47.4	23.3	36.8
Mild	26.3	16.7	26.5	31.6	40	35.3
Moderate	23.7	33.3	27.9	15.8	26.7	20.6
Severe	10.5	23.3	16.2	5.2	10	7.3
X_4^2: A vs. B = 4.1*; a vs. b = 6.4*; C vs. c = 4.5; A vs. a = 1.9; B vs. b = 2.9.						
Infectivity						
Nil	60.5	36.7	50	73.7	46.7	61.8
Mild	10.5	16.7	13.2	10.5	26.7	17.6
Moderate	10.5	20	14.7	5.3	13.3	8.8
Marked	5.3	10	7.4	2.6	6.7	4.4
Highly infectious	13.2	16.6	14.7	7.9	6.6	7.4
X_4^2: A vs. B = 4.1; a vs. b = 6.4; C vs. c = 4.5; A vs. a = 1.9; B vs. b = 2.9.						
Risk						
Nil	28.9	6.7	19.1	57.9	16.7	39.7
Life-threatening	0	20	8.8	0	13.3	5.9
Sexual power (S)	36.8	23.3	30.9	23.7	20	22.1
General health (H)	23.7	40	30.9	13.2	26.7	19.1
S+H	10.5	10	10.3	5.2	23.3	13.2
X_4^2: A vs. B = 14.4**; a vs. b = 18.1**; C vs. c = 27.7*; B vs. b = 4.2. X_3^2: A vs. a = 6.6.						

*$p < .01$; **$p < .05$

to the complete nonoccurrence. The dynamics of this social cognition reinforcement could be well convincing if we consider the associated epidemic pattern in this region **(Fig. 13)** and compare this epidemic curve with each of the factors of social perception, viz., seriousness, infectivity, and risk perception within this time frame **(Figs. 14 to 16)**. That clearly shows

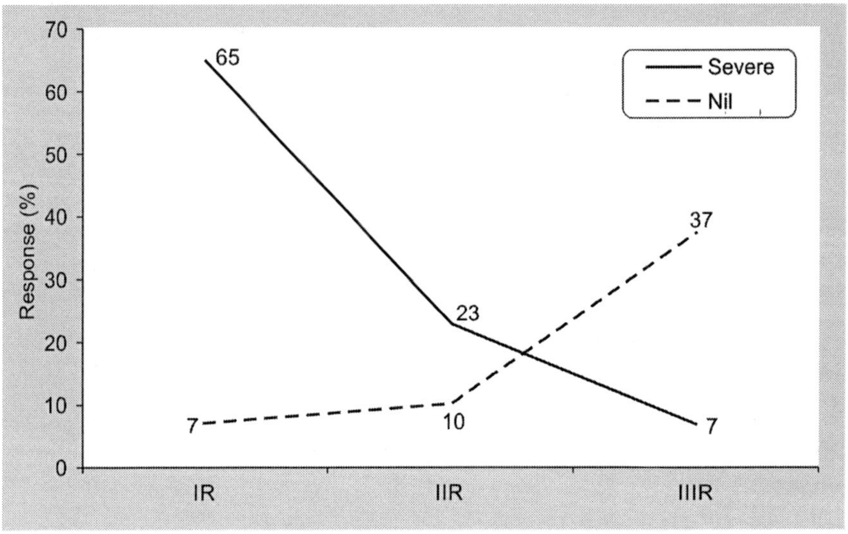

Fig. 14: Longitudinal variation in "seriousness" of Koro perception.

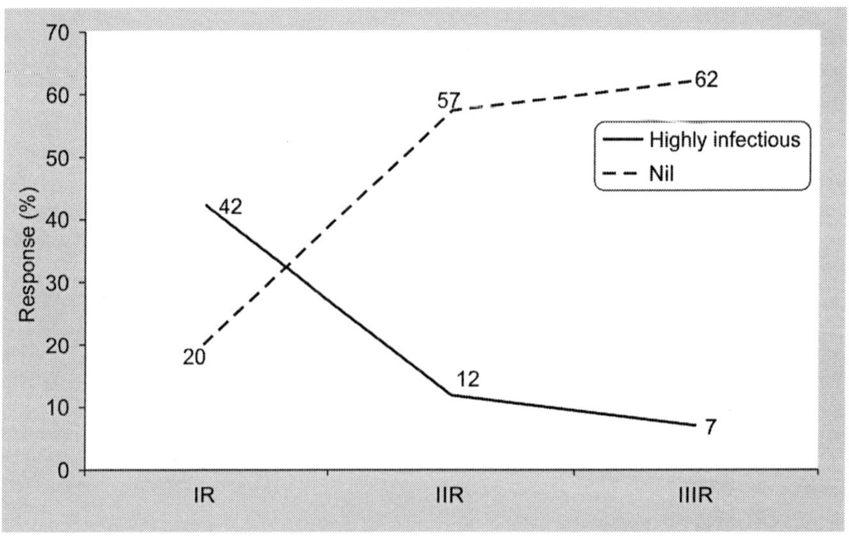

Fig. 15: Longitudinal variation in "Infectivity" of Koro perception.

how the social reinforcement turns from initially favorable to unfavorable acceptance of the illness gradually with time.

Time is the most critical variable in any cognitive appraisal, as it offers sufficient intervals for observing the natural course of the event. The social model of Koro as a *highly vulnerable* illness gradually lost its cognitive intensity over time. This is a dynamic process, started from the event's

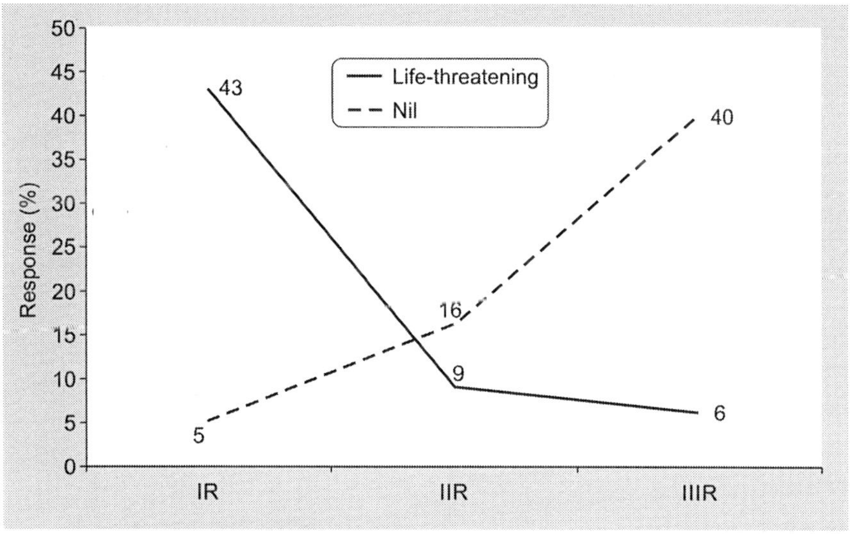

Fig. 16: Longitudinal variation in "Risk" of Koro perception.

inception in the community, but probably when it attains an arbitrary level of a shift from positive towards negative cognition, some neutralizing effects evolve, as manifested in the reduction of incidence curve of the illness. Psychiatric epidemics are well-known for their acute rise and precipitous fall with eventual weaning and incidence rate.[53-55] Thus, the social response curve influences the illness incidence curve in the psychiatric epidemic, which is evident in the present study of the Koro epidemic **(Fig. 17)**.

ILLNESS PARADIGM: STUDY OF THE PROFESSIONAL GROUP

Introduction: Illness perception and response are socially learned phenomena because the magnitudes of symptoms and disability are the products of subjective experience and social definitions.[22] The process of labeling involves the orientation of people about the sick role. The massage to the patient as how to conform a sick role is guided and reinforced by the opinion and attitude of help-providing therapists.[29] The "doctor" is essential because his opinion provides a scientific basis for social cognition.[56] The clinician should guide the social cognitive process by providing constructive explanations and not reinforcing maladaptive behavior.[22] The present investigation studied the local treatment people's opinions from physicians, surgeons, general practitioners, and paramedical staff, who were involved in treating the Koro cases during the epidemic months in the region.

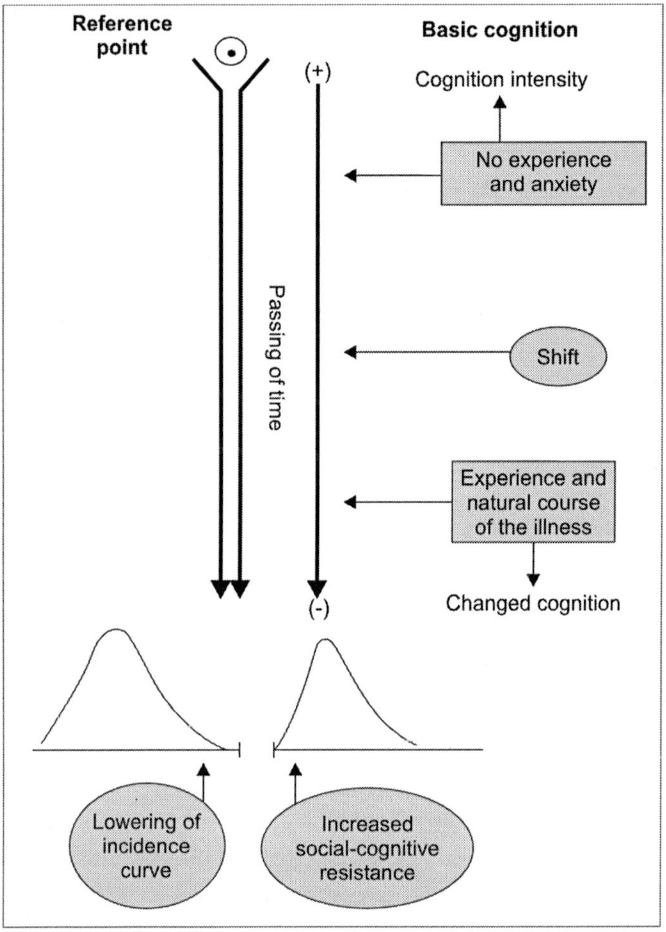

Fig. 17: Time and social perception in psychiatric epidemic.

Results

Assessment of opinions of 160 professionals (medical and paramedical personnel) was done during the Koro epidemic in North Bengal. P = Physician; GP = General Practitioner; S = Surgeon; PMS = Paramedical staff

Table 25 shows the pattern and comparison of Koro's "illness type" opinion of professional groups. The professional group significantly ($p < .001$) differed in their Koro illness type perception. Surgeons and Paramedical staff endorsed higher responses for Koro as a physical disorder and lower responses to the "nil" category ($p < .01$) compared to those of the Physicians. The difference ($p < .05$) of responses of Surgeons and Paramedics compared to those of GPs was similar. Paramedics also differed significantly ($p < .05$) from the Surgeons.

TABLE 25: Comparison of Koro's "illness type" opinion of the professionals.

Perceived cause	P		GP		S		PMS		Total				
	n: 40		40		40		40		160				
	No	%	No	%	No	%	No	%	No	%	X^2	df	p Value
Physical (P)	17	42.5	22	55.0	29	72.5	32	80.0	100	62.5	28.24	9	0.001
Mental (M)	6	15.0	4	10.0	6	15.0	–	–	16	10.0			
P + M	5	12.5	6	15.0	5	12.5	6	15	22	13.8			
Nil	12	30.0	8	20.0	–	–	2	5.0	22	13.8			

$X^2_3 = 1.93$ 15.13** 17.83**
X^2_3 9.43* 9.45*
$X^2_3 =$ 8.24

*p < .05; **p < .01
(GP: general practitioner; P: physician; PMS: paramedical staff; S: surgeon)

TABLE 26: Comparison of Koro's "seriousness" opinion of the professionals.

Perceived seriousness	P		GP		S		PMS		Total				
	n: 40		40		40		40		160				
	No	%	No	%	No	%	No	%	No	%	X^2	df	p Value
Nil	13	32.5	10	25.0	2	5	4	10.0	29	18.1	55.6	9	0.001
Mild	11	27.5	12	30.0	4	10.0	3	7.5	30	18.8			
Moderate	9	22.5	12	30.0	5	12.5	3	7.5	29	18.1			
Severe	7	17.5	6	15.0	29	72.5	30	75.0	72	45.0			

$X^2 = 0.94$ 25.92** 26.63**
X^2 27.33** 29.37*
$X^2_3 =$ 1.33

*p < .01; **p < . 001
(GP: general practitioner; P: physician; PMS: paramedical staff; S: surgeon)

Table 26 displays the opinion about Koro's "Seriousness" "by the professional group. Of the total respondents, 18% perceived Koro as a nonserious illness, while 45% considered it severe ($p < .001$). When each group's responses were compared, it was seen that significantly ($p < .01$) larger number of Physicians and smaller numbers of Surgeons considered the illness to be nonserious. Likewise, significantly ($p < .01$), more GPs and fewer PMS perceived the disease as mild and moderate. On the other hand, significantly ($p < .01$) more Surgeons and PMS considered Koro a "Severe illness" than the Physicians and GPs.

TABLE 27: Comparison of Koro's "risk" opinion by the professionals.

Perceived risk	*P*		*GP*		*S*		*PMS*		*Total*				
	n: 40		*40*		*40*		*40*		*160*				
	No	*%*	*No*	*%*	*No*	*%*	*No*	*%*	*No*	*%*	X^2	*df*	*p Value*
No danger	14	35	10	25.0	–	–	–	–	25	15	63.45	12	0.001
Life-threatening	–	–	6	15.0	7	17.5	11	27.5	24	15.0			
Sexual power loss (S)	12	30	20	50.0	22	55	25	62.5	79	49.4			
General health (H)	9	22.5	4	10.0	2	5.0	4	10.0	19	11.9			
S + H	5	12.5	–	–	9	22.5	–	–	14	8.7			

$X^2_4 = 15.59$** 29.54** 36.49**
$X^2_4 =$ 19.84** $X^2_3 = 12.03$*
X^2_3 10.75*

*p < 0.05; **p < 0.01
(GP: general practitioner; P: physician; PMS: paramedical staff; S: surgeon)

Table 27 depicts the opinion about Koro's "risk" by the professional group. They showed a significant ($p < .001$) overall difference in the response pattern. Only 15% (comprising Physicians and GPs) perceived Koro as nondangerous; 49.4% believed Koro imposes a potential risk to sexual power; 15% considered Koro a life-threatening illness, and 11.9% felt it might have a detrimental effect on general health. An intra-group comparison also showed a significant difference viz., more GPs, Surgeons, and PMS endorsed ($p < .01$) potential sexual hazard from Koro than Physicians. Similarly, more Surgeon and PMS viewed ($p < .01$) sexual risk from Koro than GPs. PMS" responses on this item were also higher ($p < .05$) than those of the Surgeons.

Table 28 exhibits the opinion about the "infectivity" of Koro by the professionals. The overall response of professionals showed significant ($p < .001$) differences, viz., 33% of the total responses marked the "non-ineffective" potential of Koro compared to 17.5% and 38% belonging to "severe" and "highly infectious" categories, respectively. An intragroup comparison also showed that the response patterns of Surgeons and PMS groups were different ($p < .01$) from those of the Physicians and GPs.

Discussion: It has been seen time and again that others significantly influence the labeling and evaluation of any distress or behavioral dysfunction in the community, viz., family and friends, community elders, and local healers. Usually, these informal labeling and evaluative processes appear to proceed

TABLE 28: Comparison of opinion about Koro's "infectivity" potential by the professionals.

	P		*GP*		*S*		*PMS*		*Total*				
	n: 40		*40*		*40*		*40*		*160*				
Perceived infectivity	***No.***	***%***	***No.***	***%***	***No.***	***%***	***No.***	***%***	***No.***	***%***	X^2	***df***	***p Value***
Nil	25	62.5	17	42.5	8	20	3	7.5	53	33.1	55.94	12	0.001
Mild	–	–	5	12.5	–	–	–	–	5	3.1			
Moderate	4	10.0	2	5	5	12.5	2	5.0	13	8.1			
Severe	4	10.0	7	17.5	8	20	9	22.5	28	17.5			
Highly infections	7	17.5	9	22.5	19	47.5	26	69.0	61	38.1			

$X^2_4 = 8.26$ $X^2_3 = 15.7$** $X^2_3 = 30.82$**
$X^2_4 =$ 13.17** 23.31**
X^2_3 4.71*

*$p < 0.05$; **$p < 0.01$
(GP: general practitioner; P: physician; PMS: paramedical staff; S: surgeon)

before medical help-seeking. These inputs from others are likely to reinforce the prevalent cultural conceptions and evaluations of symptoms since family, friends, or other significant community members share the same culture.[57-59] So, the disease model and/or its treatment perception remain completely culture-dependent till this stage. Contact with health professionals after that further influences these interpretations and evaluations. In other words, medical experts transform a patient's symptoms into a specific diagnosis and transmit relevant scientific concepts and information regarding the illness.[60] This information transmission then enters into the social network and helps society rearrange or revisit its previous cognitive appraisals about the disease.

Hafez,[61] in his study of the "mysterious gas poisoning" in the Jordan West Bank, clearly showed how the Arab medical community, being influenced by sociopolitical conflicts, expressed opinions that accelerated the epidemic. It is evident in the present study that the medical and paramedical communities of this region predominantly favored an "illness" model for Koro. They identified Koro as a physical illness of a serious nature with its health risk and infective potential. It is interesting to note that among all the professional groups, the responses of the GPs sound more rational, probably because of their free and frank mixing with the community and their first-hand opportunity to deal with many Koro cases in the community.

It is a matter of great concern to observe that the local health care providers saw Koro as "a strange sexual phenomenon" due to unfamiliarity with Koro. They lacked the skills for the appropriate management of cases. They failed to offer requisite medical explanations to meet the social curiosity at the point of extreme mass anxiety and fear. Instead, their views and opinion reinforced the social cognition of Koro as a severe disease (with life-threatening risk and high infectivity). Because of its similar nature to that of mass perception, it favored the rapid spread of Koro's illness-construct in the community through milling behavior[34] and various social communication networks.

Due to their cultural inhibitions (or ignorance?) of sexual matters, all the professional groups placed undue stress on the sexual power-loss/malfunctioning as one important aftermath of Koro. On this point, they simply reflect the ongoing mass anxiety concerning this atypical sexual-behavioral expression of Koro in the community. In the early part of the epidemic (first 2–3 weeks), Koro patients were brought to the hospital and private clinics, but later they were reluctant to visit allopathic facilities. Interestingly, a homeopath doctor, a pharmacist, and a medical student were also among the Koro sufferers. The Koro patients and their family members increasingly turned towards traditional modes of treatment. These social treatments imposed several health hazards yet were accepted by most Koro patients and their families. This study's conclusion supports the view of Sirois[28] that medical people have significant cognitive contributions insofar as the mass perception of a psychiatric epidemic is concerned. A prompt, coordinated response to resolve the widespread community anxiety is a duty of the health professionals in the face of mass episodes of psychogenic illness. Physicians in the community should be prompted to identify, diagnose, and treat the cases at their earliest so that the spread of the outbreak could be mitigated quickly.[62]

SOCIAL RESPONSE OF THE TOTAL SAMPLE (R+U+P): FIRST RATING

Summary: The beliefs and attitudes of the community, including those of the treatment people toward any behavioral abnormalities in question, usually influence the incidence, course, prognosis, or outcome of the maladaptive behavior. An analysis of social responses from the community (rural group, n = 88 + urban group, n = 118 + professional group, n = 160 = total 366) shows an identical dimension of Koro as a positive illness paradigm during the height of epidemic occurrences. Interestingly, the professional group also shared similar or even similar beliefs, so far as Koro's disease model is concerned.

Results

Table 29 and Figure 18 show that 80.6% of the total sample viewed Koro as a form of physical illness, and only 6% discarded its illness potentialities.

TABLE 29: Koro "illness type" perception of the community (n = 366).

Perceived type	*Rural + urban*		*Professional*		*Total*	
n	*206*		*160*		*366*	
	No.	*%*	*No.*	*%*	*No.*	*%*
Physical (P)	195	94.7	100	62.5	295	80.6
Mental (M)	5	2.4	16	10.0	21	5.7
P+M	6	2.9	22	13.7	28	7.7
Nil	–	–	22	13.8	22	6.0

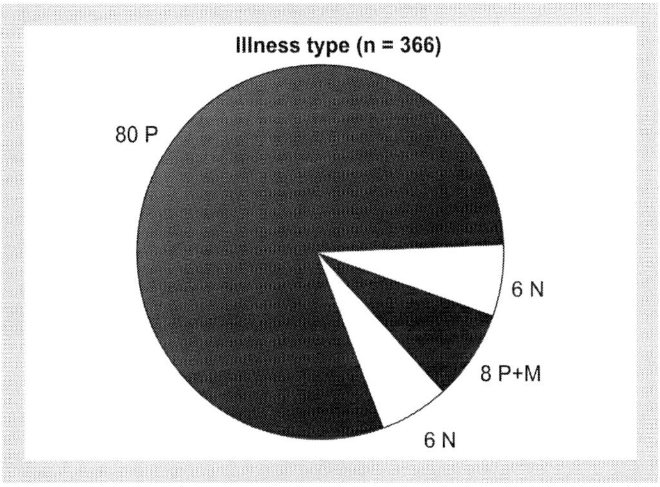

Fig. 18: Koro "Illness Type" perception of the community. P = Physical, M = Mental, P + M = Physical and Mental, N = Nil

Table 30 and Figure 19 indicate that 58.5% of the sample perceived Koro as a severe illness, while 10% endorsed its nonserious nature.

Table 31 and Figure 20 depict that only 21.6% of the sample estimated "no chance of infection" from Koro. Percentage distribution of the graded positive categories responses shows a progressively increasing endorsement, viz. mild 3.8%, moderate 13.7%, severe 17.2%, and highly infectious 43.7%.

Table 32 and Figure 21 evince that only 8.2% of the sample rejected the proposition that Koro has any dangerous risk. 32.2% perceived a "life-threatening" risk, while 38.5% viewed "loss of sexual power" as the risk of Koro illness.

Discussion: This positive illness cognition reinforces the acceptability of Koro in the community as an illness model. It is also noteworthy that although the rural and urban populations differed in their responses

TABLE 30: Koro's "seriousness" perception of the community (n = 366).

Perceived seriousness	*Rural + urban*		*Professional*		*Total*	
n	*206*		*160*		*366*	
	No.	*%*	*No.*	*%*	*No.*	*%*
Nil	8	3.9	29	18.1	37	10.1
Mild	15	7.3	30	18.8	45	12.3
Moderate	41	19.9	29	18.1	70	19.1
Severe	142	68.9	72	45	214	58.5

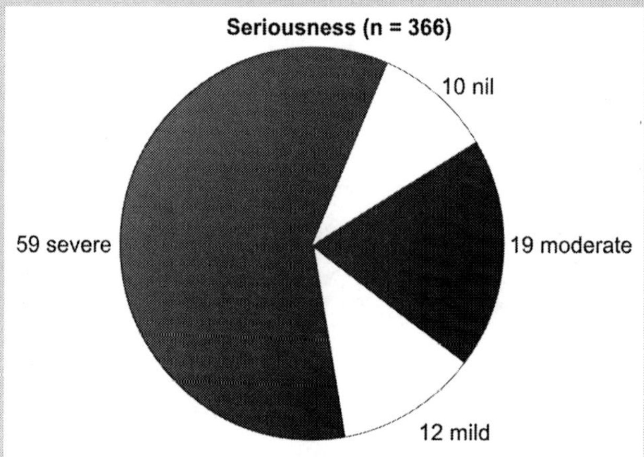

Fig. 19: Koro's "seriousness" perception (%) of the community.

TABLE 31: Koro's "infectivity" perception of the community (*n* = 366).

Perceived infectivity	*Rural + urban*		*Professional*		*Total*	
n	*206*		*160*		*366*	
	No.	*%*	*No.*	*%*	*No.*	*%*
Nil	26	12.6	53	33.1	79	21.6
Mild	9	4.4	5	3.1	14	3.8
Moderate	37	18.0	13	8.1	50	13.7
Severe	35	17.0	28	17.5	63	17.2
Highly infectious	99	48.0	61	38.1	160	43.7

to illness type or chance of infection, they showed remarkably identical responses since the seriousness and risk of Koro are concerned. Simultaneously, the medical opinion, which ought to profoundly influence the ongoing social perception, is also noteworthy in this context. Different

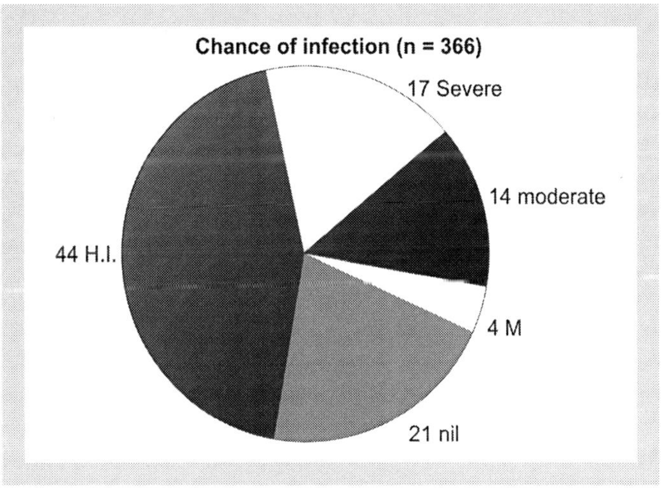

Fig. 20: Koro's "infectivity" perception (%) of the community.

TABLE 32: Koro "risk" perception of the community (n = 366).

Perceived risk	*Rural + urban*		*Professional*		*Total*	
n	*206*		*160*		*366*	
	No.	*%*	*No.*	*%*	*No.*	*%*
No danger (ND)	6	2.9	24	15	30	8.2
Life-threatening (LT)	94	45.6	24	15.0	118	32.2
Sexual power loss (LSP)	62	30.1	79	49.4	141	38.5
General health problem (GHP)	26	12.6	19	11.9	45	12.3
LSP + GHP	18	8.7	14	8.7	32	8.7

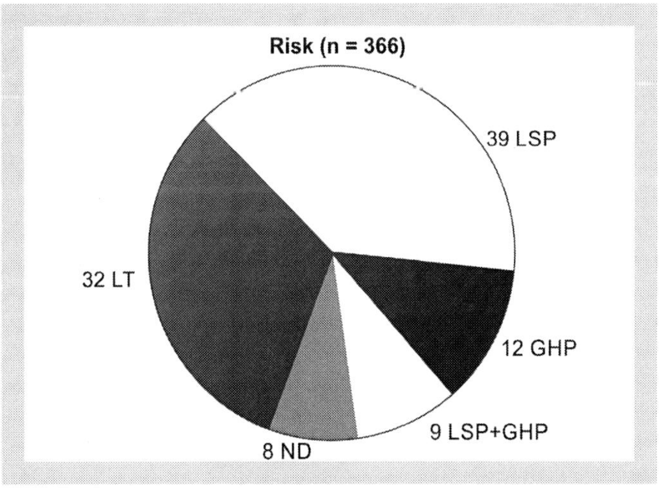

Fig. 21: Koro's "risk" perception (%) of the community.

professional groups of the medical community have expressed their Koro perception, which is very similar to social responses. The treatment people have failed to offer any rational and practical scientific explanation about the illness, which would meet the social curiosity at the time of extreme need.

There is little doubt that the region's medical community lacked the optimum knowledge and requisite skills necessary for managing such patients. Still, they also developed or framed a pseudo-scientific medical theory (sexual mischievousness). This *medical theory* reflects their rejective attitudes and, in practice, opposes social attribution. For example, the overall social understanding of its cause was "body heat" and "supernatural" (vide reference to the section on cause cognition). The confirmation of the Koro illness from social and medical communities and the unpreparedness of treatment people to offer a definite treatment options couple together and increase the uncertainty and fear about Koro that favor the atmosphere for crowd response. This accelerates contagion through the psychological mechanism of blurring rationality, highly suggestive, imitation, identification, and circular emotional reactions.[63] Hafez[61] asserts the medical community's role that contributes markedly towards elaborating the delusional system and its quasi validation in the epidemic of "mysterious gas poisoning" in the Jordan West Bank.

Time is an essential variable in any cognitive appraisal, as it offers a sufficient interval for observing the natural course of the event. Thus, the present study shows that the strength of Koro's positive illness perception parallels the incidence curve of the epidemic, viz., from high to low levels over time. Unlike the organic epidemics of infectious origin, where the density ratio of a particular virus or bacteria to the population dictates the epidemic waves (if not intervened therapeutically), the psychiatric epidemics are very well known for their acute rise and sharp fall. This is because of the rapid cognitive shifts of society from a positive to a negative direction. The social dynamics of the perceptual change regarding Koro's disease model are well illustrated in the present study. Illness modeling and human behavior are critical elements in spreading mental epidemics,[64] even in infectious disease epidemics.[65] In this regard, the prevailing sociocultural perception accelerates the emotional contagion[66] in the community and the psychological dimension of the epidemic.[67] This is evident in this study.

It is interesting to note that despite some differences in the response patterns, the total sample (rural + urban + professional) identified Koro as a *positive illness paradigm* as follows **(Fig. 22)**:

- Koro is a physical illness: 80.6%
- Koro entails a severe type of seriousness: 58.5%
- Koro is a life-threatening illness (32.2%), with a possible negative impact on sexual function (38.5%)
- Koro has a very high infective potential: 43.7%.

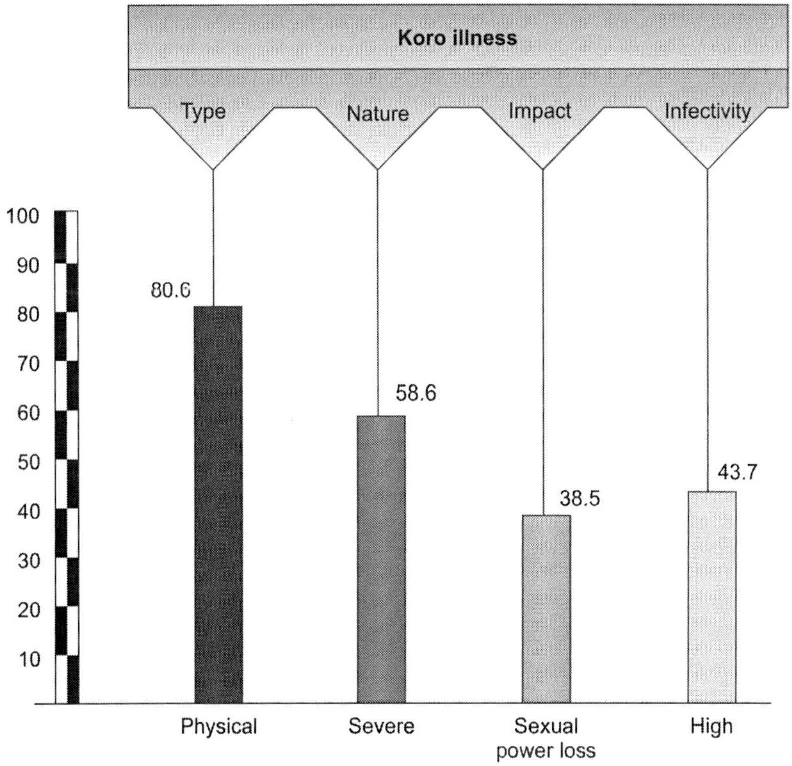

Fig. 22: Koro positive illness paradigm (%) (total social sample, n = 366).

Conclusion: The present study offered the following findings in support of the social response to Koro as a positive illness paradigm:

- The Koro illness was accepted as a definite illness by the community.
- The dangerous nature of the illness in terms of its seriousness, health risks, and contagiousness was attributed maximally during the first few weeks of the epidemic.
- The medical community responded almost identical to the general community insofar as the perception of Koro illness is concerned.
- The passage of time changed the direction of the social Koro perception from high to low vulnerability.

CAUSE COGNITION OF KORO

Introduction: Angel and Thoits[49] divided the cognitive model of illness labeling phenomena into three distinct parts, viz., positive endorsement of any physical/emotional behavior, the interpretation and evaluation of the abnormality, and the determination of the course of action (treatment decision). The category of understanding and assessment of any deviant behavior they term "second-order categorization" considers the complex nature of the illness in question, including its cause. This cognitive evaluation process is heavily influenced by cultural factors like social desirability, prevalent beliefs and knowledge, and advice from significant others in the community.

It has been seen that the individuals, and then the community, evaluate any deviant behavior following the learned dimension of health and illness construct of the society.[68] These dimensions indicate the cultural and social beliefs concerning anatomy, physiology, and the disease's etiology.[69,70] These cultural cognitive categories (about the disease cause/expression) are not fixed but are malleable and change due to experience, education, and scientific medical intervention.[71] Social cognition of psychiatric morbidity is thus fundamental because of the cultural relations with behavioral dispositions and treatment selection and compliance. This is more so because of the need for urgent intervention in stopping the process of contagiousness in the community. Media also plays an essential role in spreading the news and anxiety in the community.[72]

The present study was designed to explore Koro's etiology's cognitive dimension as perceived by the community. This study also examined Koro etiology's cognitive profile among the local treatment people to explore the similarity/difference between the cognition of the two groups.

Study sample: A social response regarding the opinion about cause of Koro was elicited from a sample (n 366: rural 88 + urban 118 + treatment people 160) by field study during the Koro epidemic.

Results

Table 33 and Figure 23 showed the distribution of Koro's different responses about its cause by the rural and urban groups. In the rural groups, the first three responses in descending order were "body heat" (30.7%); "supernatural" (21.6%), and "unknown" (18.2%). Almost a similar pattern was also observed in the urban group, viz. 33.9% "body heat"; 15.3% "unknown" and 12.7% "supernatural." Perception of "physical" causative background in Koro in terms of "fever" and "physical strain" was reported in 13.7% and 8.4% of the rural and urban groups. Psychological dysfunction, viz. fears, or mental reaction or combination of both, as a cause of Koro, was perceived more by the urban (16.9%) than the rural (7.9%) group.

Table 34 depicts the distribution and intra-group comparison of perceived cause of Koro among the professional group. The highest attribution was sexual because in each professional group, viz. 37.5%. Physicians; 40% GPs; 37.5% Surgeons and 27.5% PMS. 35% of Physicians and 7.5% GPs opined for "mischievousness" as the cause of Koro. A significant difference in the overall opinion pattern was seen in GPs ($p < .01$), in surgeons, and PMS ($p < .05$) from that of Physicians. A similar difference was also noted in the PMS response

TABLE 33: Distribution of Koro "Cause" perception of rural and urban groups.

	Rural (n = 88)		*Urban (n = 118)*	
Perceived causes	*No.*	*%*	*No.*	*%*
Not known	16	18.2	18	15.3
High fever	10	11.4	5	4.2
Physical strain	2	2.3	5	4.2
Body heat	27	30.7	40	33.3
Sexual	6	6.8	11	9.3
Supernatural	19	21.6	15	12.7
Mischievousness	1	1.1	4	3.4
Fear (F)	6	6.8	14	11.9
Mental (M)	1	1.1	3	2.5
F + M	–	–	3	2.5

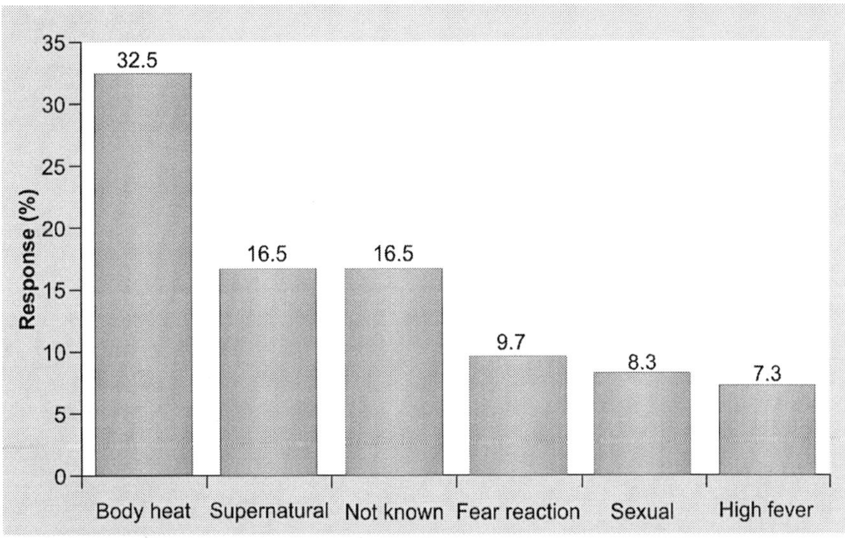

Fig. 23: First six perceived causes of Koro: Community perception (n = 206).

($p < .05$) compared to Surgeons. Interestingly, 12.5% GPs, 25% Surgeons, and 30% of the PMS group endorsed "body heat" as Koro's cause.

Table 35 compares patterns of perceived cause between the community (rural + urban) and the professional groups. The community group showed higher endorsement to "body heat" and "supernatural" causes and lower approval to "sexual" and "mischievousness" than the professional group ($p < .01$). All other responses showed no significant difference.

TABLE 34: Comparison of the "perceived cause" of Koro of different professional groups.

	P (n = 40)		*GP (n = 40)*		*S (n = 40)*		*PMS (n = 40)*	
Perceived causes	***No.***	***%***	***No.***	***%***	***No.***	***%***	***No.***	***%***
Not known	1	2.5	2	5.0	6	15.0	10	25.0
High fever	–	–	4	10.0	2	5.0	–	–
Physical strain	1	2.5	3	7.5	–	–	–	–
Body heat	–	–	5	12.5	10	25.0	12	30.0
Sexual	15	37.5	16	40.0	15	37.5	11	27.5
Supernatural	–	–	–	–	–	–	4	10.0
Mischievousness	14	35.0	3	7.5	–	–	–	–
Fear (F)	5	12.5	4	10.0	7	17.5	3	7.5
Mental (M)	3	7.5	2	5.0	–	–	–	–
F + M	1	2.5	1	2.5	–	–	–	–
	X^2_8		19.56** X^2_8		34.9* 14 X^2_5		X^2_9 9.4	43.78* 26.3*

*p < .05; **p < .01

TABLE 35: Distribution of "cause" perception of the total sample.

	Community group (n = 206)		*Professional group (n = 160)*		
Perceived causes	***No.***	***%***	***No.***	***%***	***Z score***
Not known	34	16.5	19	11.9	1.25
High fever	15	7.3	6	3.8	1.44
Physical strain	7	3.4	4	2.5	0.55
Body heat	67	32.5	27	16.9	3.44*
Sexual	17	8.3	57	35.6	–6.47*
Supernatural	34	16.5	4	2.5	4.36
Mischievousness	5	2.4	17	10.6	–3.28*
Fear (F)	20	9.7	19	11.9	–0.67
Mental (M)	4	1.9	5	3.1	–0.73
F+M	3	1.5	2	1.3	0.17

*p < .01.

Figure 24 shows the distribution of opinion about Koro's cause among the total sample (rural, urban, and professional combined). The profile of perceived cause opinion from highest to lowest categories presents the

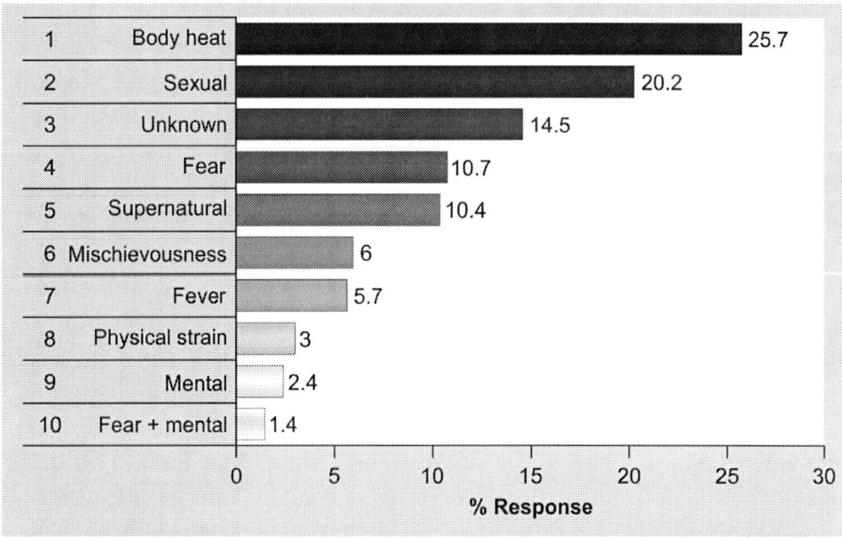

Fig. 24: Ranking of the total sample's Koro "cause" opinion (n = 366).

following distribution: body heat (25.7%), sexual (20.2%), unknown (14.5%), fear (10.7%), supernatural (10.4%), and mischievousness (6%).

Discussion: Social perception of any disease is heavily dependent on the people's cultural cognitive resources and patterns. Some prevalent traditional beliefs and theories exist in every society, and people are used to perceiving any deviant behavior in the first instance by this frame of cultural/ ethnomedical references. A good example is the Mexican categorization of any illness based on either the "hot or cold" dimension or "children's or old people's" disease—the two most prevalent Latin cultural perceptions.[73] The social cognitive evaluation of cause perception of any illness is critical for at least two reasons: Firstly, it has a severe implication for indigenous folk treatment (along with its associated health hazards). Secondly, in cases of a psychiatric epidemic, it directs and guides the symptom presentation and spread of the illness in the community. The findings of the present study are essential from this perspective.

It has to be remembered that Koro is not like other usual diseases, nor was it previously known to the community under this study. The community's primary response regarding the cognitive evaluation of its cause/effect reflects the prevalent cultural concept of illness, viz., excessive body heat generation and supernatural influence. However, many respondents frankly admitted their complete ignorance about any assessment regarding Koro's cause. This group primarily acted as a dangerous medium for spreading rumor and fear reactions in the community, thus helping spread Koro in the region. The third predominant perception is the attribution of "physical" causes like fever, physical strain, and sexual disabilities.

The cognitive spectrum of the local treatment people reveals some exciting features. Their evaluations strikingly corroborate the community's cognition almost identically. They offer Koro no new or acceptable medical cause except a heavy emphasis on the "sexual" and "mischievousness" categories. These two medical views play a crucial role in the social treatment-seeking by the affected individual or their family members during the epidemic. Although 8.3% of the community responses attributed a "sexual cause" for Koro (in contrast to 35.6% of the professionals), the conceptual disposition or meaning of this *sexual disability* is altogether different from that of the professionals. The community's cognitive categorization of this sexual cause was mainly focused on the inherent or constitutional sexual weakness, sexual abnormalities like too much nocturnal emission, or impotence. But rarely, inappropriate sexual urge or arousal. All these were viewed as involuntary disabilities of an individual, which potentiate their vulnerability to Koro affliction. So, in a very usual and modest sense, they are the persons who deserve social sympathy and help. On the other hand, the professional categorization of "sexual cause" stresses dissocial sexual behaviors primarily, e.g., sexual promiscuity/prostitute visit, too much masturbation, and excessive sexual urge or motivation (sexy). These labelings involve a negative moral overtone, and, for obvious reasons, this cause assignment gets reacted upon with psychological resentment by the Koro patients and their family members.

"Mischievousness" is another cognitive dimension where the community and the professional stand opposite. 10.6% of professionals, in contrast to 2.4% community responses, viewed the "penis symptom" of Koro as deliberate malingering, which they termed "mischievousness" believing that the patients "are exploiting the ongoing situation; by their callous and silly behavior." The validity of this professionals comment probably rests in the fact that a few cases displayed very informal complaints of penis retraction/shortening, without any accompanying features of marked anxiety, lacking acute dramatic presentation of classical Koro. Those confounding cases were either hysterical (conversion), or some of them, at least, were cases of organ dysmorphophobia, which surfaced during the epidemic. Koro's strong epidemic wave disintegrated these differences and professional inefficiency, and lack of in-depth study and examination marked this confusion. Virtually, these cases contaminated the actual Koro incidences during the epidemic time. Professionals from this experience probably generalized Koro as the manifestation of a mal intended mischievous behavior. Of course, "mischievousness" could not be at any rate a medical etiology or a diagnosis. This attribution, naturally, contradicts the positive social paradigm of Koro as a severe Illness. These inconsistencies of the professional view are probably the reason for both the facts concerning Koro treatment, viz. the professionals reluctance to treat certain Koro cases and increased preference of Koro patients/family members for folk rather than medical treatment. Strikingly, the professional groups also reinforce these cultural conceptions. It is worth noting that 16.9% of the professionals endorsed excessive body heat as Koro's cause. Thus, these cultural etiologies direct and guide the mode of social treatment, the details of which are discussed in the "treatment" section.

ETHNOMEDICAL COGNITION OF KORO: PATIENTS' PERSPECTIVE

Introduction: Koro, a psychogenic reactive state, is intimately related to the cognitive reference of the sociocultural construct of somatization with sexuality, does reflect varied types of illness beliefs in different cultural groups. There are a handful of medical hypotheses of Koro (both sporadic and epidemic forms). These are: premorbid sexual conflicts and guilt,[74,75] morbid preoccupation with sexual functioning,[76,77] heightened genital awareness and autonomic hyperarousal,[78,79] biomedical potentials,[80,81] hypochondriacal genital concern,[82] mass fear about castration anxiety[12] and cultural belief in evil fox spirit.[83,84]

But there is not a single self-report about the ethnomedical explanatory framework of Koro patients from any of the cultural groups from which Koro was reported to date. This is an essential gap in our knowledge, mostly when folk explanations and illness cognition play a significant role in disease causation.[85,86] The present study attempts to bridge this gap by exploring the ethnomedical causation of Koro illness as perceived by the patients in Indian culture.

Material and Methods

Sample: A total of 101 male Koro cases (55 from Darjeeling, 27 from Koch-Bihar, and 19 from Jalpaiguri district) were interviewed in different hospitals, private clinics, and on community visits during the epidemic.

Instrument: One-to-one interview on:

- *Perceived cause cognition:* After establishing a good rapport with each patient during the clinical interview, he was asked to designate a single cause of his Koro illness, which he considered the most important contributor. He was invited to provide a free response without any hesitation and not bothering about the correctness of his answer or worrying about whether it corresponds to the usual medical causes. It was stressed that his assessment is only required. All the collected responses were grouped according to their similarities, whereby seven categories emerged, viz., unknown origin, fever, physical strain, increased body heat, sexual cause, supernatural cause, and fear.

- *Ethnomedical explanation of perceived causes:* A detailed descriptive open-ended account of each causal factor (regarding its role in Koro causation) from each patient was recorded. As "body heat" was the prevalent idea, (Note 1-4) further probing was done regarding its detailed ethnophysiological explanations (explanatory model), which were then framed into possible distinct models and presented.

Results

Table 36 depicts the demographic character of the sample. The maximum percentage of cases were Rajbanshis, unmarried with primary education, and of agricultural occupation.

Table 37 illustrates the distribution of different ethnomedical perceptions of Koro's cause as the patients perceived. The highest proportion of cases (54.6%) attributed *excessive body heat* as the principal cause of Koro, followed by attribution to *the supernatural* (14.9%) and *sexual* (7.9%) causes.

Ethnomedical Explanations:

Body Heat: The detailed ethnophysiological narratives of body heat mechanisms for causing Koro is grouped into four models (by the author) according to their central theme and presented in **Table 38**. Interestingly, all Rajbanshi patients (100%) and most Behari Hindu cases (87.5%) perceived the body heat as the leading cause of their penile symptoms. Following is a brief description of each of the models.

Body Heat—Structural Model: The maximum (47.2%) of patients perceived that when the usual body heat becomes excessive, it destroys incoming nerves (Note 5) and blood channels from the abdomen to the penis, resulting in shrinkage.

Body Heat—Sexual Energy Model **(Fig. 25)***:* Patients (25.5%) in this group stated that sexual energy is stored inside the penis and scrotum. This energy is primarily responsible for maintaining penile girth, erotic desire, and sexual functions like erection and seminal discharge. In Koro, the pathological increase of body heat consumes this sexual energy, and the situation resembles a "low-heat" condition of old age, namely, shrinking of penis and scrotum. However, unlike in old age, where the process is slow and gradual, it is sudden, untimely in Koro. It thus gains an illness dimension with accompanied anxiety and fear of losing male potency.

Body Heat—Heat-Loss Model **(Fig. 26)***:* Proponents of this model (18.2%) expressed a well-knit homeostatic physiological explanation of heat in the body. Body heat is perceived here as beneficial inner energy for maintaining all bodily functions. Excessive body heat causes damage to the penile pathways and the seminal sac (situated under the abdomen's umbilicus).

TABLE 36: Demographic character of the sample (n = 101).

1. *Age in years:*	*Mean ± sd: 23.6 ± 7.35*	
2. *Ethnicity:*	*No.*	*%*
Rajbanshi	42	41.6
Bengali Hindu	24	23.8
Behari Hindu	8	7.9
Nepali Hindu	9	8.9
Jain	5	4.9
Muslim	8	7.9
Christian	5	4.9
3. *Marital Status:*		
Single	65	64.4
Married	33	32.7
Separated	3	2.9
4. *Education:*		
Nil	18	17.8
Primary	49	48.5
Secondary	29	28.7
College	5	4.9
5. *Occupation:*		
Nil	19	18.8
Student	18	17.8
Agriculture	33	32.7
Business	14	13.9
Tea plantation worker	8	7.9
Service	9	8.9

TABLE 37: Ethnomedical explanation of Koro etiology (n = 101).

Perceived causes of Koro	*No.*	*%*
1. Increased body heat	55	54.6
2. Supernatural	15	14.9
3. Sexual	8	7.9
4. Physical strain	6	5.9
5. Fever	5	4.9
6. Fear	4	3.9
7. Unknown	8	7.9

TABLE 38: Ethnomedical explanation of Koro etiology (n = 55).

	Ethnicity									
	Rajbanshi		*Behari Hindu*		*Nepali Hindu*		*Bengalee Hindu*		*Total (n = 55)*	
Body heat model	*No.*	*%*	*No.*	*%*	*No.*	*%*	*No.*	*%*	*No*	*%*
1. Structural	22	40	1	1.8	1	1.8	2	3.6	26	47.2
2. Sexual energy	9	16.4	2	3.6	1	1.8	2	3.6	14	25.5
3. Heat loss	7	12.7	3	5.5	0	0	0	0	10	18.2
4. Heat avoidance	4	7.3	1	1.8	0	0	0	0	5	9.1
Total	42		7		2		4			
Z of the group total	100		87.5		22.2		16.7			

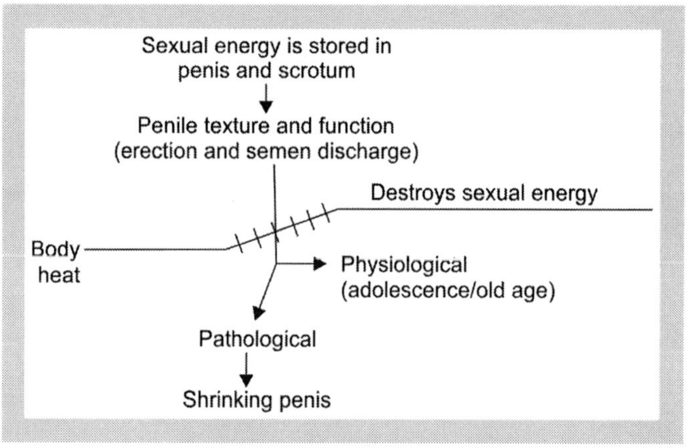

Fig. 25: Sexual-energy model.

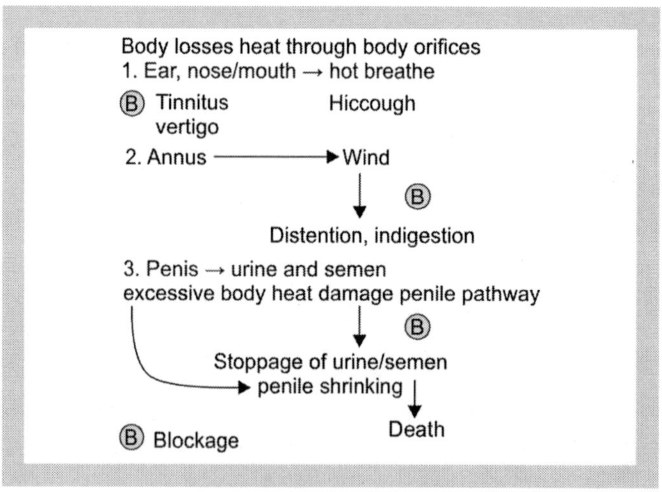

Fig. 26: Heat-loss model.

These are causing any of the following three dangerous conditions, viz., penile shrinkage, stoppage of urine, and blockage of seminal discharge, all of which have the potential to cause death if not intervened immediately.

Body Heat—Heat Avoidance Model: Patients (9.1%) in this category stated that the skin plays an essential role in the conduction of normal body heat. Fever is one such example of heat loss through the skin. Penis, a susceptible organ, is vulnerable to damage by increased body heat. So in Koro, a state of increased body heat, the penis shrinks or retracts into the abdominal cavity to avoid heat insult. Interestingly, unlike the others, this model tries to explain a protective body mechanism for the etiopathogenesis of Koro. The pathological fear and anxiety it arouses is because of the suddenness of the process and uncertainty and unpredictability regarding the reappearance of the penis and return of body heat to the average level.

Influence of body heat on other body systems: Ethnomedical perception regarding the involvement of other body systems by excessive body heat was also elicited. Forty types of ailments involving four body systems (head and neck, gastrointestinal, genitourinary, and general symptoms) have been attributed to the body heat by Koro patients. The four highest attributed distress/illness to body heat in order of decreasing frequencies were insomnia (94.5%), excessive seminal fluid liquidity (81.8%), liver damage (78.2%), and heat over the head (65.5%). Black menstruation was the highest attribution (40%) of body heat impact in the female genitourinary system.

Supernatural cause: In this category, a relatively good amount of feeling of social paranoia was evident, e.g., envious persons inflicted the illness by black magic or spell, which helped to generate an internal malevolent force inside the body (abdomen) that pulled the penis inside. Many family members collected charmed red threads from the local priest/Gunin and believed that wearing at the waist may block the supernatural influence **(Fig. 27)**. Some patients thought that the Koro malady is a punishment given by God for their excessive masturbatory habit (causing useless spoilage of valuable semen) or past sexual misdeeds. God wanted to make them sterile or sexually weak forever via Koro.

The widespread Koro preventive ritual in North Bengal is an excellent example of mass belief in occult or evil influence to cause Koro. Marking ear lobules and suprasternal fossa with slaked lime **(Fig. 28)** and wearing a fine sheathe of black-stem arum around great toes was regarded as adequate protection against the evil influence and thus against Koro.[87]

Sexual cause: In this category, a sense of intense guilt was attached to masturbation, seminal nocturnal discharge, perceived semen density (too liquid), and sexual acts like prostitute visits and illegal sexual intercourse within the bond of family kinships (incest). The resultant effects of all

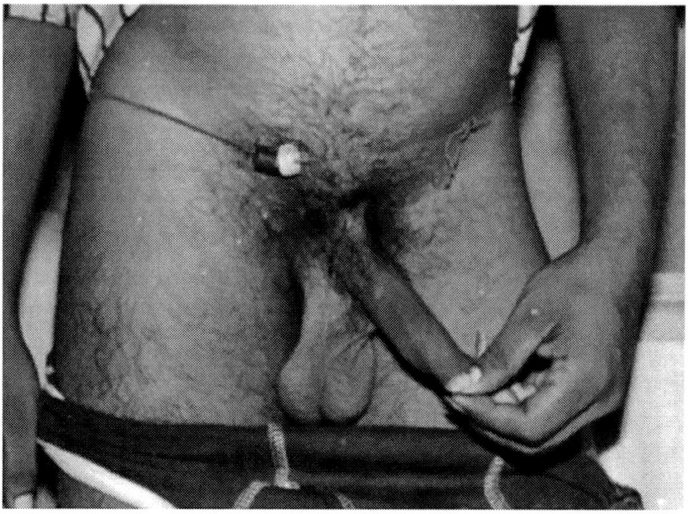

Fig. 27: Manual self-pulling of the penis by a Koro sufferer at a hospital emergency, wearing a red chanted thread with copper nuts and a cowrie shell for mitigating evil influences.

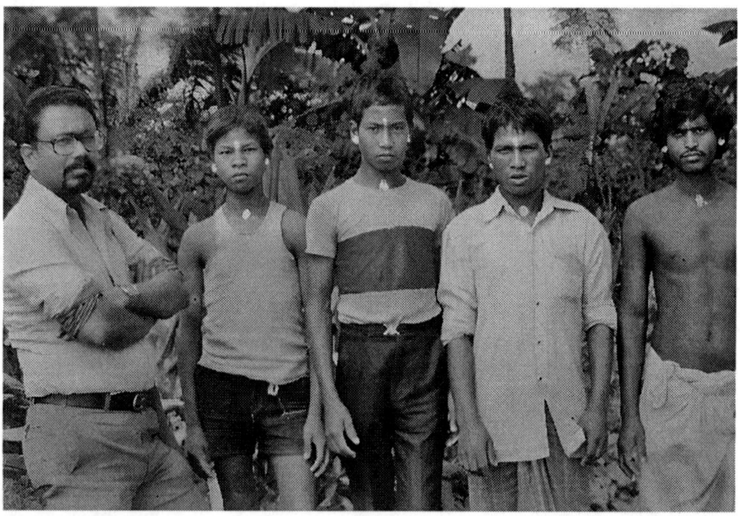

Fig. 28: The author, with a group of young persons (Sukna village, Darjeeling) during the epidemic. All smeared lime spots as a preventive measure against the potential Koro attack.

these "sexual wrong-doings" lead to sexual weakness, making the subject vulnerable to Koro illness. Recourse to Kabiraji, Homeopathic or indigenous herbal folk medicines, and special food items (Note 6) to cure nocturnal emission was not an infrequent finding among the cases (30.7%).

Physical cause: Physical disability, either from fever or physical strain, was believed to cause Koro in 10.9% of cases. Physical stress included bearing a load, working for long hours in the tea garden or agricultural field.

Fear: Fear was described as the mental reaction to the various ongoing threatening news or spreading rumors of Koro illness in the locality. (Note 7) Two crucial facts elicited from the Koro patients of Koch-Bihar district need to be mentioned at this point. First is the episodic community fears wave at one to two years, prevalent in some districts' rural areas. These highly sensitive rumors address the presence of some imaginary creature supposed to kill or cause significant harm to people if they confront them face-to-face. One that happened a few months before the Koro epidemic was the evil human-like demon, locally called "Hullu". The second phenomenon is the experience of a fearful monosyllabic mystic or magical sound, somewhat akin to a solitary auditory hallucination, just before the Koro attack. Seventeen patients of this sample (16.8%) had such personal experiences and all the cases of Koch-Bihar district acknowledge this phenomenon. The sound, lexically resembling "kottash/kattaow," (Note 8) is heard suddenly by the subject, usually in an open space (paddy field, riverbank). That invokes a dreadful feeling of impending danger in the hearer, who instantaneously develops a sense of numbness in the groin area with an intense feeling of penile pull. This "magical sound" gained a terrible fear symbol in the locality during the epidemic days. People avoided going to the field alone and took charmed amulets from local folk healers to protect themselves from this sound (to make it inaudible to them). The illness was also locally known as the attack of Kottash or "Kattaow." The precise source and intent of this perilous sound were not clear to them. Still, some patients believed it was an evil force, somewhat like a malevolent spirit cult, whose intention was to make the hearer sexually invalid or even dead if not attended to immediately.

Conclusion: The ethnomedical explanation of Koro elicited in this study reflects the age-old Indian cultural illness perception relating to physical (heat) and nonphysical (magic) etiology, which runs as a historical tradition through the centuries. It is also interesting to note how the two most ancient civilizations, Indian and Chinese, interpret the illness in terms of physical philosophy, i.e., heat and cold. The hot-cold disease theory is also a world-view of many ethnic communities worldwide.[88] Magic or supernaturalism, an answer to man's unresolved anxieties and queries; hence, constitutes an archetypal concept of illness, disability, or dysfunction.[89] and offers a folk explanation of Koro in the community. Modern medicine should consider all these ethnomedical postulations for better treatment negotiation and compliance.

NOTE

1. Kapur,[90] provides a critical ethnomedical concept of rural India concerning body heat and semen. It is believed that semen or vital essence is a refined form of life energy. The concentration of semen generates "heat" necessary for body functions. The male center of "heat" is the head, while it is the vagina for females.
2. Aho and Minott,[91] in their study of medical folk beliefs among people of Trinidad and Tobago, West Indies, noted a deep faith in the hot-cold theory of disease. In Trinidadian culture, hot or cold labels are attached to symptoms, causes, and illness remedies. Numerous descriptive lexicon titles, e.g. "getting a chill" or "throat hot," "heat in the belly," "too much heat in the body," "too heated food" are attributed as causes of illnesses. Treatment involves using (either external application or internal consumption) of "cool" medicines for "hot" diseases or vice-versa.[92]
3. The Puerto Rican folk medicine system[93] classifies disorder into hot (Caliente) and cold (Frio) groups. Foods and herbal medicine are also accordingly classified. Examples of "cold" illnesses are arthritis, common colds, menstrual period, joint pains, and *pasmo. Pasmo* refers to two different conditions. Firstly, it denotes the tonic spasm of any body's voluntary muscles exposed to cold. This condition reminds one of a similar proclamation of classical Chinese medicine regarding the spasm of the penis (retraction) from exposure to chill or cold wind. The second use of *pasmo* is for a chronic cough or stomach pain. The cold foods include avocado, bananas (in Chinese belief consumption of cold food may precipitate an attack of Koro—one Koro case was reported by Oyebode et al.,[79] who developed Koro symptoms after eating a banana); coconut, sugar cane, and white beans. The hot diseases are constipation, diarrhea, rashes, tenesmus, ulcers, and foods are alcoholic drinks, coffee, garlic, onions, and tobacco.[94]
4. *Suudu* is a culture-bound syndrome mainly reported from South India in Tamil culture.[95] The chief complaint is painful urination and feeling of pelvic "heat," attributed to increasing inner body heat (often due to dehydration). Both sexes may be affected.
5. Slot,[96] in the early part of the 19th century, attempts to elicit the ethnomedical explanation of Koro from traditional healers of the Macassaran area of Sulawesi. He stated Koro to be the affliction of nerves (nerve contracting disease). Associated fever is a bad prognostic sign. Potential precipitators for Koro mentioned were: physical labor, genital trauma (owing to a fall from horseback), and immoderate sexual practices.
6. In the Ayurvedic concept, semen generates from essential foods: chyle → blood → flesh → fat → bone marrow →, and ultimately semen is produced. So, it is a common custom of food preferences in many cultures related to perceived sexual arousal.[97] This is why many Sri Lankans prefer foods

that have imagined semen fostering quality or cultural symbolism.[46,98] Bottero,[99] discussed the psychological significance of semen loss in the Indian subcontinent.

7. Jilek,[100] describes a collective fear of ghosts in the Zhanjiang town of Guangdong province, China, during a Koro epidemic. The villagers use drum beating, bell ringing, and bursting of firecrackers to drive the ghosts out of the village. The villagers believed that the ghost made the genitals of men and women's breasts shrink and disappear into the abdomen and chest.
8. *Kattaw* is also a local syntax for small tortoises living in the riverbed.[101] In Koch-Bihar district, rural people use the lexicon Kattaw or Kura for tortoise.[7]

TREATMENT COGNITION FOR KORO

Preamble: The health care system of any society invariably bears the impression of its cultural care models at the primary level.[58,102] Popular medical care by individuals, family members, friends, and essential community members reflects the traditional beliefs and practices based primarily on the ethnophysiological cognitive evaluations of illness etiology of this particular culture.[45,103] Chrisman and Kleinman[104] thus aptly state that any society's curative practices constitute a cultural system involving three crucial variables, popular beliefs and laypersons' practices; folk medicine as practiced by indigenous people healers and modern scientific medicine. The initial identification of illness and decisions regarding treatment are primarily dependent on this social framework because it involves a vital dimension of group support, social acceptance, and the established social network system.[22] This is one of the fundamental reasons why home diagnosis and home remedies continue to play a significant "medicare" role even in today's society. Cultural modes of treatment are of particular interest in cultural-bound syndromes because various health-related rituals and practices provide care and management. There are examples in the psychiatric-anthropological literature about the "social treatments" that are significantly influenced by the ethnomedical perception of human anatomy, physiology, and folk etiology of illness.[105-107]

This study compared treatment opinion between the community (rural and urban) and local treatment people, highlighting the cultural influence on the help-giving procedure and reflecting the dimension of similarities and dissimilarities between the two mutually bonded (care seeker/caregiver) groups.

Methodology

- *Community sample:* 206 (88 rural + 118 urban) persons, as illustrated in the previous chapter.

- *Professional group:* Consisted of 160 professionals, as illustrated in the previous chapter.
- *Instrument:* Social Response Pattern Schedule, described in the previous chapter.
  The "Treatment Cognition" section includes four items: (1) Treatment option; (2) medicine option, (3) natural treatment option, and (4) mental treatment option.
- *Study Design:* Details are noted in "Time of Social Response Ratings" at the beginning of this social response study

Results

Study of Treatment Option

- *Rural Group* **(Table 39)**: Comparison of "treatment option" as advocated by members of non-Koro (NKF) and Koro family (KF) members. Both groups showed no difference in their treatment opinions. "Non-medical" or "Natural treatment" was the highest frequency of responses in both groups. Any of the groups did not endorse the "No treatment" opinion.
- *Urban Group* **(Table 40)**: Both the groups showed the highest endorsement to non-medical, i.e., natural treatment. 11.7% of non-Koro family members stated that no treatment was necessary for Koro. These differences in opinions between the groups were significant ($p < .05$).
- *Professional group* **(Table 41)**: Opinion of professional groups showed only Physicians (32.5%) and General Practitioners (5%) opined "no treatment" for Koro. G.P., Surgeons, and Paramedical staff endorsed the category of "natural treatment" than Physicians significantly. Surgeons advocated more "medical treatment" than paramedics ($p < .01$). There were no differences observed in surgeons and paramedics opinions in comparison to those of GPs.
- *Urban vs. Rural Group* **(Table 42)**: The rural group endorsed more "natural treatment" (78.4%) for Koro than the urban group (53.4%),

TABLE 39: Treatment option response between non-Koro families (NKF) and Koro families (KF) rural groups.

	NKF group (n = 45)		*KF group (n = 43)*		
Options	*No.*	*%*	*No.*	*%*	X^2
Medical (M)	3	6.7	3	6.9	*(df = 2)* 2.01 (NS)
Natural (N)	33	73.3	36	83.7	
M + N	9	20	4	9.3	
No treatment	–	–	–	–	

NS = nonsignificant.

TABLE 40: Treatment option response between non-Koro families (NKF) and Koro families (KF) urban groups.

	NKF group (n = 60)		*KF group (n = 58)*		
Options	***No.***	***%***	***No.***	***%***	X^2
Medical (M)	5	8.3	1	1.7	*(df = 3)* 12.03*
Natural (N)	32	53.3	31	53.5	
M + N	16	26.7	26	44.8	
No treatment	7	11.7	–		

*$p < .05$

TABLE 41: Treatment option responses of the different professional groups.

	P (n = 40)		*GP (n = 40)*		*S (n = 40)*		*PMS (n = 40)*	
Options	***No.***	***%***	***No.***	***%***	***No.***	***%***	***No.***	***%***
Medical (M)	12	30.0	10	25.0	12	30.0	7	17.5
Natural (N)	6	15.0	15	37.5	20	50.0	24	60.0
M + N	9	22.5	13	32.5	8	20.0	9	22.5
No treatment	13	32.5	2	5.0	–	–	–	–
	X^2_3		12.83*		20.59**		25.12**	
			X^2_3		4.09		3.33	
					X^2_2		14.79	

*$p < .05$; **$p < .01$

TABLE 42: Comparison of "treatment option" between urban and rural groups.

	Urban (n = 118)		*Rural (n = 88)*		
Options	***No.***	***%***	***No.***	***%***	X^2
Medical (M)	6	5.1	6	6.8	*(df = 3)* 18.59*
Natural (N)	63	53.4	69	78.4	
M + N	42	36.6	13	14.8	
No Treatment	7	5.9	–	–	

*$p < .01$

while the urban group was more in favor of combined medical and natural treatments (35.6%) than the rural group (14.8%). 5.9% of urban respondents also favored "no treatment" for Koro. These opinion differences between the groups were significant ($p < .01$).

- *Community vs. Professional Group* **(Table 43 and Fig. 29)**: The professional group endorsed more "medical" and "no treatment" and less "natural treatment" ($p < .01$) than the community group. There were no differences

TABLE 43: Comparison of "treatment option" responses between community (urban + rural) and professional groups.

	Community (n = 206)		*Professional (n = 160)*		*Z*
Options	*No.*	*%*	*No.*	*%*	*Score*
Medical	12	5.8	41	25.6	–5.34*
Natural	132	65.1	65	40.6	4.47*
M + N	55	26.7	39	24.4	0.51
No treatment	1	3.4	15	9.4	–2.39*

*$p < .01$

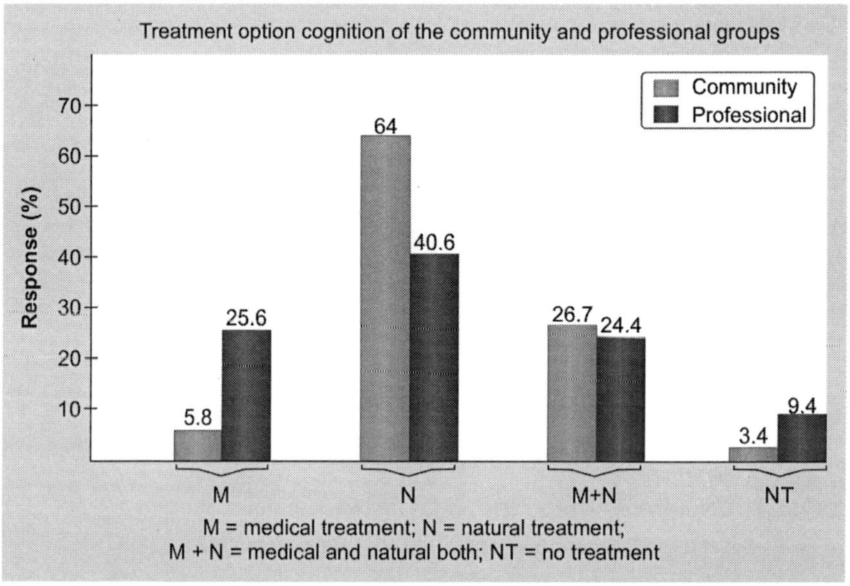

Fig. 29: Comparison of treatment options among the groups.

between the groups insofar as the opinion regarding combined treatment is concerned. Interestingly 40.6% of the professionals advocated the scope of natural therapy in Koro.

Study of Choice of Medicine Type

- *Rural Group* **(Table 44)**: Comparison of responses between NKF and KF rural group regarding the choice of the medicine type for Koro treatment. NKF members favored all medicines in different percentages, while KF members preferred only allopathic and Kabiraji medicines. There were no significant differences between their medicine choices.
- *Urban Group* **(Table 45)**: A comparison of NKF and KF urban group responses showed that NKF members advocated all medicine types in

TABLE 44: Responses for medicine type choice of non-Koro families (NKF) and Koro Families (KF) rural groups.

	NKF (n = 45)		*KF (n = 43)*		
Medicine type	***No.***	***%***	***No.***	***%***	X^2
Nil	33	73.3	36	83.7	*(df = 4)* 6.79 (NS)
Allopathic	3	6.7	2	4.7	
Homeopathic	4	8.9	0	0	
Kabiraji	3	6.7	5	11.6	
Ayurvedic	2	4.4	0	0	

NS = nonsignificant.

TABLE 45: Responses for medicine type choice of NKF and KF urban groups.

	*NKF (n = 60)**		*KF (n = 58)*		
Medicine type	***No.***	***%***	***No.***	***%***	X^2
Nil	34	56.7	31	53.4	*(df = 4)* 8.87 (NS)
Allopathic	18	30	11	18.9	
Homeopathic	3	5	5	8.6	
Kabiraji	3	5	11	18.9	
Ayurvedic	2	3.3	–	–	

*Persons of the "no treatment" category also gave an opinion regarding possible medicine choice.
NS = nonsignificant.

different percentages, like KF members except the Ayurvedic medicines. The reactions of both groups showed no difference.

- *Urban Vs. Rural Group* **(Table 46)**: Urban respondents favored maximally allopathic medicines (25.6%) followed by Kabiraji medicines (11.9%). On the other hand, the rural group stressed Kabiraji treatment (9.1%) more than allopathic medication (5.7%). Overall, more urban respondents (44.9%) preferred drug treatment than the rural group (21.6%).

Study of the Natural Treatment Option

- *Rural Group* **(Table 47)**: Showed that water pouring (WP) (100%) was the prevailing opinion in both Koro-affected and nonaffected family members. The majority in both groups also opined for penile pull (PP), while the option for salt-water (SW) feeding came low in the list.
- *Urban Group* **(Table 48)**: Here, also, the predominant option (100%) was for water pouring, but Koro family members were more in favor of

TABLE 46: Comparison of responses on medicine type choice between urban and rural groups.

	Urban (n = 118)		*Rural (n = 88)*		
Medicine type	***No.***	***%***	***No.***	***%***	***X^2***
Nil	65	55.1	69	78.4	*(df = 4)* 16.0*
Allopathic	29	25.6	5	5.7	
Homeopathic	8	6.8	4	4.5	
Kabiraji	14	11.9	8	9.1	
Ayurvedic	2	1.6	2	2.3	

*$p < .01$

TABLE 47: Natural treatment option of the rural group.

	NKF (n = 33)		*KF (n = 36)*	
Treatment options	***No.***	***%***	***No.***	***%***
WP	33	100	36	100
PP	21	63.6	28	77.8
SW	3	9.1	6	16.7

(PP: penile pull; SW: salt water; WP: water pouring)

TABLE 48: Natural treatment option of the urban group.

	NKF (n = 32)		*KF (n = 31)*	
Treatment options	***No.***	***%***	***No.***	***%***
WP	32	100	31	100
PP	10	31.3	27	87.1
SW	4	12.5	16	51.6

(PP: penile pull; SW: salt water; WP: water pouring)

penile pull (87%) and saltwater feeding (51.6%) than the non-Koro family members.

- *Urban vs. Rural Group* **(Table 49)**: Comparing the responses for natural treatment options showed that both groups prevailing opinion was water pouring (100%). However, the rural and urban groups viewed a higher penile pull and salt water feeding.
- *Community Vs. Professional Group* **(Table 50)**: Comparing responses between community (urban + rural) and professional groups showed that 72.3% of the professional responses favored water pouring. They also endorsed less response regarding penile pull and equal reaction to saltwater feeding than community options.

TABLE 49: Comparison of natural treatment opinions between urban and rural groups.

	Urban (n = 63)		*Rural (n = 31)*	
Treatment options	*No.*	*%*	*No.*	*%*
WP	63	100	69	100
PP	37	58.7	49	71
SW	20	31.7	9	13

(PP: penile pull; SW: salt water; WP: water pouring)

TABLE 50: Comparison of natural treatment options between the community and professional groups.

	Community (n = 132)		*Professional (n = 65)*	
Treatment options	*No.*	*%*	*No.*	*%*
WP	132	100	47	72.3
PP	86	65.2	22	33.3
SW	29	21.9	14	21.5

(PP: penile pull; SW: salt water; WP: water pouring)

Opinion Regarding Mental Treatment in Koro

- *Rural Group* **(Table 51)**: Distribution of NKF and KF members' responses regarding their opinion about "mental treatment" in Koro. Both the groups discarded such a treatment scope for Koro.
- *Urban Group* **(Table 52)**: This compared NKF and KF members' responses regarding their opinion about mental treatment in Koro. 16.7% of NFK and 10.3% of KF members endorsed positively.
- *Urban vs. Rural Group* **(Table 53)**: A comparison of responses between urban and rural respondents showed that 13.6% of urban respondents advocated mental treatment than rural groups ($p < .01$).

Discussion: The previous section pointed out how people have used social ritualistic healing methods to treat the Koro illness. In this study of treatment cognition, this trend has been substantiated by the urban and rural people's higher option for natural treatment-seeking, viz. water pouring on the patient, manual or mechanical penile pull, or forced salt-water (often mixed with lemon juice) feeding. Urban groups, due possibly to their increased exposure to health care facilities and acquaintance with allopathic drugs, showed a higher response for a combined treatment for Koro, i.e., natural therapy with medicines, than rural groups. Professionals responses to treatment options reveal an exciting situation. GP, Surgeon, and PMS groups were more in favor of natural treatment than the physicians. All the groups also

TABLE 51: Response regarding mental treatment in Koro of the rural group.

	NKF (n = 45)		*KF (n = 43)*	
Mental treatment	*No.*	*%*	*No.*	*%*
No	45	100	43	100
Yes	0		0	0

TABLE 52: Response regarding mental treatment in Koro of the urban group.

	NKF (n = 60)		*KF (n = 58)*		
Mental treatment	*No.*	*%*	*No.*	*%*	X^2
No	50	83.3	52	89.7	*(df = 1)* 1.01 (NS)
Yes	10	16.7	6	10.3	

NS = nonsignificant.

TABLE 53: Comparison of "mental treatment" response between urban and rural groups.

	Urban (n = 118)		*Rural (n = 88)*		
Mental treatment	*No.*	*%*	*No.*	*%*	X^2_1
No	102	86.4	88	100	*(df = 1)* 12.94*
Yes	16	13.6	0	0	

*$p < .01$

advocated the need for a combined treatment. In reality, this response is almost identical to that of the community.

No differences were noted between Koro-affected or nonaffected families in rural and urban settings in choosing the medicine type. But in totality, the urban groups favored medicines, particularly allopathic medicines, than the rural groups. Kabiraji was seen to be a popular treatment option in both groups.

In the choice of natural treatment, water pouring is the most popular treatment advocated by both Koro-affected and nonaffected family members of rural and urban groups. Members of the Koro-affected families were more in favors of penile pull than their non-Koro counterparts. This practice was also more frequent in rural responses. Interestingly, 72% of the professionals endorsed water pouring as a natural treatment method in Koro. However, more surprising is the finding that 33.8% of them opined for penile pull as a treatment method. The option for salt water, astonishingly, revealed an identical response. 13.6% of urban respondents favored scope for some mental treatment, viz. persuasion to make the patient fear-free, and some psychotropic medicine to relieve anxiety and insomnia.

Four respondents mentioned the effectiveness of diazepam injection in such cases.

The popularity of indigenous/folk treatment methods was related to the failure of any provision for medical management by the treatment people during the epidemic and their identical views about treatment. Medical indecisiveness, or rather echoing social cognition, is an essential social dynamic in the genesis, spread, and increased indigenous treatment-seeking by the people in distress. A very similar situation was observed in Singapore during a massive Koro epidemic there. The Chinese Physician' Association of Singapore held a seminar during the epidemic. It was declared that the Shook Yang epidemic was due to "fear, rumor-mongering, climatic conditions and imbalance between Heart and Kidneys."[11]

Thus, the Chinese Physicians' Association believed that penile retraction is a reality with a genuinely high risk to life, although no authentic, verified cases had ever been reported.[11]

A survey of the world Koro literature also provides various modes of indigenous healing rituals to treat Koro. Some notable examples are: the manual traction of the penis with iron pincer followed by a medical drink, made up from "masculine" substance like a mixture of alcoholic beverage, powdered deer horn, bamboo chip, also mammelong, flower shoot of the male palmyra (*Borassus flabelliformis*) and stalk of the arenga palm (*Arenga saccharifera*) among the Macassaran people of Sulawesi (Slot, 1935).[96] Permanent anchoring down the penis with hooks on board or encasing of the penis in the longitudinal groove of "lie teng hok," a jeweler's scale, followed by a drink, is the usual treatment. The glass is "panas" (Warm)—a mixture of hot or yang principles, composed of arak, gunpowder, powered tin with sulfur, and different herbs was reported by Palthe[108] as the indigenous treatment found among the Malay-speaking Chinese of Old Batavia. Palthe[109] also described the use of "penis rods" or sharp perforation of glans with a quilt as a preventive method against the shooting of the penis within body.

In reality, all the indigenous treatment methods express Koro's ethno-medical concept among the population groups. Since body heat is the prevalent social concept of Koro in the North Bengal epidemic (vide the Cause Cognition section), water pouring constitutes a significant treatment modality. Penile pull, of diverse nature, is a universal finding and dictates an area where medical intervention is necessary because of the risk of infection and injury. Medical input and help are crucial for information transmission and safety management of Koro.

STUDY OF KORO ACQUAINTANCE SOURCE

Introduction: LeBon,[110] suggested that in mass response to the psychiatric outbreak, the people tend to feel and behave in the same way because one person's emotions and actions spread through a group reaction—a process he termed "contagion." Conformity is one crucial variable in this contagion process, where the individual does what other members of the group or community do because of social pressure.[111] In conformity, it is the majority that affects the rest. In the process of conformity again, the role of crowd response is operative because it is evident that not all persons in a community get the chance or scope to see or examine the cases in question personally or directly. Then how does the illness information spread in the sociometric channel in the community? It is enacted by crowd response, where some emotional identification with others in the same setting works.[112] Or some identical cultural beliefs for the "new disease" is sufficient to make one person's experience meaningful to another, irrespective of the direct witnessing of the illness in question for proof. This proposition is also proved by the construct of "emotional contagion and collective behavior."[66] Thus Tseng and Hsu[113] defined mass hysterical behavior as "a sociological-psychological phenomenon in which a group of people through social cognition, collectively manifest psychological disorder within a brief period of time" (p. 77).

There is no research data in the literature to assume the specific ratio distribution between direct witnessing and indirect information gathering (hearing) component of a crowd response in the spread of a mental outbreak. Nor do we know which division of people plays a significant role in crowd response over the other. The initial cognitive assessment of threat and atypicality of the illness in question positively influences this direct-indirect (information gathering) ratio. In the event of alleged high-threat illness assessment, both the information sources probably act synonymously and help contagion of a psychiatric outbreak in a community. This exciting research area may highlight valuable social-communicative variables operative in psychiatric outbreaks.

The present study was designed to explore how many people in a community could witness Koro cases personally. It is evident in the Social Response study (discussed above) that the members of Koro-affected (KF) and non-Koro affected (NKF) families did not show any significant differences in their perception about the illness type, seriousness, risk, and infectivity of Koro during the epidemic time. So this investigation will help us understand the ratio of persons with direct and indirect Koro acquaintance and their role in the information transmission (about Koro) during the epidemic.

Materials and methods: This study dealt with the elicitation of the Koro acquaintance source of 366 individuals of the Social Response Study sample (88 rural + 118 urban + 160 professionals). Koro acquaintance source was divided into two types: Direct, who personally saw or handled Koro case (s), and Indirect, who never witnessed any such case face-to-face but gathered the information from their family or friends or from community discussions/ or who has firsthand experience.

Results

Table 54 displays the Koro acquaintance source of the study population. Out of 366 individuals, 59.3% acquired the Koro information directly. 40.7% of persons had no direct exposure to the Koro cases. They gathered the information through indirect sources. Among the three groups, in the professional sample, persons with indirect Koro information were more (46.9%) in contrast to rural (28.4%) and urban (41.5%) examples. It is interesting to note that in the professional group, GPs had the highest percentage (80%) of direct Koro information while the Paramedical Staffs (PMS) had the least (35%).

Ratio percentage analysis between Direct: Indirect acquaintance source of these three groups shows the following distribution:

Discussion: Psychiatric epidemic is a social phenomenon that affects a proportion of the overtly "normal" population with some covert vulnerability that develops or unfolds under certain specific psychosocial situations.[26] The dissipation of illness information is an essential variable in the social cognitive circuit. The social communication networks help develop a circumscribed environment where illness messages spread via direct-indirect pathways. At this point, visual proof or hearing from others serves the same purpose as transmitting illness information in the community.

TABLE 54: Koro acquaintance source of the social response study sample (n = 366).

	Koro acquaintance source				
	Direct		*Indirect*		*Direct-indirect ratio*
Study population	*No.*	*%*	*No.*	*%*	
Rural sample (n = 88)	63	71.6	25	28.4	7 : 3
NKF (n = 45)	26	57.8	19	42.2	
KF (n = 43)	37	86.1	6	13.9	
Urban sample (n = 118)	69	58.5	49	41.5	3 : 2
NKF (n = 60)	28	46.7	32	53.3	
KF (n = 58)	41	70.7	17	29.3	
Professional sample (160)	85	53.1	75	46.9	11 : 9
Physician (n = 40)	22	55.0	18	45.0	
GP (n = 40)	32	80.0	8	20.0	
Surgeon (n = 40)	17	42.5	23	57.5	
PMS (n = 40)	14	35.0	26	65.0	
Total	217	59.3	149	40.7	3 : 2

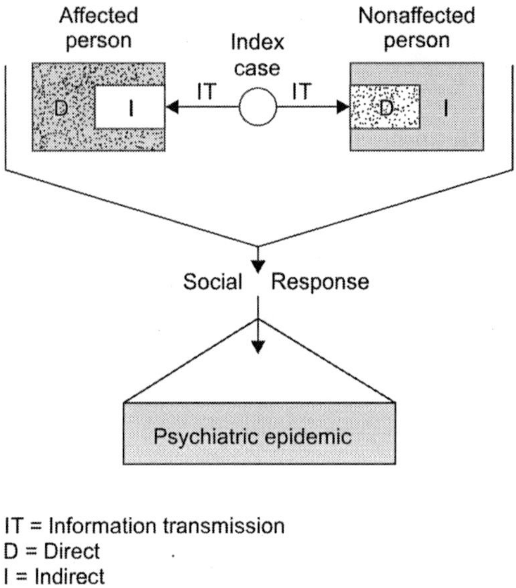

Fig. 30: Dynamics of information transmission in psychiatric epidemic.

A person with indirect details may be a suitable medium for rumor transmission. Simultaneously, those with direct exposure may exaggerate the phenomenon with personal bias, thus facilitating rumor transmission. Affected persons are also vulnerable to these direct-indirect information networks. Colligan et al.,[114] found that nonaffected workers in an industrial mass psychogenic illness reported hearing of more people becoming ill than affected, while affected reported witnessing more people becoming ill. So it is seen that in the psychiatric epidemic, both direct and indirect information transmission takes place in the social network system. Both types of communication are equally important in as much as the social response to the illness and the consequent spread of the epidemic is concerned **(Fig. 30)**. Ngui[11] in his survey of the Singapore Koro epidemic, found among a patient cohort of 226 cases (males 220; females 6), previous knowledge of Koro was quite prevalent: among the males- 24.5% had past knowledge of Koro illness. Among all the cases, 76.4% had either direct or indirect knowledge of Koro with eating pork.

PART FIVE: MEDICAL AND SOCIAL TREATMENT OF KORO

Summary: An account of the medical treatment that was offered to the Koro patients by the local general practitioners, hospital doctors, private specialists, and by the author himself is briefly documented. The "social" or folk treatments, i.e., the ritualistic healing method advocated by priest-healers, village medicine man (*jikri* or *Gunin*), was the most popular treatment choice, adopted by most Koro patients and their families.

MEDICAL TREATMENT OF KORO

A brief account of medical (allopathic) treatment offered to Koro patients during the Koro Epidemic is presented. An extraordinary placebo effect of "injection treatment" as an emergency medical intervention was noted in the patient and their family and friends. Craving for vitamin "tonics" by Koro patients was noteworthy. An account of these medical treatments, along with their psychotherapeutic effects, are discussed.

Injection treatment: Koro patients were usually brought to the hospital/private clinics by a group of over-anxious relatives, friends, and community people. Relatives or friends insisted on the urgent demand for an emergency medical intervention, as they believed the treatment would be a life-saving measure. This "compelling emergency" invoked by the awaiting over-anxious and potentially "hazardous" mob coupled with the ignorance of the attending physician promoted the latter to institute a "medicine injection" protocol instantaneously: which ranged from an intramuscular injection of diazepam 5 mg as well as promethazine 50 mg, or Chlorpromazine 25 mg, or an anabolic steroid, vitamin B_1, B_6 , B_{12} , or nikethamide, tetanus toxoid to intravenous infusion of a bottle of 5% dextrose solution. The immediate effects of these "emergency injection treatment regimens" were dramatic. In some cases of dextrose infusion, the patient felt "ok", and only after transfusion of a quarter bottle of fluid they urge for discontinuation of the same. Intramuscular diazepam, chlorpromazine, though not so dramatic, yielded an excellent clinical response. Some general practitioners reported a combination of two or three injections one after another in different shots (e.g., diazepam 5 mg, promethazine 50 mg, and 2 mL of B_1, B_6, B_{12}) yielded promising results (probably reflecting the emergency intervention). The patients usually become free of genital retraction symptoms and heightened anxiety within 20–30 minutes. One general practitioner reported that he cured his six male Koro patients by an emergency intramuscular injection of one ampule of vitamin B_6 deeply in the gluteal region.

Craving for "vitamin tonic" was remarkable due to both general perceptions of masses about the "strength-giving property" of the vitamin liquid and indiscriminate prescribing of the same by the few general medical practitioners. It is worthwhile to recall here one such example of an Ayurvedic rejuvenating tonic that claims to offer "secret strength and regaining of lost power" (pointing covertly to sexual arousal) printed a picture of a galloping horse on its packing box. This tonic was in high demand during the epidemic months, and one of the medicine shops sold 200 bottles on average daily during the early part of the epidemic. Also on high sale, other topics such as B-complex, liver extracts, glycerophosphate, and cyproheptadine syrups were in high demand.

It was observed that Koro patients, either in a hospital or at private clinics, were regarded as an unwelcome burden. This was primarily due to ignorance of physicians about Koro and secondarily, because of the accompaniment of a chaotic and disturbing mini-crowd with each patient. The compulsion of emergency was present at both ends of the spectrum: the physician wants to eliminate this vexing problem at his earliest. The patient party demands immediate medical intervention and recovery. Quick injection and/or dextrose infusion in that sequence reflects the demonstration of "emergency" intervention (something has been done to the patient). It also helps the patient reorganize his coping attempt to get free of his Koro symptoms to facilitate the earliest discharge from the stressful hospital environment. Though "Injection treatment" is nonspecific from a medical point of view but has a demonstrable spectacular synergistic placebo effect on the whole scenario. These medical interventions somehow had a positive psychotherapeutic impact on Koro's psychodynamics, be it hysterical somatization or panic-stricken Koro reaction. This holds for the female Koro patients as well.

Psychiatric treatment of Koro: The treatment experience of the author of 64 Koro cases (55 male and 9 female) has shown that the following treatment regimen offered an excellent clinical response. Of these cases, 21 were (19 males and 2 females) treated at the North Bengal Medical College (5 males were inpatient at the Department of Medicine), and the rest 43 at the community level.

Treatment Steps at Medical College OPD/A and E:

- All the accompanying persons were requested to remain outside the clinical room.
- Strong assurance that this illness is not life-threatening helps alleviate the patient's anxiety and relatives. The next step is the prompt physical examination, including inspection and palpation of the genital organ and pulse and blood pressure recording. These necessary steps at the initial contact were found helpful in establishing a good rapport with the patient and alleviating the relatives' anxiety.
- In cases with extreme anxiety and panic, intramuscular 10 mg diazepam injection, sometimes with intramuscular promethazine 50 mg, offered good recovery from their Koro pang.
- Oral day-time oxazepam tablet, 15–30 mg BID or TID, and diazepam 5 or 10 mg at bedtime for 2–3 days made the patients normal in the majority of the cases.
- The patients with pre-existing psychiatric illness, e.g., depression or schizophrenia, responded nicely to doxepin hydrochloride (25–50 mg BID) and haloperidol (5 mg BID/QID), respectively, for 7–14 days.

- Educational psychotherapy and an elaborate discussion on genital morphology and functions helped alleviate Koro patients' fear of losing sexual virility or a future attack.
- Two female cases, one with agitated depression and the other with varied hypochondriacal symptoms, responded well within a week to treatment with doxepin hydrochloride (50 mg BID) and oxazepam (30 mg BID). However, they had to continue treatment for their primary illness for a few more weeks or months.
- In some cases (16 males), follow-up (up to 3–4 months) supportive psychotherapy was needed to boost their "masculine morale" and self-esteem.

SOCIAL TREATMENT OF KORO

The community's various healing modalities with social sanction reflected the societal cultural attribution to Koro perception. In this region, the local faith healers, called "Jhirkri" or "Gunin", also endorsed similar healing methods to cure genital retraction in Koro. This cultural Koro perception could be viewed from three broad categories insofar as its folk-etiology is concerned, viz., body heat concept, supernatural causation, and organ pathology. The respective curative treatment methods advocated were: Water pouring to cool the body from heat; force-counterforce paradigm leading to penile traction and care of the sex organ (penis) **(Fig. 31)**.

Another cultural understanding of body heat dissolution was the forced feeding of common salt (NaCl) solution with lemon juice. This idea was that salt facilitates vomiting and thereby relieves the patients from "distension" caused by "excessive body heat. Common salt and lemon juice are believed to have medicinal value and are often used in different home remedial measures, e.g., gargle with salt-water in throat infection; bandage with salt and ice in sprains or blunt injury of the limbs, etc. Lemon water has excellent digestive properties and is regarded as a cooling (of body heat) agent.

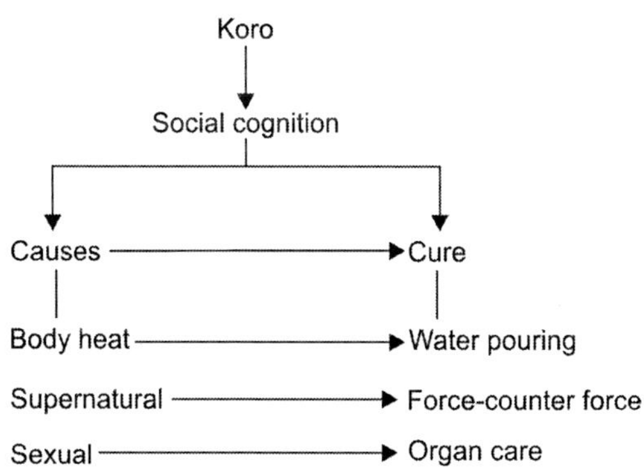

Fig. 31: Cultural cognition and its interaction between cause and cure of Koro.

Ripe lemon (golden yellow in color) is used in several religions and domestic rituals. Lemon is also believed to have a protective property from envious neighbors" unholy magical influence or evil intent. So a thread containing 3 or 4 yellow lemons interspersed with red chilies was usually kept hanging at the entrance door of many houses or in front of shops during the epidemic in the region.

Sociritualistic Healing of Koro

Curative Methods

During the epidemic, the primary healing ritual was cooling the body by pouring several buckets of water over the Koro-affected person or immersing him up to the neck in a pond or river, irrespective of his/her will or the time of the day. Pouring water over Koro-affected persons became a social event of great enthusiasm during this time. Many known or unknown neighbors or passersby volunteered to carry the patient and pour water in a certain jovial mood. The whole sequence often took a ceremonial character. A brief account of social curative "treatment" of 104 male and one female Koro cases is reported. Medical and surgical fatalities involving 4 deaths from such social "treatment" is also reported.

Table 55 shows the account of four deaths (all males) arising out of such "treatment" of Koro patients from West Bengal. Three were the victims of water-pouring and its consequent profound hypothermic shock.

Table 56 shows the account of medical complications of water pouring (WP)/immersion of 28 Koro cases and salt-water feeding of 4 patients, of which one was a female Koro (with breast symptom). The cases were treated at different hospitals, e.g., Siliguri sub-divisional hospital (16); Jalpaiguri Sub-divisional hospital (6); Mal Rural hospital (3); Dinhata Block hospital (2), and North Bengal Medical College hospital (5). The figures in parentheses indicate the number of cases treated at each hospital.

TABLE 55: Deaths from Koro social "treatment."

Case	1	2*	3**	4
Age (years)	17	38	32	27
Marital status	Single	Married	Married	Single
Ethnicity	Behari Hindu	Oraon (Tribe)	Bengali Hindu	Bengali Hindu
Clinical presentation	Profound hypothermic shock			Brought dead
Forced immersion	9 hours (in a river)	12 hours (in a pond)	10 hours (in a pond)	Forced feeding of 5 Kg. Salt (NaCl) Soln

*A tea plantation worker, treated by a Jhikri. **Also inhaled water.

TABLE 56: Medical complications of Koro social "treatment."

n	*Sex*	*Age in years Mean (SD)*	*Length of water-pouring in hours Mean (SD)*	*Clinical features*
9	Male	26 (6.7)	6.1 (4.3)	Hypothermic shock, bronchopneumonia
13	Male	21 (9.2)	2.3 (2.8)	Hyperpyrexia, pneumonitis
6	Male	24 (10.7)	4.4 (2.8)	Cough, mild temperature, muscular pain, weakness
4	3 Males 1 Female	18 (3.8) 18	Salt-feeding/4 hours/ 2.1 (1.2) Kg	Nausea, vomiting, loose motion, drowsy state, muscular pain

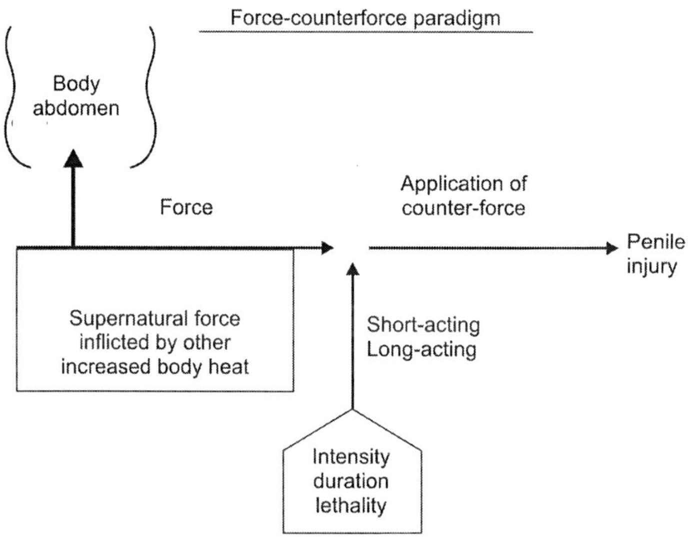

Fig. 32: Social perception of "force-counterforce" in the prevention of penile retraction.

Figure 32 shows the force-counterforce paradigm's social cognitive construct in the context of "supernatural" causation (malevolent intra-abdominal penile pull) of Koro illness. The sudden onset of supernatural force was not precisely understood by the patient or the community's people. Still, as suggested, the probable causes were related to the transgression of social sex-norms or inappropriate (or forbidden) sexual desire, wishes, or thoughts (that increases body heat) of the incumbent or inflicted by others through black magic. Whatever may be the primary cause, the supernatural force creates an internal pressure within the body (abdomen) that pulls the penis towards the abdomen. This pull's intensity, duration, and lethality were thought to be the determinant variables for Koro distress's and clinical "severity". The indrawing of the penis in Koro, they perceived as a reflection of a dynamic force acting from within with a mal-intent to dissolute the organ (and ultimately leading to death or sexual disability). The folk prescription advocated was the application of counterforce, either manual or mechanical penile traction, to prevent the fatal penile indrawing. The application and the nature of external counterforce (short or long-acting) was determined by the hypothetical assessment of the degree of strength of the internal pull (usually by the local healer or a community elder). All these maneuvers could potentially lead to penile injury **(Fig. 33)**.

The account of penile traction in 65 male Koro cases showed 16 cases had manual traction and 49 cases had mechanical traction **(Table 57)**. Manual traction sometimes was induced by the patient himself, but others always imposed mechanical traction.

Table 58 shows the account of various sex-organ (penis) care methods in four Koro cases.

Preventive Method

Fear of Koro infectivity affected rural and urban people, predominantly illiterate, unskilled laborers, and youths of urban slum areas. The people of this region practiced two types of preventive social rituals during this epidemic. The predominant pattern was the forehead's marking, ear lobules, and suprasternal fossa with white lime spots **(Fig. 37)**.

Lime and local culture: White lime ($CaCO_3$) is a substance of much social importance because of its multiple usage and ritualistic significances. White lime is used to prepare betel leaf (*Piper betle-Paan*) for chewing; slaked lime is mixed with tobacco for chewing, both of which constitute a prevalent habit of people of this region. Lime is believed to have a medicinal

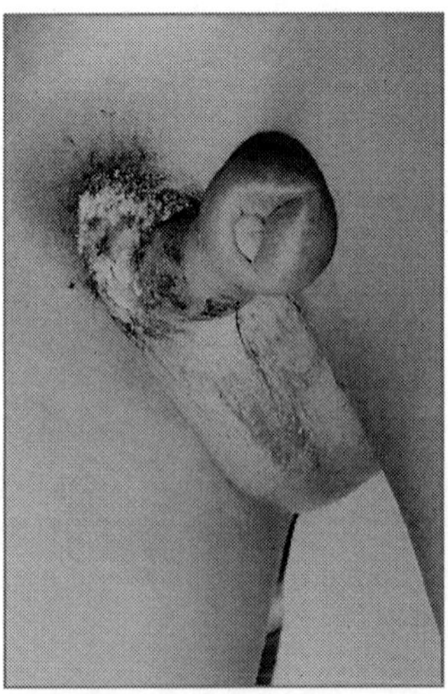

Fig. 33: Infected balanitis after an injury from mechanical traction.

property for which the drinking of supernatant clear lime water is a frequent home remedy for indigestion, especially in children. The application of a paste of hot lime and turmeric dust over the site of joint sprain or fracture is a widely practiced traditional healing aid. Lime (with betel leaf) is an essential ingredient in worship and in black magic and spells by *Tantricks* or

TABLE 57: Various types of mechanical penile tractions used in Koro cases (n = 49).

Type	*Number of cases*	*Method of traction*
I.	16	Hanging traction—by pulling the penis with a rope or clout, and a weight (brick or iron bar or stone piece or iron weight used in weighting was tied at the hanging end, and the patient was kept standing **(Fig. 34)**
II.	12	By clothing materials like a dhoti, lungi, towel or shari, etc.
III.	9	By wire—naked iron wire or insulted electric wire
IV.	7	By rope—coconut rope **(Fig. 35)** synthetic plastic cord or fishing thread, etc.
		The traction cord's free end is either fixed with a stand (window bar, cot leg, bamboo post) or others held manually by others
V.	4	By iron cooking pincer manfully held by others **(Fig. 36)**
VI.	1	By pricking the prepuce with a fishing hook and the other end is fixed with the right great toe, others straight the leg

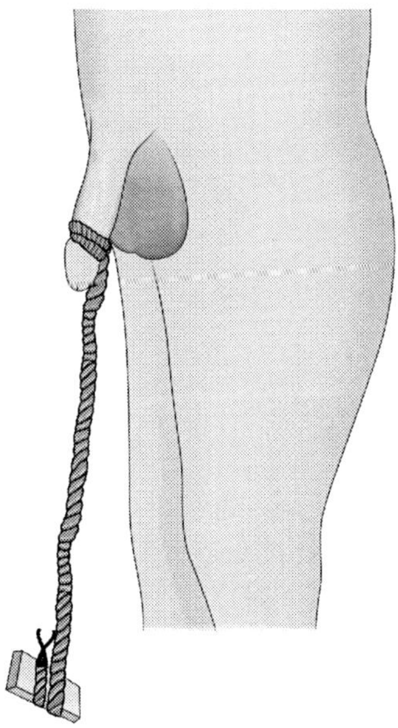

Fig. 34: Hanging traction.

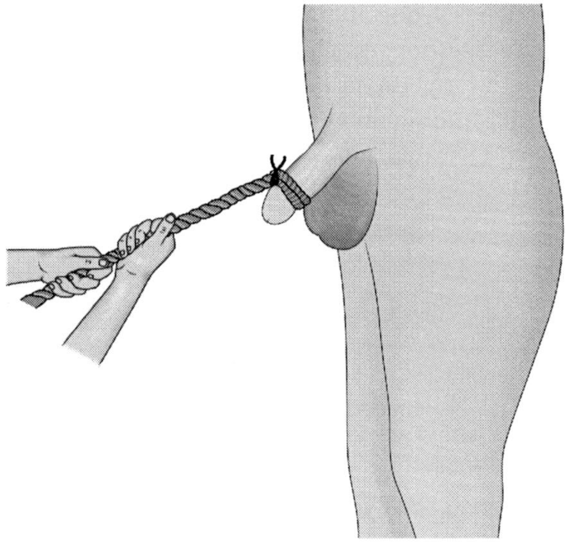

Fig. 35: Rope traction.

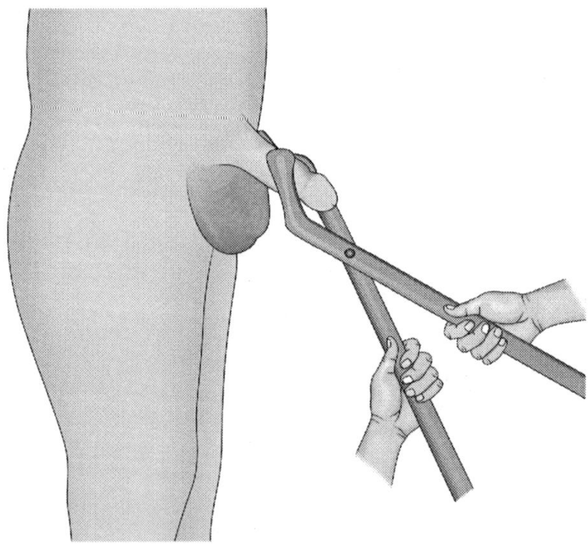

Fig. 36: Mechanical traction.

TABLE 58: Account of various sex-organ (penis) care methods in four Koro cases.

- *Potassium permanganate solution:* 46 years, a homeopathic practitioner (Rural)
- *Raw "Dettol" (an antiseptic) solution:* 27 years, Public Health Engineering Worker (Rural)
- *Washing soda (NaOH) solution;* 26 years, North Bengal State Transport Cleaner (Urban)
- *Common salt (NaCl) solution* with ice chips and manual traction: 14 years, tea plantation worker (Urban)

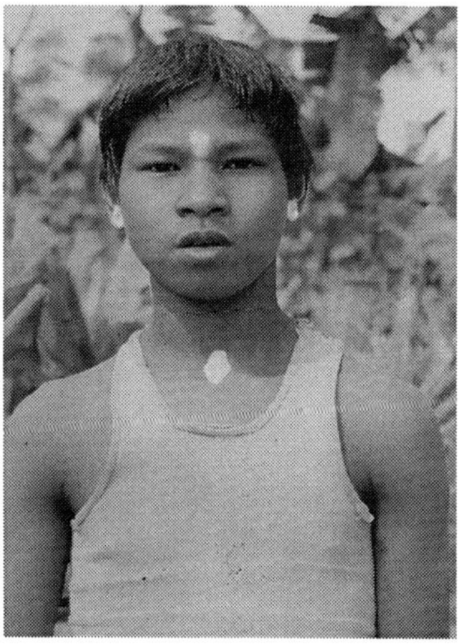

Fig. 37: Lime smearing on ear lobule and front of the neck to prevent Koro.

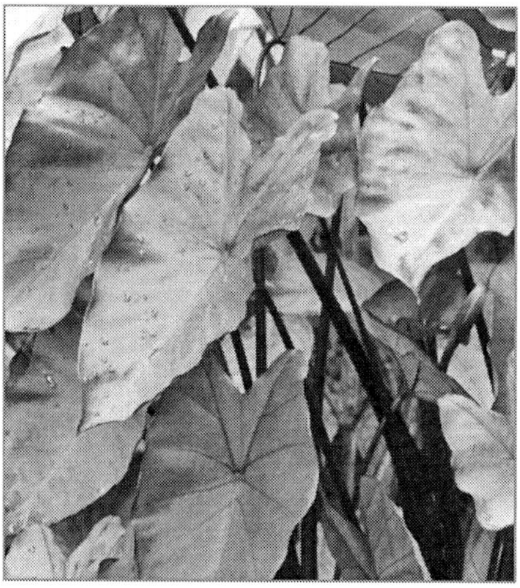

Fig. 38: Black-stem Arum.

folk healers. Lime and vermilion spots over earthen pots *(Ghat)* carry marks of magical and supernatural influence or force during the process of sprit-driven rituals in possession cases by folk healers. Charmed slaked lime is frequently used with evil intent to harm others (either by mixing it with food secretly or keeping it within the house boundary).

The second preventive practice was rapping great toes with a thon scale or sheath of black stem arum (*Typhonium trilobatum*) **(Fig. 38)**. It is also an edible vegetable in certain sections of the population. It is also known as *Bengal Arum* and has many home-medicinal uses among communities. These plants are usually associated with ghost tales and religious, tribal rituals. One of the *Jhikris* (local folk healers), a tea plantation worker, said that the arum scale offers invisible protection to the wearer from any unholy or ghostly or envious infliction of bodily harm, including genital retraction.

REFERENCES

1. Chowdhury AN, Pal P, Chatterjee A, Roy Das M, Chowdhury, BB. Analysis of North Bengal Koro epidemic with three years follow-up. Ind J Psychiat. 1988;30:69-72.
2. Biswal P. Personal communication. 1984
3. Chattopadhyaya A. Atisa and Tibet. 1967; Calcutta Indian Studies.
4. Banerjee AK (Ed.). West Bengal District Gazetteers, Darjeeling. 1980; Government of West Bengal.
5. Sanyal CC. Tista-Karatoyyar Ruprekha (in Bengali). Jalpaiguri District Centenary Souvenir. Jalpaiguri. 1970;pp. 348.
6. Ghosh B (Ed.). Census 1971, Series 22, 1974. West Bengal District Census Handbook: Jalpaiguri District, Calcutta.
7. Mazumder D. West Bengal District Gazetteers: Koch Bihar, Calcutta: 1977; West Bengal Government Press.
8. Census of India. 1971, Series 22, West Bengal, Part IIA, General Population Table. 1973; Delhi.
9. Hamilton FB. History of Cooch-Bihar. J Asiatic Soc Bengal, Vol. VII, Part-I. 1838; Calcutta.
10. Gwee AL. Koro—Its origin and nature as a disease entity. Singapore Med J. 1968;9:3-6.
11. Ngui PW. The Koro epidemic in Singapore. Aust NZ J Psychiat. 1969; 3: 263-6.
12. Suwanlert S, Coates D. Epidemic Koro in Thailand: Clinical and social aspects. Transcul Psychiatric Res Rev. 1978;16:64-6.
13. Chowdhury AN. Clinical analysis of 101 Koro cases. Ind J Soc Psychiat. 1992;8:67-70.
14. Dutta D, Phookun HR, Das PD. The Koro epidemic in Lower Assam. Ind J Psychiat. 1982;24:370-4.
15. Chakrabarty A, Das S, Mukherjee A. Koro makes an epidemic appearance in India. Transcul Newsletter III, 1982; 3-4 December.
16. Chakrabarty A, Bag DC. Genesis of the Koro Epidemic in West Bengal and Assam: Implication of Turtle Cults. Human Sc. 1989;38:142-9.
17. Chowdhury AN. Koro in Females—An analysis of 48 cases. Transcul Psychiatric Res Rev. 1994;31:369-80.
18. Chowdhury AN. Koro in Schizophrenia with a case report from an Industrial set up. Indust Psychiat J. 1992;51:47-59.
19. Chowdhury AN. Koro in affective disorder with a case report from industrial set up. Indust Psychiat J. 1992;52:71-83.
20. Chowdhury AN. Koro among Kinship. Ind J Soc Psychiat. 19895: 24-6.
21. Kaplan BH, Cassel JC, Gore S. Social support and health. Medical Care. 1977;15:47-58.
22. Mechanic D. Illness behaviour, social adaptation and management of illness. J Nerv Ment Dis. 1977;165:79-87.
23. Waxler NE. Culture and mental illness. A social labeling perspective. J Nerv Ment Dis. 1974;159:379-95.

24. Stahl SM. Illness as an emergent norm or doing what comes naturally. In: Colligan MJ, Pennebaker JW, Murthy LR (Eds.). Mass Psychogenic Illness. A Social Psychological Analysis. New Jersey: Lawrence Erlbaum Associates Publisher; 1982. pp. 183-98.
25. Colligan MJ, Smith MJ. A methodological approach for evaluating outbreaks of Mass Psychogenic Illness in industry. J Occup Med. 1978;20:401-8.
26. Colligan MJ, Murphy LR. Mass Psychogenic Illness in Organizations: An Overview. J Occup Psychol. 1979;52:77-90.
27. Scheff T. Being mentally ill. Chicago: Aldine;1966.
28. Sirois F. Perspective of Epidemic Hysteria. In: Colligan MJ, Pennebaker JW, Murphy LR (Eds.) Mass Psychogenic Illness. A Social Psychological Analysis. New Jersey: Lawrence Erlbaum Associates Publisher; 1982. pp. 217-36.
29. Raman AC, Murphy HBM. Failure of traditional prognostic indicators in Afro-Asian psychotics: Results of a long term follow-up survey. J Nerv Ment Dis. 1972;154:238-47.
30. Denitz S, Lefton M, Augrist S, Pasamanick B. Psychiatric and social attributes as predictors of case outcome in mental hospitalization. Social Problem. 1961;8:322-8.
31. Mechanic D. Social psychologic factors affecting the presentation of bodily complaints. New Engl J Med. 1972;286:1132-9.
32. Mechanic D. Sociocultural and social psychological factors affecting personal response to psychological disorders. J Health Soc Behav. 1975;16:394-404.
33. Cobb S. Social support as a moderator of life stress. Psychosom Med. 1976;38(5):300-14.
34. Turner RH, Killian LM. Collective Behaviour. 2nd edition. New Jersey: Prentice-Hall; 1972.
35. Smelser NJ. Theory of Collective Behaviour. New York. The Free Press; 1963. p. 48.
36. Lang K, Lang GE. Collective Dynamics. New York: Thomas Y Crowell Company; 1961. p.16.
37. Kerckhoff AC. Analyzing a Case of Mass Psychogenic Illness. In: Colligan MJ, Pennebaker JW, Murphy LR (Eds.) Mass Psychogenic Illness. New Jersey: Lawrence Erlbaum Associates Publisher; 1982. pp. 5-20.
38. Sirois F. Epidemic hysteria. In: Roy A (Ed). Hysteria. London: John Wiley and Sons Limited; 1982. pp. 101-5.
39. Sirois F. Epidemic Hysteria. Acta Psychiatrica Scand. 1974;(Suppl 252):1-45.
40. Champion FP, Taylor R, Joseph PR, Hedden JC. Mass hysteria associated with insect bites. J South Carolina Med Assoc. 1963;59:351-3.
41. Jacobs N. The Phantom Slasher of Taipei: Mass Hysteria in a Non-Western Society. Soc Problems. 1965;12:318-28.
42. Knight JA, Friedman TI, Sulianti J. Epidemic Hysteria: A field study. Amer J Pub Health. 1965;55:858-65.
43. Mechanic D. The experience and reporting of common physical complaints. J Health Soc Behav. 1980;21:146-55.
44. Zola I. Culture and symptoms: An analysis of patient's presenting complaints. Amer Sociol Rev. 1966;31:615-30.
45. Kleinman A. Patients and Healers in the Context of Culture. Berkley: California University Press; 1980.

46. Obeyeskere G. The Impact of Ayurvedic Ideas on the Culture and the Individual in Sri Lanka. In: Leslie C (Ed.) Asian Medical Systems: A Comparative Study. Berkley: University of California Press;1977. pp. 201-26.
47. Karckhoff AC, Back AW. Sociometric patterns in hysterical contagion. Sociometry. 1965;28:2-15.
48. Hocking B. Anthropological aspect of occupational Illness epidemics.' J Occup Med. 1987;29:526-30.
49. Angel R, Thoits P. The impact of culture on the cognitive structure of illness. Cul Med Psychiat. 1987;11:465-94.
50. Thoits PA. Self-labeling processes in mental illness: The role of emotional deviance. Amer J Sociol. 1985;91:221-49.
51. Eisenberg L. Disease and illness: Distinctions between professional and popular ideas of sickness. Cul Med Psychiat. 1977;1:9-3.
52. Markush RE. Mental Epidemics: A review of the old to prepare for the new. Pub Health Rev. 1973;2:353-442.
53. Editorial: Epidemic Hysteria. BMJ. 1979;2:408-9.
54. Small GH, Borus JF. Outbreak of illness in a school chorus: Toxic poisoning or mass hysteria. New Engl J Med. 1983;308:632-5.
55. Moffatt MEK. Epidemic hysteria in a Montreal train station. Pediatrics. 1982;70:308-9.
56. Menzel H. Innovation, integration, and marginality: A survey of Physicians. Amer Sociol Rev. 1960;25:707-8.
57. Kadushin C. Why People Go to Psychiatrist. New York: Atherton Press; 1969.
58. Febrega H Jr. Disease and social behaviour. An Interdisciplinary Perspective. Massachusetts: M. I. T. Press; 1974.
59. Kessler RC, Brown RL, Broman CL. Sex differences in psychiatric help-seeking: Evidence from four large-scale surveys. J Health Social Behav. 1981;22:29-64.
60. Frank J. Persuasion and healing. New York: Schocken Books; 1961.
61. Hafez A. The role of the press and the medical community in the epidemic of "Mysterious Gas Poisoning" in the Jordan West Bank. Amer J Psychiat. 1985;142:833-7.
62. Jones FT. Mass psychogenic illness: Role of the individual physician. Am Fam Physician, 2000;15:62(12):2649-53.
63. Spence M. Foundation of Modern Sociology. New Jersey: Prentice-Hall; 1979. pp. 312-4.
64. Boss LP. Epidemic hysteria: A review of the published literature. Epidemiologic Rev. 1997;19(2):233-43.
65. Funk S, Salthe M, Jansen VAA. Modeling the influence of human behavior on the spread of infectious diseases: a review. J Royal Soc Interface. 2010;7:1247-6.
66. Hatfield E, Rapson RL, Le Y L. Emotional contagion and empathy. In: Decety J, W Lckes (Eds). The Social Neuroscience of Empathy. Boston: MIT Press; 2009. pp. 19-30.
67. Strong P. Epidemic psychology: A model. Sociol Health & Illness. 1990; 12(3):249-59.
68. Markus H. Self-schemata and processing information about the self. J Personality Soc Psychol. 1977;35(2):63-78.
69. Kleinman A. Neurasthenia and depression: A study of somatization and culture in China. Cul Med Psychiat. 1982;6:117-90.

70. Nichter M. Idioms of distress: Alternatives in the expression of psychosocial distress: A case study from South India. Cul Med Psychiat. 1981;5:379-408.
71. DiMaggio P. Culture and cognition. Annual Rev Sociol. 1997;23:263-87.
72. Small GW, Borus JF. The influence of newspaper reports on outbreaks of mass hysteria. Psychiatric Quart. 1987;58(4):269-78.
73. D' Andrade RG, Quinn NR, Nerlove SB, Romney AK. Categories of Diseases in American-English and Mexican-Spanish. In: Romney AK, Shepard RN, Nerlove SB (Eds.). Multidimensional Scaling: New York: Seminar Press; 1972. pp. 9-54.
74. Gwee AL. Koro—A cultural disease. Singapore Med J. 1963;4:119-22.
75. Rin H. A Study of the aetiology of Koro in respect to the Chinese concept of illness. Int J Soc Psychiat. 1965;11.7-13.
76. Yap PM. Koro—A Culture-bound Depersonalization Syndrome. Brit J Psychiat. 1965;111:43-50.
77. Yap PM. Koro in a Briton. Brit J Psychiat. 1965;111:774-5.
78. Chowdhury AN. Psychic infectivity: The role of positive illness cognition in psychiatric epidemic. J Personality Clin Studies. 1992;8:125-8.
79. Oyebode F, Jamieson R, Mullaney J, Davison K. Koro: A psychophysiological dysfunction? Brit J Psychiat. 1986;148:212-4.
80. Edwards JW. Indigenous Koro: A genital retraction syndrome of insular south east Asia: A critical review. Cul Med Psychiat. 1984;8:1-24.
81. Chowdhury AN. Dysmorphic Penis-image perception: the Root of Koro Vulnerability. A longitudinal study. Acta Pschiatrica Scand. 1989;80:518-20.
82. Rosenthal S, Rosenthal PA. Koro in an adolescent: Hypochondriasis as a stress response. Adolescent Psychiat. 1982;10:523-31.
83. Price RH. A symposium on the vulnerable male: cultural variations on the castration theme. Transcul Psychiatric Res Rev. 1992;29:87-90.
84. Chowdhury AN. Psychiatric morbidity and the Fox connection. Transcul Psychiatric Res Rev. 1993;30:399-401.
85. Kirmayer LJ. Culture, Affect and Somatization. Part I. Transcul Psychiatric Res Rev. 1984;21:159-88.
86. Kirmayer LJ. Culture, Affect and Somatization. Part II. Transcul Psychiatric Res Rev. 1984; 21: 237-262.
87. Chowdhury AN. Role of medical cognition in psychiatric outbreaks: Study from North Bengal Koro Epidemic. Ind J Behavioural Sc. 1991;1:64-7.
88. Hardwood A. The Hot-Cold theory of disease. J Amer Med Assoc. 1971;216:1153-8.
89. Frazer JG. The Golden Bough: A study in magic and religion. London: Macmillan and Company Limited; 1950. pp. 18, 217, 495, 502.
90. Kapur RL. The role of traditional healers in mental health care in Rural India. Soc Sc Med Anthropol. 1979;13(B1):27-31.
91. Aho WR, Minott K. Cerole and Doctor Medicine: Folk Beliefs, practices, and orientations to modern medicine in a rural and an industrial suburban setting in Trinidad and Tobago, The West Indies. Soc Sc Med. 1977;11:349-55.
92. Currier R. The Hot-Cold Syndrome and symbolic balance in Mexican and Spanish-American folk medicine. Ethnology. 1966;3:251-63.
93. Martinez C, Martin HW. Folk diseases among Mexican-American: Etiology, symptoms, treatment. J Amer Med Assoc. 1966;196:161-4.
94. Abad B, Boyce E. Issues in psychiatric evaluations of Puerto Ricans: A social-cultural perspective. J Operational Psychiat. 1979;10:28-39.

95. Chhabra V, Bhatia MS, Gupta R. Culture bound syndromes in India. Delhi Psychiat. 2008;11(1):15-8.
96. Slot JA. Koro in Central Celebes. Geneeskundig Tijdschrift voor Nederlandsch-Indie. 1935;75:811-20.
97. Zimmer HR. Hindu Medicine. Baltimore: The Johns Hopkins Press; 1948. p. 184.
98. Obeyeskere G. Symbolic food, pregnancy cravings and the envious female. J Psychol. 1985;20:637-62.
99. Bottero A. Consumption by semen loss in India and elsewhere. Cul Med Psychiat. 1991;15303-320.
100. Jilek WG. Epidemic of "Genital Shrinking" (Koro): Historical review and report of a recent outbreak in South China. Curare. 1986;9:269-82.
101. Chowdhury AN. Tortoise: A psycho-anthropological perspective. Eastern Anthropologist. 2003;56 51-9.
102. Demers R, Altamore R, Mustin H, Kleinman A, Leonardi D. An exploration of the death and dimensions of illness behaviour. J Family Pract. 1980;11:1085-92.
103. Hulka BS, Kupper LL, Cassel JC. Departments of physician utilization. Medical Care. 1972;10:300-9.
104. Chrisman N, Kleinman A. Popular health care and lay referral network. In: Mechanic D (Ed.). Handbook of Health, Health Care, and Health Professionals. New York: Free Press; 1983.
105. Kleinman A. Depression, somatization and the "New Cross-cultural" Psychiatry. Soc Sc Med. 1977;11:3-10.
106. Young A. Some Implications of medical beliefs and practices for Social Anthropology. Am Anthropologist. 1976;78:5024-31.
107. Suchman EA. Social patterns of illness and medical care. J Health Hum Behav. 1965;6:2-16.
108. Palthe van PMW. Koro: Eine Merkwurdige Angsthysterie. Internationale Zeitschrift fur Psychoanalyse. 1935;21:249-57.
109. Palthe van PMW. Anauvulling op Het Artikel "Koro", een Eigenaardige Angstneurose. Geneeskundig Tijdschrift voor Nederlandsch-Indie. 1935;75: 836-7.
110. LeBon G. The Crowd. London: F. Unwin; 1895.
111. Freedman, JL. Theories of Contagion as they relate to Mass Psychogenic Illness. In: Colligen MJ, Pennebaker JW, Murphy LR (Eds). Mass Psychogenic Illness. A Social Psychological Analysis. New Jersy: Lawrence Erlbaum Associates Publisher; 1982. pp. 171-82.
112. Kerckhoff AC. A Social Psychological View of Mass Psychogenic Illness. In: Colligen MJ, Pennebaker JW, Murphy LR (Eds). Mass Psychogenic Illness. A Social Psychological Analysis. New Jersey: Lawrence Erlbaum Associates Publisher; 1982. pp.199-216.
113. Tseng WS, Hsu J. Minor psychological disturbances of everyday life. In: Triandis HC, Draguns JG (Eds). Handbook of Cross-cultural Psychology, Psychopathology, Vol VI. Boston: Allyn and Bacon; 1980. pp. 61-98.
114. Colligan MJ, Urtes, MA, Wisseman C, Rosenstell RF, Anania TL. An investigation of apparent Mass Psychogenic Illness in an electronics plant. J Behavioral Med. 1979;5:297-309.

APPENDIX I

SOCIAL RESPONSE PATTERN SCHEDULE

Introduction: Following are a few questions about the recent illness in the region. We are interested to know your opinion about this illness. We expect you to answer honestly the way you feel. There is no response as right or wrong. Your answers will remain confidential, and you can withdraw from answering at any time.

This is voluntary participation, and we thank you for your cooperation and help.

Name/ Serial Number			*Date:*
Age:	*Sex: M/F*	*Marital Status: S/M/W/D/S*	*Religion: H/M/C/O*
Address:			
Ed		*Oc*	*Income Rs/month*

1. *Is it an illness?* Yes/ No.
2. *How serious is the condition?*
   0 = Nil
   1 = Mild
   2 = Moderate
   3 = Severe
3. *What are the risks involved?*
   0 = No danger
   1 = Life and death question
   2 = Loss of sexual power
   3 = Weakness and general health problems
4. *What is the type of illness?* Physical disease/Mental disease/Both
5. *Is it infective?* Yes/No.
6. *What is the chance of infection?*
   1 = Mild
   2 = Moderate
   3 = Severe
   4 = Highly infectious
7. *What is/are the cause of the illness?*
   1 = Not known
   2 = High fever
   3 = Physical exhaustion
   4 = Increased body heat
   5 = Sexual cause
   6 = Supernatural cause
   7 = Mischievousness
   8 = Fearfulness
   9 = Mental cause
8. *What should be the treatment of the condition?*
   1 = Medicinal
   2 = Non-medicinal (Natural treatment)
   3 = 1 + 2
   4 = No treatment
9. *What type of medicine will help?*
   1 = Allopathy
   2 = Homeopathy
   3 = Kabiraji
   4 = Ayurvedic
10. *What type of natural treatment will help?*
    1 = Water pouring
    2 = Pulling out of the penis
    3 = Wearing "*kachu*" leaf scale
    4 = All of the above
11. *Is there any scope of mental treatment?* Yes/No.
12. *How you know about the illness?*
    1 = Eyewitness
    2 = Hearing from others
13. *What is the local name for the illness?*

APPENDIX II

KORO SYMPOSIUM

The author organized a symposium on Koro at the Psychiatry Department of North Bengal Medical College and Hospital, Siliguri, Darjeeling district, on 20–21 December 1986 **(Fig. 1)**. Koro study team, other medical officers, and general practitioners of the region were invited to present their experiences about Koro and the epidemic. Dr Alain Bottero of Salpetriere Hospital, Paris, France, was the special guest in the seminar. Koro's report from other districts (Hooghly and Murshidabad) of the state was also presented **(Figs. 2 to 6)**. There was a field visit in adjoining Tea Estates to meet some *Gunin* and *Jhakri* who treated Koro illness during the epidemic.

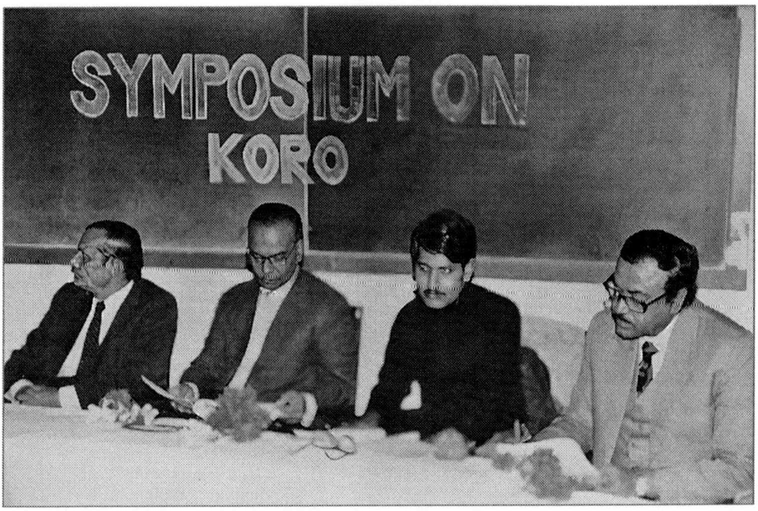

Fig. 1: From left: Professor NC Chowdhury, HOD, Department of Sociology and Social Anthropology, NB University; Professor SM Nandi, HOD, Department of Medicine, NB Medical College and Hospital; Professor SP Banerjee, Principal, NB Medial College Dr A Chakraborty, Administrator-Superintendent, NB Medical College Hospital.

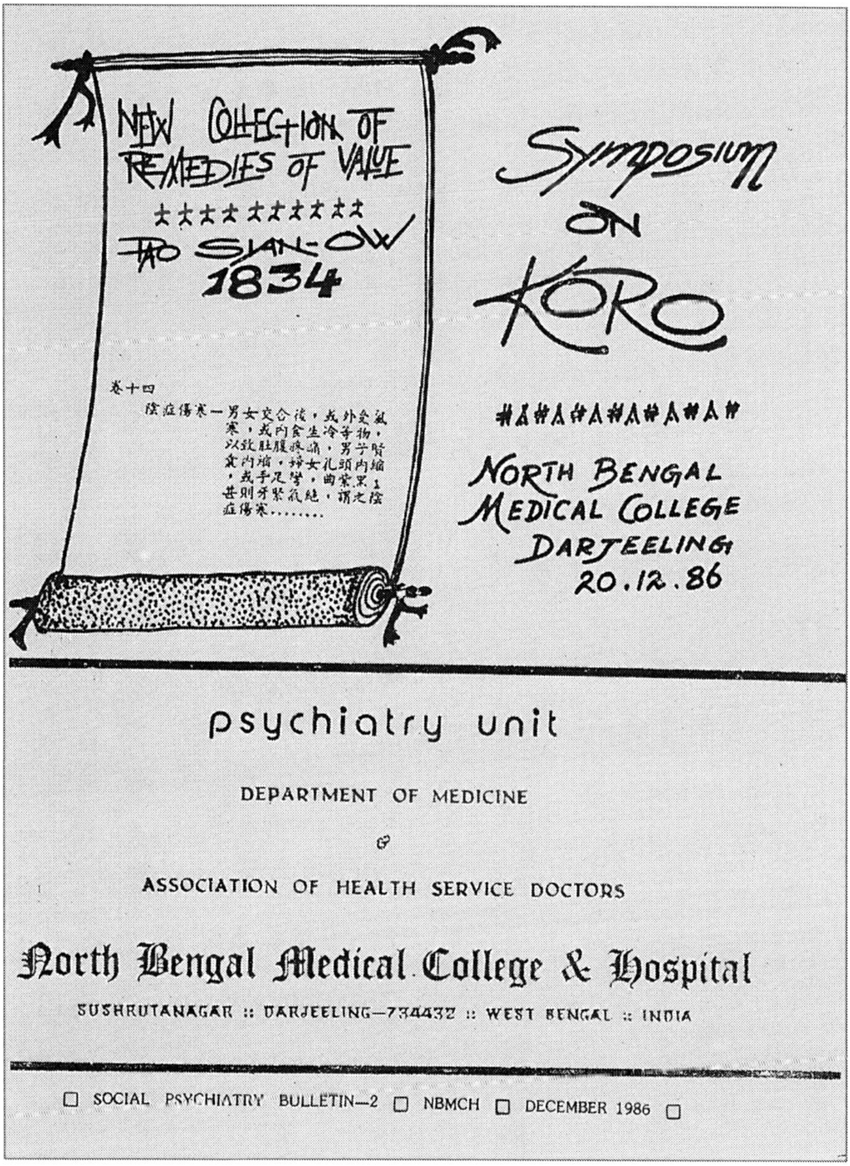

Fig. 2: Cover page of the brochure designed by the author.

PSYCHIATRY UNIT

Department of Medicine

&

Association of Health Service Doctors

NORTH BENGAL MEDICAL COLLEGE & HOSPITAL

SUSHRUTANAGAR, DARJEELING

WEST BENGAL, INDIA

INVITING YOU AT THE

☐ **KORO-SYMPOSIUM**

20th December, 1986 : 9-30 am. — 1-30 pm.

N. B. Medical College & Hospital.

☐ **POST-SYMPOSIUM FIELD VISITS**

- 20th December, 1986 : 2-30 pm. — 6 pm.
  Interview with koro affected persons at
  Gaya Ganga Tea Estate and Nischinta Pore Tea
  Estate of Dirjeeling District.

- 21st December, 1986 : 8-30 am. — 6 pm.
  Interview with Traditional Healers
  ('Gunin' & 'Jhakri') of
  Dudhia at Mirik Hill base of Darjeeling district and
  of Balapara and Mondalghat community of
  Jalpaiguri district

Dr. (Mrs.) S Biswas
Dr. S. P. Banerjee
Joint Convenor

Dr. A. N. Chowdhury
Dr. A. Mukherjee
Joint Orgz. Secretary

Fig. 3: Invitation.

PROGRAMME

Inaugural Session : 9-30 a m.

Note of Introduction	:	**Dr. A. N. Chowdhury**, *Assistant Professor, Psychiatry Unit.*
Welcome Address	:	**Dr. (Mrs) S. Biswas**, *Associate Professor Head, Psychiatry Unit.*
		Dr. S. P. Banerjee, *President, Association of Health Service Doctors, NBMCH.*
Inaugural Address	:	**Professor D. B. Dutta**, *Vice-Chancellor, N. B. University*
Address by Guest-in-Chief	:	**Dr. Alain Rottero**, *Salpetriere Hospital, Paris, France. (Sexual Neurosis in French Culture)*
Address by Guest-in-Honour	:	**Professor N. C. Chowdhury**, *Department of Sociology & Social Anthropology, North Bengal University.*
Presidential Address	:	**Professor S. M. Nandi**, *Head, Department of Medicine.*
Vote of Thanks	:	**Dr. A. Mukherjee**, *General Secretary, Association of Health Service Doctors, NBMCH.*

Coffee Break : 10.30 a.m.

Koro Symposium : 10·40 a.m.

Time & Title of the Paper	Speaker
10-40 am : Koro Outbreak in Siliguri Town : Few Remarks.	**Dr. A. Chatterjee, MD.** *Specialist Physician, S. D. Hospital, Siliguri.*
10-50 am : Koro Epidemic in Jalpaiguri District.	**Dr. S. Das, MD.** *Psychiatrist, District Hospital, Jalpaiguri.*
11 am : Koro Outbreak in Uttarpara Town (Hooghly District)	**Dr. R. Bhattacharya, MD.** *Registrar, Department of Medicine, N. B. Medical College*
11-10 am : Comprehensive study of Koro phenomenon including the ethnohystorical analysis of world Koro with special reference to 1982 North Bengal Koro Epidemic. And presentation of two male Koro Cases.	**Dr. A. N. Chowdhury, MD.** *Assistant Professor, Psychiatry Unit, North Bengal Medical College*
12-20 pm : Psychosexual instability in North Bengal region in relation to emerging socio-economic changes.	**Dr. M. Das Gupta, Ph. D.** *Professor & Head, Department of Economics Nort Bengal University.*
12-40 pm : Koro Epidemic in Murshidabad District : Report from Uttar Mohammodpur and Anupnagar area of Jongipore Subdivision.	**Dr. C. Sarkar, DCH.** *SHMO., Paediatric Unit, North Bengal Medical College*
12-50 pm : Koró in the Hills.	**Dr. B. B. Das Chowdhury, MBBS.** *General Practitioner, Siliguri Town.*

Discussion : 1·00 p.m.

Fig. 4A

KORO OUTBREAK IN SILIGURI TOWN: FEW REMARKS

Dr. Amalendu Chatterjee, MD.
Specialist Physician
Sub-Divisional Hospital, Siliguri
Senior Medical Member of the Koro Study Team.

Koro, a peculiar psychogenic disorder, took place in an epidemic form in the Siliguri Town at the second week of July 1982. The first case was reported (a 18 years boy) at about 2 A.M. at S.D. Hospital while I was on emergency duty. I never saw such cases before, so I immediately called Dr. A.N. Chowdhury (he was staying at S.D. Hospital campus during this time) and he also with his wonder examined the case. With utter surprise, from the following morning Koro cases (locally they called it 'Jhin Jhini') in groups came to the hospital and we were completely puzzeled to entertain all the cases at a time. I think we have seen more than 200 cases at the hospital and in the town but due to our ignorance about the whole phenomena we, I must say, lacked proper clinical evaluation and acceptance of the cases. Dr. Chowdhury with all his vigor and enthusiasm as a young psychiatrist, formed a Koro Study Team in which I was also included, and attempted to study the Koro cases systematically, both in the hospital and in the community. Gradually the news of more Koro cases, almost from all over the North Bengal region is coming to us and Dr. Chowdhury made an excellent attempt to study as much cases as possible with his limited capacity and I know he collected good amount of research data on Koro cases, not only from Siliguri town but also from other districts of North Bengal. He also made a good followup of some of my Koro cases. In fact during those days he was called among us as 'Master of Koro' and he developed a very well knit communicative channel through out this region to catch the Koro cases. I think you all will enjoy some of our Koro research findings, which will be presented by Dr. Chowdhury after a little while.

I will draw your attention regarding few important points which seems me very strange about Koro cases. Firstly most of the cases were single, ill educated, youth & adolescent, and had history of multiple socially forbidden sexual habits. Sexual pathology definetely has a great role to play in the Koro manifestations. Secondly, the patients displayed a bit peculiar behavior, for example they showed no shame or custsey while exhibiting their penis publicly. In fact many of them should no clinical anxiety as such, rather, it seemed to me,

Fig. 4B

they were making ugly jokes with the organ. Many of them also gave false address, so we failed to trace them afterwards. Thirdly, quite a few cases had febrile episode, e. g. malarial fever, viral fever, amoebic hepatitis, chest infections and the like. So what striked us, that physical exhausion may have some relation with penile shortening. Fourthly, community beliefs in traditional treatment rituals of Koro—that posed a dangerous physical threat including death. I think Dr. Chowdhury will present this paper of treatment seeking of Koro's today. At this point, we the physicians must have to take the leading role to accept the cases for treatment. As you probably know, that during the later part of Koro Epidemic, health personnels showed no interest or rather resented to take the responsibility to treat the cases as a genuine illness. Some unfortunate situations also occured in some health clinics and hospitals. I can remember Dr. Chowdhury was also severly criticized by a local physician at Mondal ghat village of Jalpaiguri District and in another occasion all his Koro photograph-negatives was snatched by a group of angry local people near the Chakchaka village of Coochbihar district on the issue that hospitals did not provide any assistance or care to the cases. Anyway, the cases gradually turned to local healers for treatment, many a time with fatal outcome.

With these few words I conclude here and hope that you all will enjoy today the detail Koro reportings to be presented by the other speakers afterwords.

Koro Epidemic in Jalpaiguri District

Dr. Sujit Kumar Das, M.D.
Psychiatrist,
District Hospital, Jalpaiguri.

The emergency Medical Officer of Jalpaiguri Sadar Hospital on the night of 2nd July 1982 received a radiogram message from the Health Department of Writers' Building Calcutta mentioning the breakout of an epidemic of a peculiar deases of Jalpaiguri District.

The EMO being a phychiatric identified it immediately as Koro a culture-bound syndrom previously unknown in Indian sub-continent. The author rushed to Dhupguri, the nucleus of this epidemic.

In the following weeks the author witnessed hundreds of people affected in an epidemic form in the District. The District Health Authority although acknowledged it as purely phychological deases but they did not consult any mental health personnel.

The cause of this cultural-bound syndrom is an epidemic form could be due to synergistic action of prevalent cultural beliefs (mythis) about sex and a fear about the encephalitis epidemic during this period in this area. In author's opinion investigations and research about the epidemic as a whole and not isolated case detection, is more important.

Koro Outbreak in Uttarpara (Hooghly) Town.

Dr. Ratneswar Bhattacharya, M.D.
Registrar,
Department of Medicine.
North Bengal Medical College & Hospitals.

In the third week of November 1982 there was a sudden outbreak of Koro in Uttarpara area of Hooghly District of West Bengal. Eleven Koro affected cases (10 male and one female) were seen by the author during his posting as a Physician in Uttarpara General Hospital. The different aspects of the Koro clinical profile was discussed.

Fig. 4C

Koro Epidemic in Murshedabad District :

Report from Uttar Mohammodpore and Anupnagar block Jongipore Subdivision.

Dr. Chirabikash Sarkar, DCH.
SHMO, Paediatric Unit,
Department of Medicine,
North Bengal Medical College & Hospital.

A total of 21 Koro cases (19 male and 2 female) were seen by the author during his posting as Medical Officer in Uttar Mohammodpure SHC of Jongipore subdivision of Murshedabad district. The different aspects of mass-behavioral profile around Koro onset and commonly used traditional healing rituals including penile and breast tie with ropes, are discussed. The placebo effect of injections other than diazepam in Koro remission is also discussed. The total Koro atmosphere of this region including the adjoining Anup Nagar Primary Health Centre area is also discussed.

Koro in the Hills.

Dr. Bidyut Baran Das Chowdhury, M.B.B.S.
General Practitioner,
Siliguri Town
Medical member of Koro Study Team.

The different clinico-social aspects of Koro cases of the hills e.g. Sonada, Mirik, Kurseong and Darjeeling area of Darjeeling district is discussed. The miraculous Koro escape of tebeto-buddhist ethnicity is also discussed.

Fig. 4D

Figs. 4A to D: Some transcripts from the Brochure.

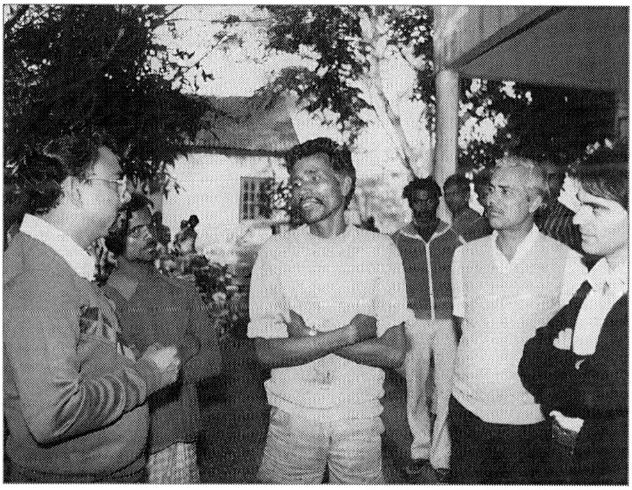

Fig. 5: Dr Alain Bottero of Salpetriere Hospital, Paris, (right) and the author at Gaya-Ganga Tea Estate, discussing with a Traditional healer (Jhakri) who treated many Koro cases in Tea Gardens of Siliguri.

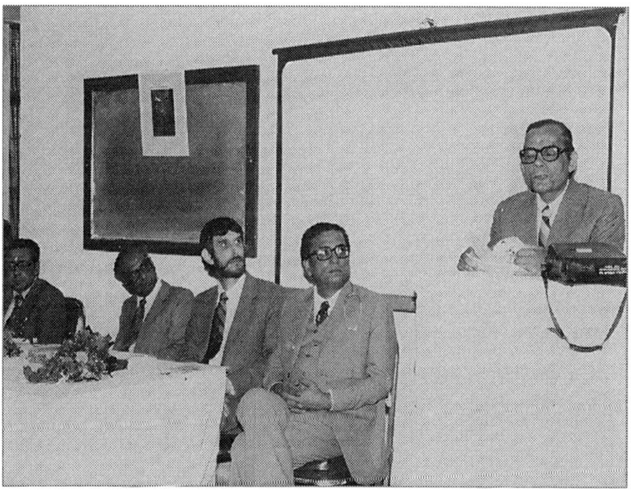

Fig. 6: Professor NC Chowdhury, Head, Department of Social Anthropology, North Bengal University, delivered his experience on the Koro epidemic in the region at the Social Psychiatry Seminar, 1984. From right to left: Professor M Sen (HOD Medicine), Dr MG Weiss, Professor DB Dutta, Vice-Chancellor NBU, and Professor DN Bhaduri, Principal, NBMCH and the author.

APPENDIX III: ABSTRACT OF PUBLISHED STUDIES OF 1982 KORO EPIDEMIC

1. S Chakraborty, S Das, A Mukherjee: Koro Makes an Epidemic Appearance in India

Transcultural Newsletter, 1982, III, 3-4 December

It is an abstracted review of the Koro epidemic of Northeastern India. It provides a brief account of the epidemic scenario with evidence of extreme panic created in this region. They provided a typical scenario as follows: "Parents who were convinced their sons" penises were shrinking had tied string thread to the foreskin and secured it to another thread tied around the waist. As a result, ulcers formed on the foreskin. In the hilly Darjeeling district, doctors had to measure boys penises at intervals to show parents there was no shrinkage.

The authors suggest that mass fear and panic may relate to the previous "mysterious disease" epidemic involving death in this region, which turned out to be cerebral malaria. Koro was termed "Kattao" in some districts, meaning "cut off."

2. DN Nandi, G Banerjee, H Saha, GC Boral: Epidemic Koro in West Bengal, India

International Journal of Social Psychiatry, 1983; 29(4): 265-268

This is a brief report of the West Bengal Koro epidemic with three case reports from rural areas. The first case was a single Hindu male (19-year-old) resident of a village on the outskirts of Kolkata. After hearing a discussion on Koro illness, while traveling on a train, he developed the disease on returning home. The second case (18-year-old) single Muslim female of Beldanga, Murshidabad district, developed Koro breast symptoms (shrinkage of the breast followed by burning and trembling) during an attempt to see some male Koro cases of her village on that day. The third one, a Hindu unmarried female (16-year-old) from a village of Howrah district, developed breast symptoms. She had a history of anxiety neurosis a year back. The authors suggested that Koro is an acute anxiety reaction where suggestion plays a key role.

3. A Chakraborty: An Epidemic of Koro in West Bengal, India

Indian Journal of Psychiatry, 1983; 25: 138-139

It is a brief report of the West Bengal Koro epidemic, with a special mention of the North Bengal region. The author traced the epidemic wave from the adjoining part of Assam to the North Bengal region of West Bengal state and further spread to South Bengal. She reported a case of Koro in a young boy with a frank psychotic attack. During the epidemic, she mentioned different local syntaxes to name Koro, e.g., Kattao in North Bengal, Jhin-Jhini in lower

Bengal, and Disco in Calcutta. She attempts to explain North Bengal epidemic in terms of social stress, the existing tension between local inhabitants and immigrant refugees from Bangladesh. Koro's dramatic presentation and associated traditional healing rituals (cold water pouring), including prevention with lime paste marking and wearing black arum slices, have been reported.

4. DN Nandi, G Banerjee, S Bera, S Nandi: Mode of Spread of Epidemic Koro in a Village of West Bengal, India

Indian Journal of Psychiatry, 1984; 26: 331-334

This is a report of the 1982 West Bengal Koro epidemic in December in South Bengal. The authors provided an excellent psychoanalytical study of mass response to illness rumors in a village in Malda district. The five reported cases (age range was 18–22 years): Three unmarried men and two married women. Both the female cases had a history of hysterical attack, and one male patient had a concurrent affective disorder. In the last portion, the authors gave an upbeat picture of the 1982 Darjeeling epidemic through a narrative of a local doctor.

It describes a case (index) of a businessman of a village of Malda district, who acted as the critical messenger of the illness news. He dissipated this information among the villagers on his way back home. He first discussed the news of this terrifying penis disease in a shop where four persons fall victim to Koro instantaneously in a chain reaction. Some panicky customers carried this news into a nearby village where, upon hearing from them, two married women were struck by the sickness. The businessman's younger brother underwent a Koro attack when the family listened to the man's news of this dangerous and highly infectious disease. This is an excellent account of social contagion where a terrified businessman terrorized others and helped spread the illness in the community. This example illustrates the dynamics of group psychology in disseminating rumors by the process of ego identification among people with suggestible personalities. They describe a unique incident of mass fear where a group of people came with their little sons, whose penises were tightly tied with rope. The fathers, not the sons, made the complaint of penile shrinkage. The authors thus commented: "Psychologically the fathers were the real victims of the epidemic. But the symptoms were not centered on their own organs (i.e., mutilation of the self). It spilled over the organs of those whom they hold as dear as the self" (p. 333).

Note: A list of 53 Koro and related research publications including North Bengal Koro epidemic by Dr AN Chowdhury and colleagues is referenced in Chapter 5 (page 93–140) in the book written by the Editor, 'Koro: Clinical and Historical Developments of the Culturally Defied Genital Retraction Disorder' Palgrave Macmillan, 2021.

Chapter 3

Mini-Koro Epidemic in South 24 Parganas, 1993

Arabinda N Chowdhury

There was a mini-Koro epidemic in the South 24 Parganas district of West Bengal, India, in 1993 (June 23 to July 8), involving 11 male persons (9 single and two married) in two hamlets of a village called Taldi, located in South 24 Parganas district, West Bengal. The index case discussed here is a young boy aged 14 years, who heard something about this "penis illness" in his school from a neighboring town, Canning; a few cases had already occurred, and people were terrified of losing their male organs. People also saw a few cases that happened on the Canning railway station platform in the broad daylight. They were primarily young persons. The same evening that 14-year-old boy had the Koro attack. The following week others were affected in a chain reaction. The clinical presentation was typical: Anxious preoccupation and fear about this disease were followed by a feeling of retraction of the penis (no scrotum) for a few minutes and then extreme exhaustion. Some

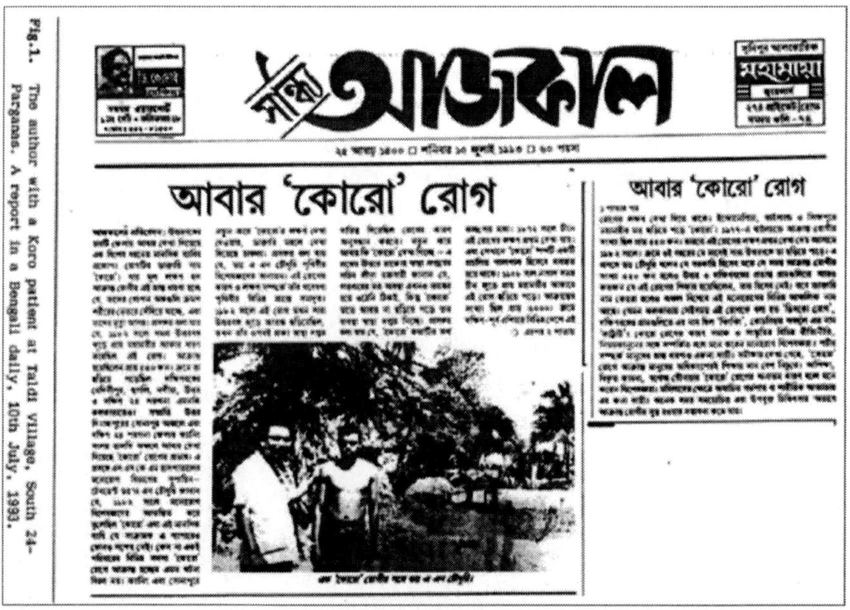
আজকাল
আবার 'কোরো' রোগ
আবার 'কোরো' রোগ
Fig.1. The author with a Koro patient at Taldi village, South 24-Parganas. A report in a Bengali daily, 10th July, 1993.

Fig. 1: Reporting of new Koro (Koro illness again) cases in West Bengal, in a Bengali Newspaper "EVENING AJKAL" (July 1993).

relatives and friends helped in manual traction of the penis (in three cases). The local "quack" (Mr Z) successfully treated two males by giving vitamin B_6 IM injection. Locally, they called it "virus illness." A few months ago, these villages experienced a bird flu epidemic, and many poultry birds were sacrificed. The author discussed with a group of villagers and the local "quack doctor" (Mr Z), who took the author to the houses of the affected persons. The author interviewed the index case and seven affected people who were available at that time. They looked anxious and fearful. The index case had the Koro attack in the morning on his way to school. The school was closed after the news reached there. Five cases (age range 18–27 years) the Koro attack in the evening (around 6–8 PM). Two patients had their attack in midnoon while working in the vegetable garden. All the victims consulted a local priest afterward and wore chanted red cotton threads around their wrists. They believe that these chanted threads offer protection from further attack or influence of any evil eye. There is a belief that someone with a mal-intent might cast a spell on some victims' families. No female was affected, and no further incidents were reported. The State Health Department entrusted the author to visit this area for the investigation. This mini epidemic was self-contained within these two village hamlets only. This news appeared in a local newspaper **(Fig. 1)**.

Chapter 4

Koro Epidemic in West Bengal, 2010

Amitava Dan, Debjit Misra

ABSTRACT

Koro is an enigmatic culture-bound or culture-related syndrome predominantly reported from Southeast Asia. Since the 18th century, several epidemics of Koro were reported in the literature from various parts of the Asia-Pacific region. In the last few decades, several states of India, including West Bengal, Assam, Tripura, and Orissa, repeatedly became the target of this sociocultural malady. One such recent epidemic of Koro hit West Bengal at the end of 2010. Initially, it was distributed predominantly in the North Bengal districts of West Bengal, districts of South and North 24 Parganas, and rural Assam. From November 2011, the epidemic unfolded in the districts of South Bengal, which was a relatively and reportedly low-prevalence zone for Koro to date. In the next few months, many cases started appearing in different hospitals with symptoms of Koro with associated physical and psychological complications. The epidemic prevailed for the next 1 year with its massive toll of morbidity in the southern part of West Bengal. This article focused on the clinical profile of Koro reported from the South Bengal part of the epidemic.

From a tertiary care Government Hospital of South Bengal, data was collected from consecutive 64 consenting patients with Koro, reported in different disciplines of the hospital for 3-month period during the epidemic. All of them were managed by standard treatment protocol and followed up for the next 3 months. Majority of the proportions of the subjects were young (mean age 17.28 years), single (81%), male (77%), educated up to primary standard (42%), agricultural workers (42%) by occupation, and belonging to Hindu (58%) rural (88%) joint (53%) family. The female proportion (23%) was also significant. Most of them were reported first at nonpsychiatric OPDs. A substantial proportion of the subjects had comorbid psychiatric (41%) and physical (23%) illnesses. Among psychiatric comorbidities, sexual dysfunctions comprised significant percentages, especially in males. One-fifth of all the patients needed indoor admission; the rest were managed at OPD. They were managed by oral anxiolytics (75%), injectable tranquilizers (9%), and other psychosocial interventions (31%). On a small proportion (12%) of patients, a new modality of psychosexual intervention, "sex education in vivo" was applied with a favorable response. Supportive medical or surgical treatment was needed for associated medical and surgical complications in 19% of subjects. Though more than one-fourth (28%) of the patients dropped out from follow-up, the rest noted a good treatment outcome.

PREAMBLE

Koro is a psycho-socio-cultural phenomenon described in the literature as an episode of sudden and intense anxiety that the penis (or, in females, the vulva and the nipples) will recede into the body, possibly causing death.[1] In Southeast Asia, people reported this illness predominantly in an epidemic form. Since the 18th century, several such epidemics of Koro have been reported in the literature from various parts of the Asia-Pacific region. As a part of Southeast Asia, in India, most of the koro epidemics were reported from West Bengal[2-9] and surrounding states of Northeast India,[10] e.g., Assam,[11,12] Tripura.[13] In the last three decades, several districts of West Bengal often became the target of this sociocultural malady, where Koro became almost pandemic.

River Ganges carries an important sociocultural significance in India, including West Bengal. West Bengal is broadly divided by the river Ganges into North Bengal and South Bengal parts. In the last few decades, there has been a higher trend of frequent migration among the people for their occupational, residential, and other purposes. A significant proportion of the population is from the districts of North Bengal (i.e., districts of Darjeeling, Jalpaiguri, Cooch Behar, Uttar, and Dakshin Dinajpur, Malda), and sections of South and North 24 Parganas immigrate people. Socioeconomic and geographical adversities are more frequent in these regions than in South Bengal part (i.e., districts of Purva and Paschim Medinipur, Bankura, Bardhaman, Birbhum, Nadia, and the capital city of the state, Kolkata) **(Fig. 1)**. Despite significant differences in socioeconomic and geographical adversities in their lives, after the state's advancement in conveyance, people from these two parts (North vs. South Bengal) started mixing up in many important social, religious, and national festivals year. They also share common media services (both social and news media) in their vernacular language **(Fig. 1)**.

With this sociocultural background, we want to narrate the Koro epidemic experienced by West Bengal, which started in October 2010. Index incident was reported from the state of Maharashtra in migrant laborers, who originally belonged to West Bengal, Assam, Orissa, etc. At the end of October 2010, both social media and electronic/print media covered the story with vivid case descriptions.[14,15] At that time, a large proportion of the migratory laborers went to their native states on festival leave. In the next few weeks, a vast surge of Koro cases was reported from the North-Bengal districts of West Bengal, the district of South and North 24 Parganas, and rural Assam. From November 2011, the epidemic extended to the districts of South Bengal, where no major

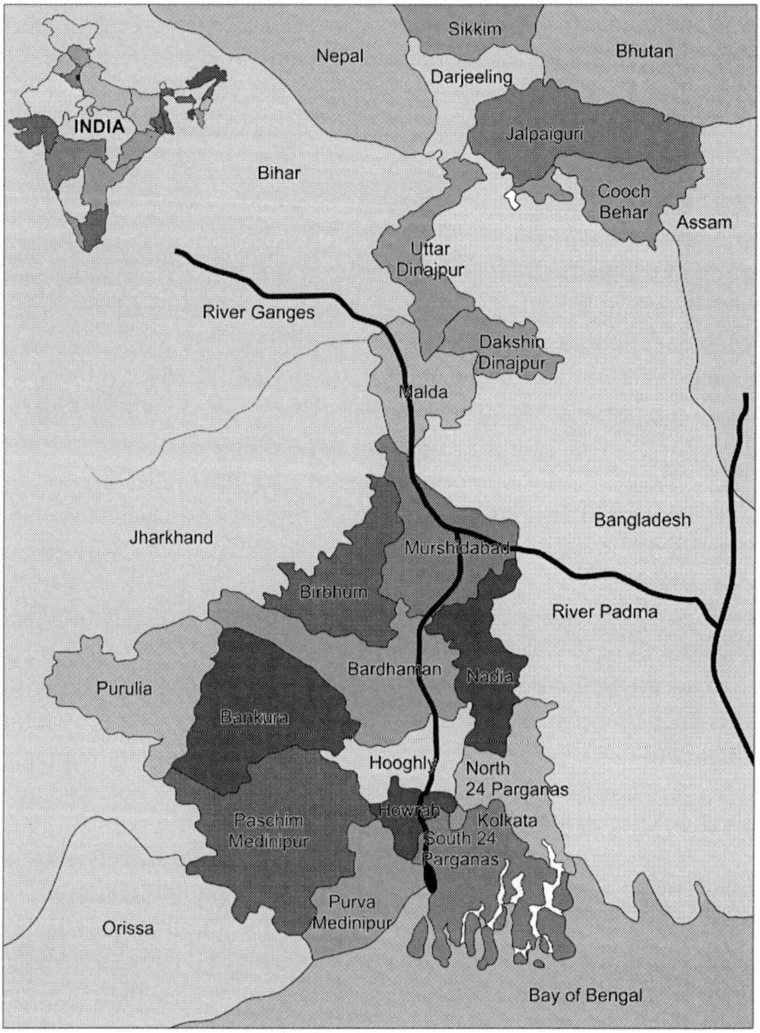

Fig. 1: West Bengal map (not to scale).

Koro epidemic has been reported to date. The epidemic trampled on almost the whole of West Bengal for the next year with its massive medical and social impact. In the entire rural West Bengal and part of the urban population, especially in the slum areas, vulnerable individuals were perturbed by the fear of being victimized by this terrible disease.

Most of the subjects had an abrupt onset of panic anxiety state, and various nonspecific somatic symptoms involving multiple parts of the body with a sense of retraction of the penis (for male) or vulva or breast (for female). General people called the illness locally "Disco Roge."[2-6] In the North Bengal region, in the initially reported epidemics of Koro, the disease was locally named "Kattao"[2] and in Assam as "Jhinjhini Bemar"[2,10,12] which indicates a disease characterized by a tingling sensation of the body. But in recent years, people of West Bengal, especially in the south Bengal part, know the disease as "Disco Roge." Locally, the term "Disco" refers to "New Fashion," and "Roge" means "disease."[3] Similarly, people of other Southeast Asian regions identified the Koro syndrome by different indigenous names according to their cultural concept of the genesis of the disease. In China, it was named "suoyang," in Cantonese as "suk-yeong,"[16] in Thai "rook-joo,"[17] etc.

In western literature, the term "koro" and the syndrome was first introduced by JC Blonk[18] as a disorder indigenous to southern Sulawesi. After that, a few case reports and psychoanalytical descriptions of koro came into the literature. Later, Koro was included in DSM-IV [(Diagnostic and Statistical Manual of Mental Disorders (fourth edition)][19] and DSM-IV-TR [Diagnostic and Statistical Manual of Mental Disorders (fourth edition), text revision][20] in Appendix I and described as "an episode of sudden and intense anxiety that the penis (or, in females, the vulva and the nipples) will recede into the body and possibly cause death." In DSM-5 (Diagnostic and Statistical Manual of Mental Disorders, Fifth Edition),[21] the term "Culture-Bound Syndromes" was changed to "Cultural Concepts of Distress," and Koro was mentioned in "Other Specified Obsessive-Compulsive and Related Disorder (300.3)" as a specifier of the phenomenon.[21] In ICD-10 (International Classification of Diseases, 10th revision),[22] Koro was described in the block of "Neurotic, stress-related and somatoform disorders" under the heading of "Other specified neurotic disorders (F48.8)."

Interestingly, these cases often appeared in clusters in a community in the form of a "mini-epidemic," and the whole epidemic resulted from several such "mini-epidemics." In a large community, the members of that specific microsociety (the portion of a society where some people were closer to each other for their social-cultural, geographical, and occupational connections) were more vulnerable during that "mini-epidemic" which terminated after a few days or weeks. Multiple such "mini-epidemics" occurred in West Bengal in almost 1-year period. Recurrences of symptoms of Koro were also observed at individual or community levels. Sometimes the index cases for these "mini-epidemics" could be traced, sometimes not. The trigger factors for the index cases mainly were social rumor and sensational news by media in the background of psychosocial and sexual vulnerability. Social and print/electronic media had an essential role in disseminating the community's waves of rumor and panics by spreading sensational messages and information, especially in their vernacular languages.[13,23-25] Terrified by panic, most of the people tried to seek help either to get relief from the symptoms or to prevent the deadly symptoms. Many of them were guided by community healers to adopt some form of indigenous treatment. Some of them attended local practitioners or quacks at the primary care level. Those they could not manage were referred to the nearest hospital or qualified specialist doctors.

A few patients and their family members also came to them directly on their own. Though most hospitals received many cases during the epidemic, only a tiny percentage of patients in the whole community could attend hospitals. This indicates the massive magnitude of the epidemic.

CURRENT STUDY

The current study was conducted at Nil Ratan Sircar Medical College, Kolkata, a tertiary care government medical college situated in the South Bengal part of West Bengal. The study was conducted by a multidisciplinary team that comprised the department of emergency, psychiatry, internal medicine, gynecology, uro surgery, etc., for 3 months, during the index epidemic.

Methodology

The department of psychiatry, in liaison with other related disciplines of the tertiary care hospital, had conducted the current study. This research was an institution-based study. Patients with symptoms of Koro and its different medical or surgical complications who attended the department of emergency, psychiatry, internal medicine, gynecology, uro surgery, etc., underwent a detailed psychiatric evaluation by a psychiatric team. Data were collected from consecutive 64 consenting patients with Koro, reported in the hospital for 3 months during the epidemic period. They were treated by standard psychiatric management and followed up for the next 3 months. All the data was collected from the patients and their family members who attended the hospital. Data was also collected from them in a narrative form regarding their understanding and perception and other persons' beliefs prevailing in the community about the illness, pattern, mode of spread of the epidemic, community response to the disease or epidemic, etc. Part of this research work was published previously as original research papers.[5,6] We have put these data together as a book chapter in this article.

Instruments Used

A self-structured proforma was used for getting data on sociodemographic profile, psychiatric and physical comorbidities, the pattern of treatment-seeking behaviors, and various modes and methods of treatment, etc. The ICD-10 was used to diagnose comorbid psychiatric illness.

Significant Observations from the Current Study

General Demography

The majority of the subjects were single (81%), male (77%), with a mean age of 17.28 years (SD 7.92) **(Fig. 2)**, educated up to the primary level (42%), agriculture workers (42%) by occupation, belonging to rural (88%) Hindu

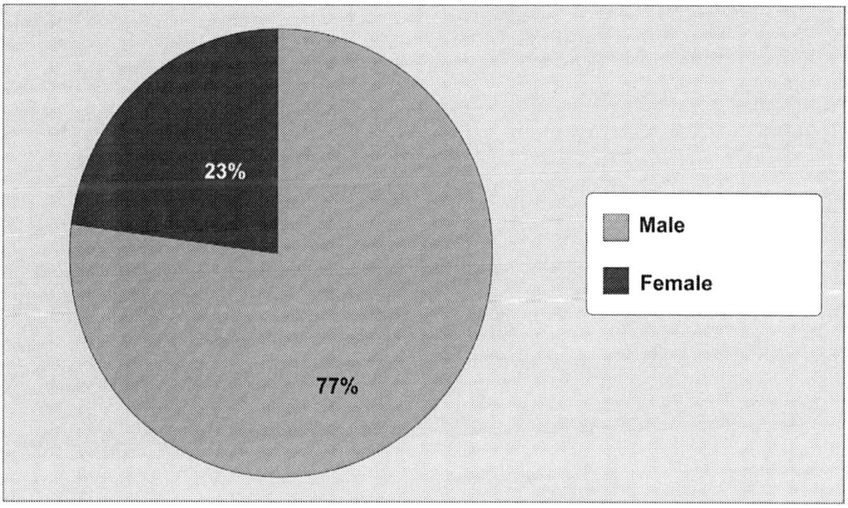

Fig. 2: Gender distribution of the sample.

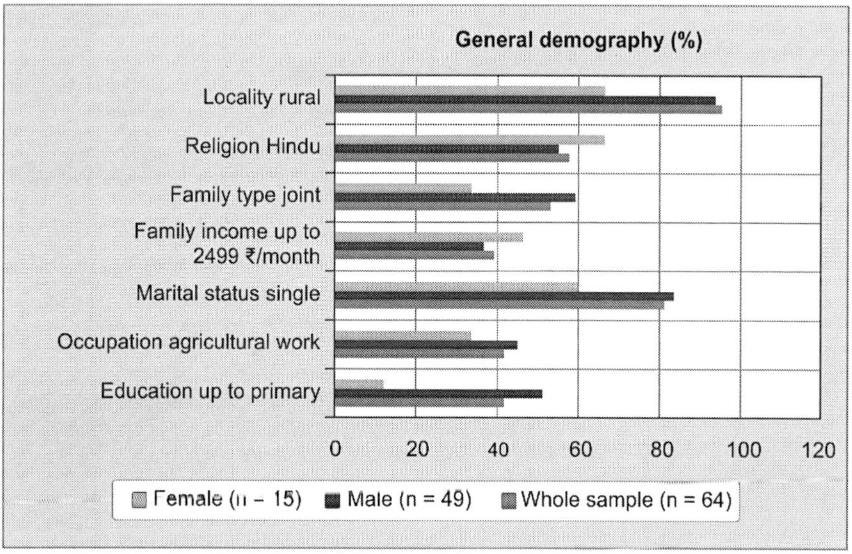

Fig. 3: Socio-demographic distribution of the sample.

(58%) joint (53%) families **(Fig. 3)**. A significant proportion of the whole study population was female (23%) **(Fig. 4)** and Muslim (39%).

Referral Pattern

A majority of patients were referred by private doctors or private hospitals (30%), other government hospitals (17%), local quacks (15.62%), community healers (13%), Homeopathy or Ayurvedic or Unani doctors (3%), schools or NGOs (2%), etc. Among the whole study population, about 11% of cases were

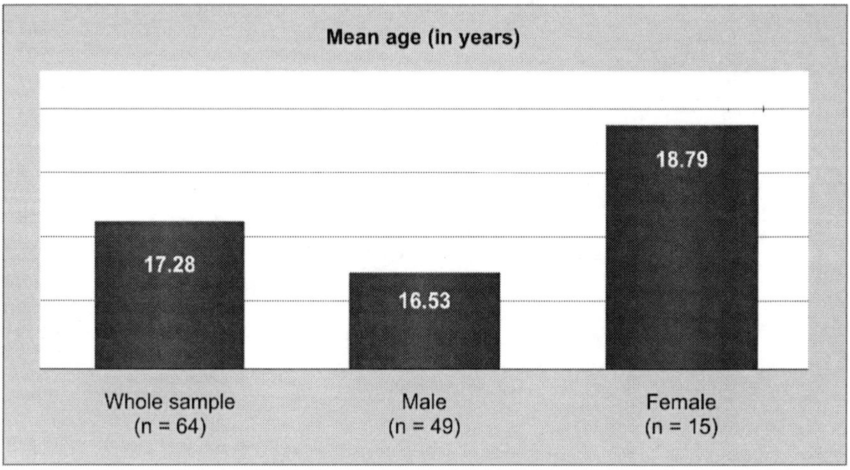

Fig. 4: Age distribution of the sample.

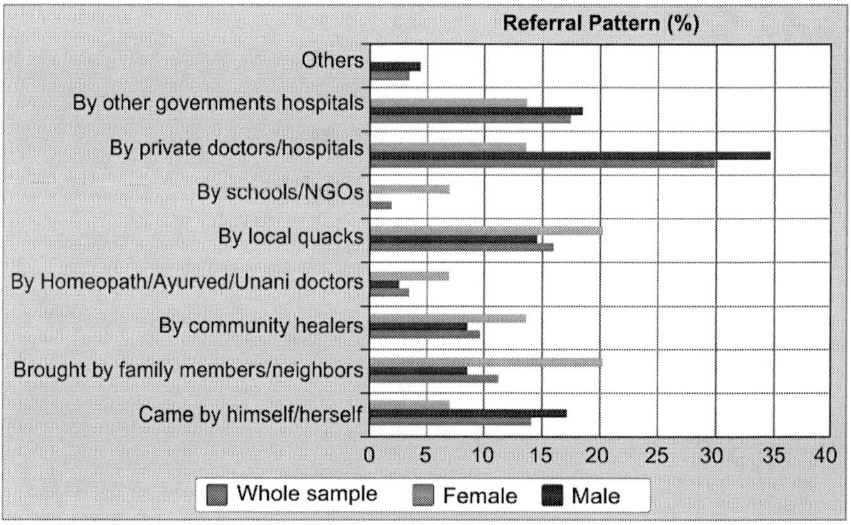

Fig. 5: Referral pattern.

brought by family members or neighbors, and only 9% came by themselves **(Fig. 5)**.

It is apparent from the above observation that a good proportion of patients in the study population sought treatment from professional medical personnel and ultimately reached up to the tertiary care hospitals of the state through the referral chain. This indicates a better health-related awareness and treatment-seeking pattern among the patients and their family members for this illness. A better economic status, availability of healthcare resources, and people's trend to utilize them in this geographical area (i.e., South Bengal) made it possible to reduce the magnitude of the treatment gap.

First Reporting at the Hospital

About 60% of the population reported first in hospital emergency, 20% at the medical or surgical OPD, and 11% at urology or gynecology OPD. While a majority of male patients reported first at emergency OPD (69.39%), the female patients (40%) reported first at the medical or surgical OPD of the hospital **(Fig. 6)**. Only a small percentage (11%) of cases directly came to the psychiatry outpatient department.

People's acceptance of psychiatric illness remains a social taboo in our society. Moreover, the apparent symptoms of Koro mimic many physical symptoms or diseases. As a result, the understanding of general people about the perceived cause of Koro and its way-out remedies are grossly misdirected. So, it is very much explainable why people with symptoms of Koro, rushed to either emergency or medical/surgical/gynecological units of the hospital rather than psychiatric unit.

Community Response to the Epidemic and any Social Treatments/Rituals done in the Community

The way people identify an illness and the style they perceive the distress from their sociocultural milieu is one of the major determinants in shaping the contour of their help-seeking behaviors. Based on the prevailing cultural concept of the physical and sexual potential of the individual, various types of indigenous and folk methods were practiced by community healers to get relief from the symptoms of Koro.[26,27] Susceptible individuals became terrified

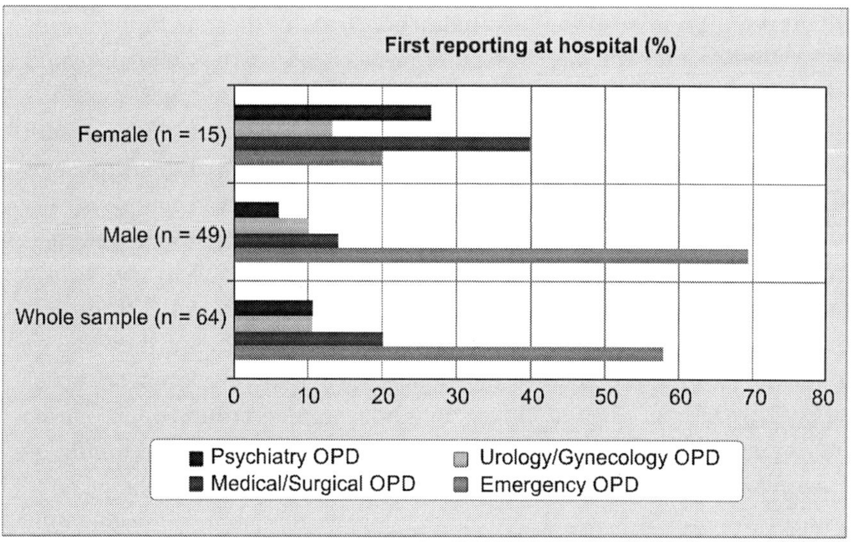

Fig. 6: First reporting at hospital.

by the widely prevailing waves of rumors, suggestions, and motives.[3] They tried to catch at a straw in drowning by obeying the rituals blindly advised by the community healers. As a part of EMIC model, several ethnomedical explanatory concepts had emerged in the mind of community people as an important causative factor for the occurrence of Koro. For example, society considered increased body heat a primary cause of this disorder.[28] Based on this concept, "water therapy"[4-6] became a commonly practiced intervention advised by the community healers and accepted by common people. In this method, victims were advised to be drowned in the cold water of a pond or well, covering their affected body parts for several hours, not even considering the other physical and detrimental psychological sides of this method. Other measures such as pouring cold water or ice taking, "cold drinks" such as sugar water and medicinal water, prescribed by community healers or obtained from places of worship, were taken to reduce excessive body heat.[4,6,28] Supplementary modes were also practiced by manipulation of the penis or breast with some ligature or by manual ways to prevent the retraction. Several other rituals were adopted as prophylactic measures, e.g., wearing chanted "dhaga," which was a single or bunch of cotton thread(s), usually red in color, to wear on the upper arm, wrist, or around the waist, usually chanted with mantras by a priest or herbal amulets around the penis or on the arm, smearing of lime over forehead, neck, ear, etc.[4,6,13,29]

More than 90% of patients reported receiving some home remedies for Koro in the study population. Among them, the most widely (44%) adopted and deleterious mode of treatment was reported to be an application of ligature around the genitalia. Adopting this method often led to surgical complications, e.g., infective and gangrenous changes in genitalia. Several patients were brought to the hospital primarily with these complications. Another detrimental way was "water therapy," i.e., to keep the victim drowned in the cold water of a pond or a well covering the genitalia or breast for hours together, even on winter nights. About 6% of subjects had practiced this deadly method on several occasions among the whole study population. Almost all of them developed severe pneumonia or other related medical complications and attended hospitals with these complications. Among female patients, manual manipulation of the breast by the patient herself or the family members was a common (11%) method to prevent its retraction. For young females, though the procedure was very embarrassing socially, they had to adopt it in an extremely anxious state. Smearing of lime over forehead, neck, ear (41%), wearing of chanted "dhaga" or herbal amulets around penis or arm (30%), application of herbal massage oil (22%) were other popular modes of preventive and curative methods people practiced. A small percentage (6%) of patients reportedly showed some faith in the modern medical system and came directly to the hospital without trying any indigenous method **(Fig. 7)**.

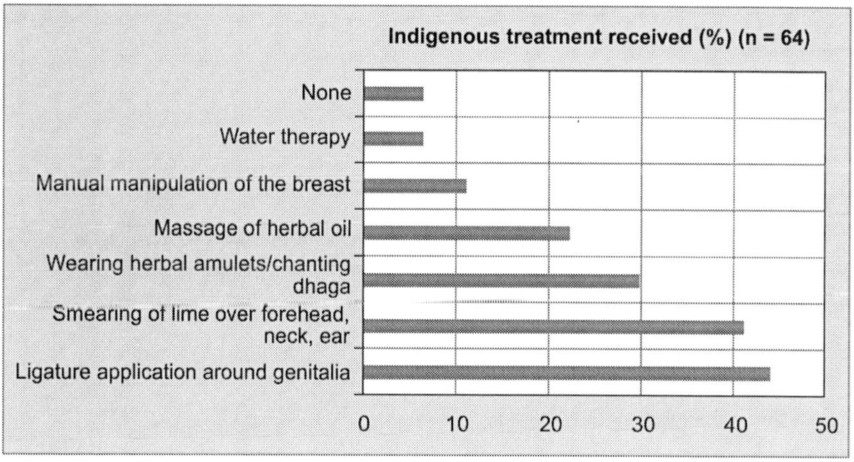

Fig. 7: Indigenous treatment received.

Comorbidities

Comorbid psychiatric illnesses: 47% of patients have a comorbid psychiatric illness among the study population. In the male population, 41% (20 out of 49) and 60% (9 out of 15) had comorbid psychiatric illnesses in females. 12% of males and 20% of females had sexual dysfunctions as psychiatric comorbidities. Among the males, 6% had premature ejaculation, 4% had erectile dysfunction, and 2% had decreased libido. Dhat syndrome was observed among 8% of male individuals. Decreased libido was present in 13% of females **(Fig. 8)**. Among the whole population, other psychiatric comorbidities were alcohol dependence syndrome (5%), major depressive disorder (3%), obsessive compulsive disorder (2%), generalized anxiety disorder (2%), agoraphobia (2%), social phobia (2%), somatoform disorder (2%), harmful use of Cannabis (2%), etc. One female patient had attempted suicide once during Koro symptoms **(Fig. 9)**.

Different types of anxiety disorders were expressed as important psychiatric comorbidity with Koro. The literature observed significantly in the research that Koro patients had a higher level of trait anxiety than the usual subjects.[30] This factor might expose their vulnerability to Koro during an epidemic. We also observed different types of sexual dysfunctions as significant psychiatric comorbidity among Koro victims. How can it be explained? A community's cultural values can strongly and intricately influence the concept of sexuality of that community. Culture even defines what is normal, what is deviant, how much it is deviant, and from where help can be sought.[31] On the other hand, the genesis of this culture-bound syndrome can be explained by individual proneness to Koro, in the background of community vulnerability. Psychodynamic conflicts, especially with sexual content, were identified as important predisposing factors for

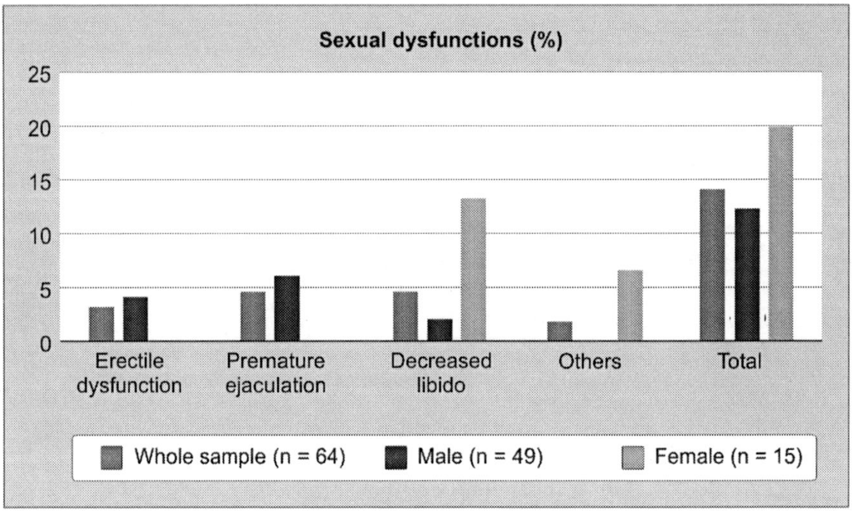

Fig. 8: Sexual dysfunctions

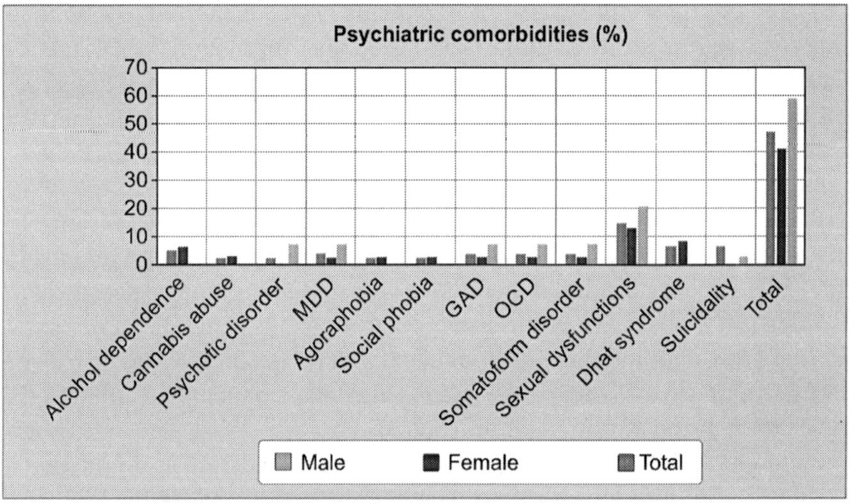

Fig. 9: Comorbid psychiatric illnesses. (GAD: generalized anxiety disorder; MDD: major depressive disorder; OCD: obsessive-compulsive disorder)

the genesis of Koro.[17,32-37] Significant masturbatory guilt, apprehension for actual or anticipatory sexual inadequacy, individual aberrant perception of genital organ image, and related psychological elaboration were considered to have substantial pathogenic and pathoplastic effects on the genesis of Koro psychopathology.[38-42] So, the sociocultural milieu of an individual plays a typical role in the occurrence of both Koro psychopathology and the pattern of sexual dysfunctions. The use of substances (e.g., alcohol, cannabis, heroin, amphetamine) and their withdrawal states was shown in the literature to be closely associated with the occurrence of Koro.[43-51] A small percentage of the current study sample also had alcohol dependence syndrome and harmful use of Cannabis.

Comorbid physical illnesses: A significant proportion (23%) of patients had comorbid physical illnesses **(Fig. 10)**. Those were either preexisting or appeared as complications of various indigenous methods of treatment for Koro. In males, 22% (11 out 49) and females, 33% (5 out of 15) had comorbid physical illnesses. Among them, genitourinary or breast symptoms comprised the major share. Of 14% of males and 27% of females had some form of recent or past genitourinary or breast symptoms before the onset of current Koro symptoms. Different genitourinary symptoms were also reported in the literature as comorbid physical illnesses associated with Koro, e.g., venereal diseases,[52-54] scrotal filarial,[55] genital pain,[53,56] infertility,[57] etc.

From the major epidemics of Koro reported worldwide a homogeneity in the phenomenology and demographic pattern was observed in the literature.[4-6,9,12,28,39] From literature, we have a prototypical impression in our mind about the presentation of a case of Koro is "an young unmarried poorly educated male subject from the lower socioeconomic status of rural background, either unemployed or engaged in nonprofessional occupation" manifested with an abrupt onset and short-lasting symptoms. In the current study, the phenomenology and demography of the majority of subjects were going similar to the literature. Only one exception was that a significant proportion (23%) of the study sample was female. This vital contradiction in gender distribution became a rule rather than the exception in several recent epidemics, especially were reported in West Bengal and surrounding states.[4-6,9,10,12,28,58-60] This replicability in the observation among the studies,

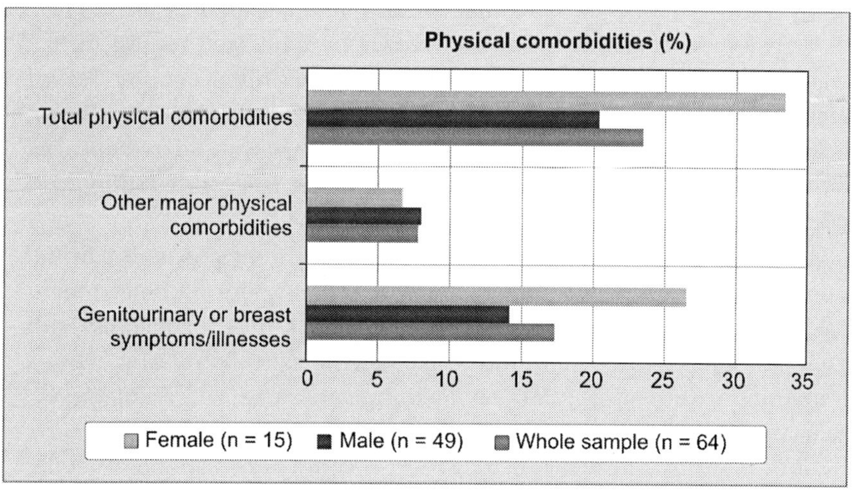

Fig. 10: Comorbid physical illnesses.

even from populations with different geographical and cultural regions, validates the construct's stability of the "Cultural" or "Epidemic" or "Classical" form of Koro.

Conversely, the mode of presentation of the sporadic and chronic cases of Koro is phenomenologically scattered and somewhat atypical. They were reported worldwide and not restricted to any specific geographical or cultural region and were often associated with one or more mental or physical comorbidities.[33,61-68] In the literature, these cases were diversely described as "Atypical Koro" or "Secondary Koro" or "Koro Like Symptom/Syndrome" (KLS), Chronic Koro, etc.[69-71] Although these converse findings are not very stable in the literature, researchers got the strength to raise the debate against the nosological position of Koro as a culture-related syndrome.

Treatment received in this hospital: All patients were managed with standard treatment guidelines supporting the current literature. In the initial step, they were educated on sex education and reassured regarding their symptoms and related distress. Pharmacological agents were also used for symptomatic relief. Specific treatment for associated psychological and physical comorbidities were also provided in liaison with respective hospital disciplines, e.g., antidepressants and psychological therapy for comorbid depressive disorder, surgical management for associated infective and gangrenous changes in genitalia, and medical management for associated pneumonia, etc.

The majority (80%) of the patients were treated in an outpatient setting. The remaining 20% required indoor admission initially, either psychiatric indoor or other medical or surgical indoors. After managing their psychiatric/medical/surgical emergencies, they were also followed up with psychiatric OPD during the rest of the study period. Most of them (75%) needed oral anxiolytics in the form of benzodiazepines (56%), antidepressants (11%), etc. A small percentage (9%) of cases were very agitated and restless during the initial acute state; they needed low-dose oral antipsychotics (AS) or injectable tranquilizers to control their acute state. For comorbid psychiatric illnesses, 31% of subjects required specific pharmacological and psychosocial treatment, and for associated physical complications, 19% needed supportive medical treatment.

The prevalence of Koro is high in those ethnic, religious, and cultural groups where reproductive ability is considered a significant determinant of a young person's worth.[1,72] Psychological conflicts, especially with sexual contents, significant guilt for excessive masturbatory practices or maintaining extramarital relations, a strong sense of sexual inadequacy, either anticipatory or in actual sense, etc., are the predisposing factors described in the literature for ensuing Koro. Individual perception of genital organ image, especially for males' dysmorphic penis image perception and related cognitive distortion, was also essential in Koro symptoms' occurrence and maintenance.[40,38] With this background, a new modality of psychosexual intervention named "sex education in vivo" was planned for patients who presented with Koro symptoms. On 11 indoor admitted male patients, this modality of intervention was tried. In the initial few days of admission, their overall level of anxiety was controlled by giving anxiolytic medications. After explaining the procedure to the patients, the intervention was started.

Each patient was separately allowed to be sexually aroused by watching pornography books, pictures or movies, etc., maintaining their privacy during ward stay at psychiatric indoor. Each of them was advised to measure the size of the penis in sexually excited state by themselves and to note the measurements on a paper. Thereafter, they were allowed to masturbate. Due to noncompliance, three patients were excluded from this psychosexual intervention and managed by other modes of treatment. For the rest of the eight patients, the procedure of sexual arousal was repeated on alternate days, and they were advised to meet the therapist separately in a session every time on the same day in the ward. During the sessions, the therapist gave him sex education, including corrections to his misconception and myths, then patients were reassured of their sexual potency by citing the records that he was advised to maintain. For each patient, the procedure was continued for the next 6–10 days according to his need. With the help of a cognitive paradigm, the therapist attempted to correct their cognitive distortions regarding their misperception of genital organ image and thus reduce their apprehension related to castration anxiety, sexual inadequacy, or disappearance of the penis with subsequent sexual jeopardy. Combining with the other treatment modalities, the symptoms of Koro and associated psychological distress significantly improved in all eight subjects. After discharge during OPD follow-up, a few booster sessions were also needed for two patients to prevent the recurrence of Koro symptoms.

Outcome of treatment: In a 3-month follow-up period, 18 patients (n = 64, 28%) dropped out of follow-up **(Fig. 11)**. The rest, 46 patients (n = 64, 72%) completed follow-up. The drop-out rate was higher among males (n = 49, 33%) compared to females (n = 15, 13%). During follow-up, it was observed that 41 patients (n = 64, 89%) completely recovered from symptoms of Koro. The recovery rate among male (n = 49, 89%) and female (n = 15, 92%) patients was comparable. The mean days to recovery were 18 (SD 5.67). Males (22 + 5.85 SD) took slightly longer time than females (15 + 4.91 SD) to recover. Two male patients had a recurrence of Koro symptoms during the follow-up period for which they were readmitted. Considering the previous epidemics and lifetime occurrence, 9% of the individuals had a Koro history. Koro symptoms were reported in other family members in 11% of the individuals. The majority (77%) of the individuals had either witnessed closely or heard about

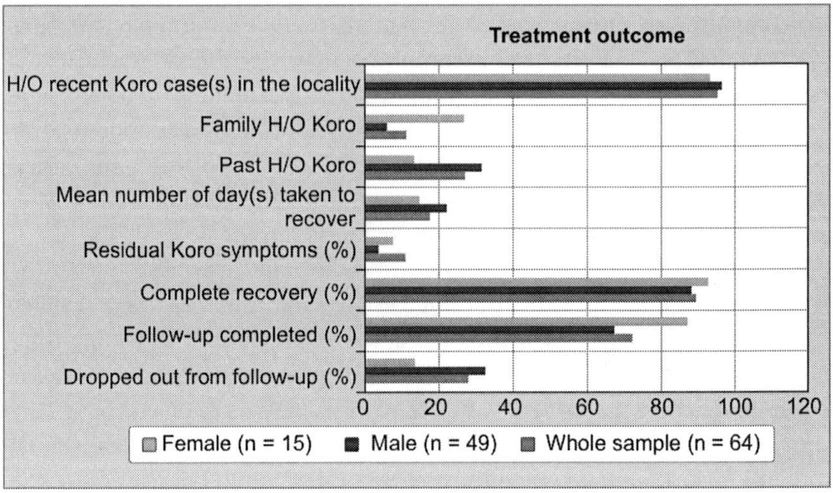

Fig. 11: Treatment outcome.

Koro case(s) occurrence in the vicinity of their locality. A small proportion of subjects (n = 64, 11%) had residual Koro symptoms at the end of 3-month follow-up period.

Female variant and gender difference: In most of the large Koro epidemics reported worldwide, the uttermost description was confined to the male gender. People have a prototypical impression in their minds that Koro means a young male victim. Much discussion was going on in the literature on the male counterpart's prevalence, phenomenology, and predisposition. Interestingly, it was observed that gender demography for Koro which was reported from West Bengal and surrounding states, was quite different. A good proportion of female subjects was recorded from almost all major epidemics from its initial reporting in this geographical region.[5-7,9-11,13,28] Even several research papers were published by Professor Chowdhury separately for female cases to explore the demographical and phenomenological characteristics of the female variant of Koro,[73,74] and he observed several essential differences in the demographic and phenomenological pattern between the genders.

A similar observation was also replicated from the current study which was conducted in a socioculturally and geographically different community, i.e., South Bengal part of West Bengal. Almost one fourth (n = 15, 23%) of the subjects were females **(Fig. 2)**. Though analogically, female phenomenology is similar to a male, most females were presented with predominantly breast symptoms rather than genital symptoms in the current study. We also found few differences between the two genders in the manifestation of symptoms of Koro. Though they were not significant statistically, they might have some clinical implications. The mean age (male 16.53 years vs. female 18.79 years) and formal education (male up to primary vs. female up to matric) of the females was slightly higher than males **(Figs. 3 and 4)**. We also found that the occupation of the majority (45%) of the males was agricultural work, whereas females were mostly students (40%) **(Fig. 3)**. There was a difference in the pattern of treatment-seeking behavior among the two genders. Males attended to the emergency on an urgent basis, even at night, which was more accessible to males. Whereas for females, family members waited for the next day's scheduled medical or surgical OPDs **(Fig. 6)**. These observations also reflect the social position of the two genders in society. In a study conducted by Prof AN Chowdhury, it was also observed that the onset time of female Koro episodes was mostly during the day, unlike that of males who reported a nighttime preponderance.[74,75]

Almost every subject (95%) had reported the occurrence of recent Koro case(s) in the close vicinity of their community, with a comparable proportion for both genders. They were well aware of these cases. Some of them even witnessed these cases. Interestingly, the current study observed that about 27% of cases of the whole sample had a history of (H/O) occurrence of Koro symptoms in the past (other than the current epidemic). Male subjects (31%) had a more substantial possibility of recurrence than female subjects (13%). On the other hand, the occurrence of Koro symptoms in the family member(s) made the females (27%) more vulnerable to Koro symptoms than males (6%), with overall family H/O of the whole sample was 11% in the current study **(Fig. 12)**. Prof Chowdhury observed that almost all the female cases were reported from epidemic settings, and very few sporadic female

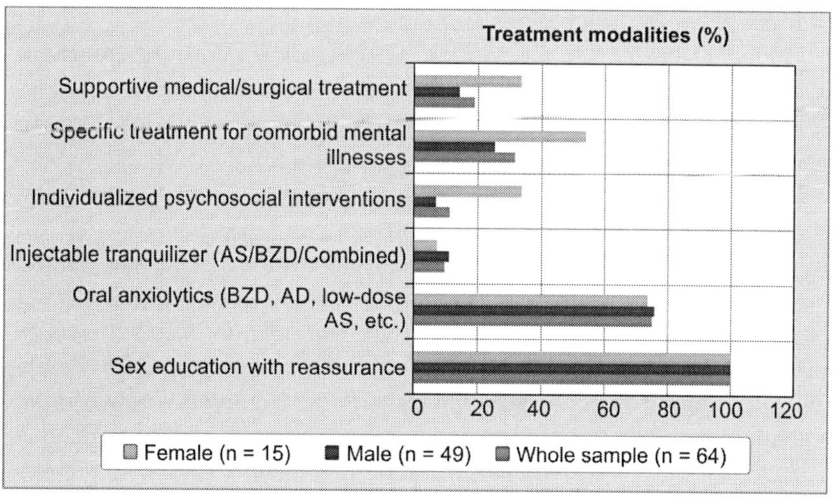

Fig. 12: Treatment modalities.

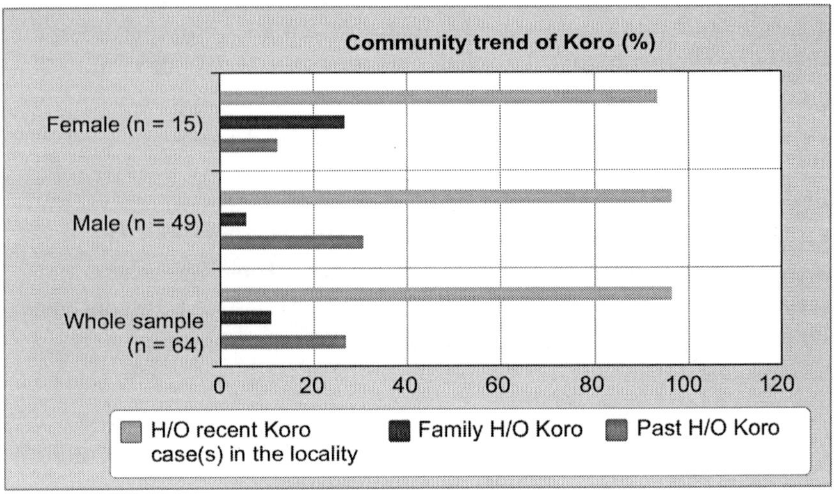

Fig. 13: Community trend of Koro.

patients were reported. This observation can be explained that epidemics provide social sanction of Koro as an illness and may also loosen cultural inhibitions in females.[1] Observation from the current study also strengthens the explanation. The effect of "loosening of cultural inhibitions" becomes more prominent when one or more male or female cases of Koro happen inside a family, and other family members try to adopt various indigenous modes of remedies, forgetting the cultural norms. Thus, the process of social sanctioning perpetuates starting a new case or maintaining it in a family and at large in a community **(Fig. 13)**.

The pattern of sexual dysfunctions in males was different from females. Predominant sexual dysfunctions found in male subjects were either erectile dysfunction or premature ejaculation. On the other hand, predominant sexual dysfunctions in females were found to be decreased libido **(Fig. 8)**. This pattern is also found in the general population without Koro. To implicate this finding clinically, we should explore the psychopathogenesis of whether sexual dysfunction in patients with Koro is either a cause or an effect or just a cooccurrence of two illnesses in an individualized way. No significant difference was noted in the current study in treatment-related parameters between the two genders, except that the new psychosexual intervention (sex education in vivo) was applied only on male subjects as it might not be socioculturally psychodynamically appropriate for female individuals. Among outcome parameters, we found a difference between the two genders in taking time to recover from Koro symptoms. On average, a male subject took 22 days, whereas a female subject took 15 days to recover entirely from Koro symptoms **(Fig. 14)**.

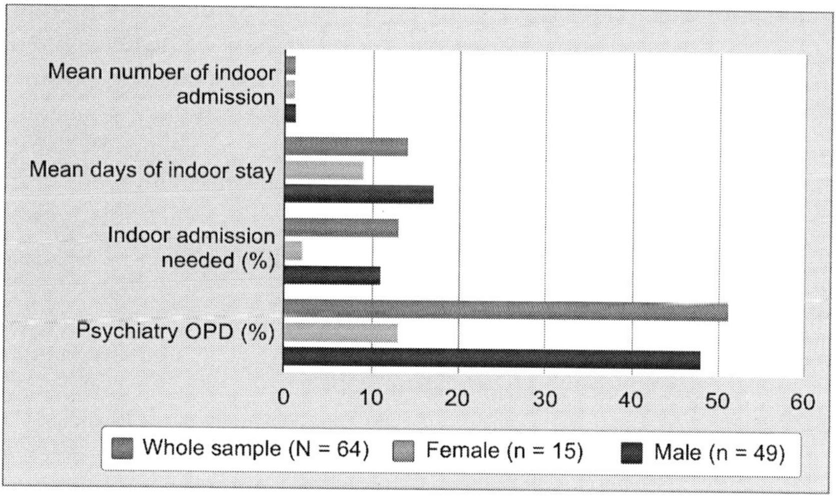

Fig. 14: Treatment settings.

CONCLUSION

The last major Koro epidemic extended to the South Bengal part of West Bengal, which was previously considered a low-vulnerable zone. Despite the significant prevailing variance in sociocultural, economic, and geographical terrain in the different parts of West Bengal, acculturation and migration of the people assist in extending the sovereignty of disease to its new geographical area. Moreover, sensational media coverages in vernacular language had an essential role in disseminating the wave of rumors and panic to start and maintain the epidemic. In the current study, the young, unmarried, low educated males who belonged to low socioeconomic joint rural families were the most affected population, identical to a prototype case of a Koro, described in the literature. Similar to the other recent major Koro epidemics reported from West Bengal and surrounding states, there was a significant female proportion in the study population. The illness was manifested with an abrupt-onset short-lasting symptoms in male and female subjects. Analogically, male phenomenology was similar to female, and breast symptoms rather than genital symptoms were predominant in females. In several clinical parameters, the two genders differed, e.g., mean age of presentation, education level, occupation, first reporting pattern in the hospital, the pattern of comorbid sexual dysfunctions, mean time taken to recover, etc. Most of them had taken the initial help from community healers in terms of indigenous modes of interventions (e.g., water therapy, ligature application), which often became socially and medically detrimental for the people. For prevailing taboos and stigma in society to mental illnesses, a skeptical attitude toward psychiatrists was very apparent in help-seeking behavior among people. However, a better attitude was noticed for other disciplines of healthcare facilities among the study population. Comorbid psychiatric illnesses, especially sexual dysfunction, were higher among Koro-affected persons. With individualized symptomatic treatment applying standard pharmacological and psychological interventions, the overall favorable outcome of the disease was noted among most affected persons. We hope observations from the current study will help clinicians and researchers conceptualize the dynamics of a Koro epidemic in the future and intervene at the individual or community level optimally.

REFERENCES

1. Chowdhury AN. Hundred years of Koro: The history of a culture-bound syndrome. Int J Social Psychiat. 1998; 44(3):181-8.
2. Chakraborty A, Das S, Mukherji A. Koro epidemic in India. Transcul Psychiat Res Rev. 1983;20:150-1.
3. Nandi DN, Banerjee G, Saha H, Boral GC. Epidemic Koro in West Bengal, India. Inter J Soc Psychiat. 1983;29:265-8.
4. Ghosh S, Nath S, Brahma A, Chowdhury AN. Fifth Koro epidemic in India: A review report. World Cul Psychiatr Res Rev. 2013; 8(1):8-20.
5. Dan A, Chaudhuri A, Patra P, Chakraborty K, Debnath A, De S, et al. Socio-demographic Profile and Treatment Seeking Behaviour of Koro Patients in an Epidemic Reported from West Bengal, India. Inter J Innov Res Develop. 2016;5(1):8-13.
6. Dan A, Mondal T, Chakraborty K, Chaudhuri A, Biswas A. Clinical course and treatment outcome of Koro: A follow up study from a Koro epidemic reported from West Bengal, India. Asian J Psychiat. 2017;26:14-20.
7. Chowdhury AN, Pal P, Chatterjee A, Roy M, Das Chowdhury BB. Analysis of North Bengal Koro epidemic with three years follow up. Ind J Psychiat. 1988;30:60-72.
8. Chowdhury AN, Banerjee G, Sen KD, Bera NK, Sharma NK. Koro in West Bengal again. Ind J Soc Psychiat. 1994;10:27-30.
9. Chakraborty S, Sanyal D. An outbreak of Koro among 19 workers in a jute mill in South Bengal. Ind J Psychiat. 2011;20(1):58-60.
10. Sachdev PS. Koro epidemic in north-east India. Aust N Z J Psychiat. 1985;19(4): 433-8.
11. Dutta D, Phookan HR, Das PD. The koro epidemic in lower Assam. Indian J Psychiat. 1982;24:370-4.
12. Dutta D. Koro epidemic in Assam. Brit J Psychiat. 1983;143:309-10.
13. Debbarma S, Das SK, Kumar A, Debbarma D, Das A, Reang T. Koro epidemic: a descriptive study. J. Evolution Med Dent Sci. 2016;5(76):5634-563.
14. Ranga K. The curious cases of shrinking genitalia: Mass panic at labour camp in Goergaon as twenty five men suffer from 'retracting' genitalia. Mid-Day, 26.10.2010. Available from http://www.mid- day.com/news/2010/oct/261010-labour-camp-Goregaon-Aarey-ColonyKoro-mumbai.htm. [Last accessed March, 2023].
15. Assam Tribune. It's a cultural syndrome, say doctors. 30.11.2010. Available from http://www.assamtribune.com/scripts/detailsnew.asp?id=sep3010/city06. [Last accessed March, 2023].

16. Bernstein RL, Gaw AC. Koro: Proposed classification for DSM-IV. Am J Psychiatry. 1990;12:1670-4.
17. Ungvari GS, Mullen RS. Koro: The delusion of penile retraction. Urology. 1994;43:883-5.
18. Blonk J C. Koro. Geneeskundig Tijdschriftvoor. Nederlands-Indië. 1895;35:150-68.
19. American Psychiatric Association. Diagnostic and Statistical Manual of Mental Disorders, 4th edition. (DSM-IV). Washington, DC: American Psychiatric Association; 1994.
20. American Psychiatric Association. Diagnostic and Statistical Manual of Mental Disorders, 4th edition. Text Revision (DSM-IV-TR). Washington, DC: American Psychiatric Association; 2000.
21. American Psychiatric Association. Diagnostic and Statistical Manual of Mental Disorders, 5th edition. (DSM-5). Arlington, VA: American Psychiatric Association; 2013.
22. World Health Organization. ICD-10 Classification of Mental and Behavioural Disorders. Diagnostic Criteria for Research. Geneva: WHO; 1993.
23. Kumar R, Phookun HR, Datta A. Epidemic of Koro in North East India: an observational cross-sectional study. Asian J Psychiat. 2014;12:113-7.
24. Small GW, Borus JF. The influence of newspaper reports on outbreaks of mass hysteria. Psychiatric Quarterly. 1987;58(4):269-78.
25. Bartaman. The state is struggling with unusual 'illness' but health department is still unalert. Kolkata edition. p.6. 12.11.2010b
26. Ceraldi S. A comparison of primary and secondary Koro. Chrestomathy. 2011;10:19-26.
27. Mitchell D. Curing koro, the shrinking penis disease. Proceedings of 1st Annual Conference of the Monash Asia Institute, Mumbai, India, 9-13 February 2004.
28. Chowdhury AN. Ethnomedical concept of heat and cold in Koro: Study from Indian patients. World Cult Psychiatry Res Rev. 2008;3:146-58.
29. Nandi DN, Banerjee G, Bera S, Nandi S. Mode of spread of epidemic koro in a village in West Bengal. Ind J Psychiat. 1984;26(4):331-4.
30. Chowdhury AN. Trait anxiety profile of koro patients. Ind J Psychiat. 1990;32(4):330-3.
31. Dan A, Ghosh A, Barai S. Research on culture-bound syndromes and sexual disorders from West Bengal. In: Chakraborty K, Bhattacharya, Neogi R (Eds). West Bengal: Its contribution to Indian Psychiatry, 1st edition.
32. Yap PM. Koro—a culture-bound depersonalization syndrome. Br J Psychiat. 1965;111:43-50.
33. Modai I, Munitz H, Aizenberg D. Koro in an Israeli Male. Brit J Psychiat. 1986;149:503-5.
34. Tseng WS, Kan-Ming M, Hsu J, Li-Shuen L, Li-Wah O, Guo-Qian C, et al. A sociocultural study of Koro epidemics in Guangdong, China. Amer J Psychiat. 1988;145:1538-43.
35. Fishbain DA, Barsky S, Goldberg M. "Koro" (Genital retraction syndrome): Psychotherapeutic interventions. Amer J Psychotherapy. 1989;43:87-91.
36. Adeniran RA, Jones JR. Koro: Culture-bound disorder or universal symptom? Brit J Psychiat. 1994;164:559-61.
37. Rosaca-Rebaudengo P, Durst R, Minuchin-Itzigsohn S. Transculturation, psychosis and Koro syndromes. Isr J Relat Sci. 1996;33:54-62.

38. Chowdhury AN. Glans penis perception of Koro patients. Acta Psychiatr Scand 1993;87:355-7.
39. Chowdhury AN. Penile perception of Koro patients. Acta Psychiatr Scand. 1989;80:183-6.
40. Chowdhury AN. Dysmorphic penis image perception: the root of Koro vulnerability. A longitudinal study. Acta Psychiatr Scand. 1989;80:518-20.
41. Chowdhury AN. Penis-root perception of Koro patients. Acta Psychiatr Scand. 1991;84:12-3.
42. Chowdhury AN. Neuroticism, extraversion and sex-guilt cognition in the genesis of koro. Samiksa. 1989;43:57-65.
43. Chowdhury AN, Bera NK. Koro following cannabis smoking: two case reports. Addiction. 1994;89:1017-20.
44. Chowdhury AN. Cannabis: a note from Bengal. Addiction. 1996;91:766-7.
45. Earlywine M. Cannabis-induced Koro in Americans. Addiction. 2001;11:1663-6.
46. Kalaitzi CK, Kalantzis A. Cannabis-induced Koro-like syndrome. Urol Int. 2005;76:278-80.
47. Holden TJ. Koro syndrome associated with alcohol induced systemic disease in a Zulu. Brit J Psychiat. 1987;151:695-7.
48. Al-Sinawi H, Al-Adawi S, Al-Guenedi A. Ramadan fasting triggering koro-like symptoms during acute alcohol withdrawal: a case report from Oman. Transcul Psychiat. 2008; 45(4):695-704.
49. Chowdhury AN, Bagchi DJ. Koro in heroin withdrawal. J Psychoactive Drugs. 1993;25:257-8.
50. Dow TW, Silver D. A drug induced Koro Syndrome. J Florida Med Assoc. 1973;60:32-3.
51. Chen E. Drug-induced Koro in a non-Chinese man. Br J Psychiat. 1991;158:721.
52. Kovács A, Osváth P. Genital retraction syndrome in a Korean woman. A case of Koro in Hungary. Psychopathology. 1998;31:220-4.
53. Heymann I, Fahy TA. Koro-like symptoms in a man infected with human immunodeficiency virus. Brit J Psychiat. 1992;160:119-21.
54. Chand SP. Koro associated with phobia for AIDS. Int J Psychiatry Med. 1998;28:353-256.
55. Keshavan MS. Epidemic psychoses or epidemic Koro? Br J Psychiat. 1983;142: 100-1.
56. Wilson S, Agin C. Genital pain associated with genital retraction: a case of Koro syndrome. J Pain Symp Management. 1997;13:176-8.
57. Cohen S, Tennenbaum SY, Teitelbaum A, Durst R. The Koro (genital retraction) syndrome and its association with infertility: a case report. J Urology. 1995;153:427-8.
58. Bartholomew E. The social psychology of "epidemic" Koro. Int J Social Psychiat. 1994;40:46-60.
59. Koro Study Team. The koro epidemic in Singapore. Singapore Med J. 1969;10:234-7.
60. Tseng WS, Kan-ming M, Hsu J, Li-shuen L, Li-wah O, Guo-qian C, et al. A sociocultural study of koro epidemics in Guangdong, China. Amer J Psychiat. 1988;145:1538-43.
61. Kendall EM, Jenkins PL. Koro in an American man. Amer J Psychiat. 1987;60(4):32-3.

62. Kumar H V. Koro in an Israeli man. Brit J Psychiat. 1987;150(1):133.
63. Bayer RS. Koro-like symptoms and transient post-ictal psychosis. Qatar Med J. 2000;9(2):68-9.
64. Srivastava M, Pandit B. Koro—A Case Report and Review. Int J Physiol. 2013; 1(1):37-40.
65. Damodaran SS, Haque Nizamie S. "Incomplete Koro"—A forerunner for mood disorder: Two case reports. Ind J Psychiat. 1993;35(1):60-2.
66. Panigrahi M, Padhy SK, Behere PB. Understanding and managing complete form of sporadic Koro syndrome associated with depression. J Postgrad Med Edu Res. 2012;46(2):104-5.
67. Agarwal SM, Divakara PG, Pramanik KB. Koro in an industrial setting. Ind J Psychiat. 1994;36(1):36-8.
68. Praharaj SK. Koro and psychosis following steroid abuse. Germ J Psychiat. 2004;7(3):49-50.
69. Shukla GD, Mishra DN. Koro like syndrome: A case report. Ind J Psychiat. 1981;23(1):96-7.
70. Kranzler HR, Shah PJ. Atypical Koro. Brit J Psychiatry. 1988;152:579-80.
71. Chowdhury AN. Cultural Koro and Koro-Like Symptom (KLS). Germ J Psychiat. 2008;11:81-2.
72. Mattelaer JJ, Jilek W. Koro—the psychological disappearance of the penis. J Sex Med. 2007;4(5):1509-515.
73. Chowdhury AN. Koro in females: An analysis of 48 cases. Transcul Psychiatric Res Rev. 1994;31:369-80.
74. Chowdhury AN, Chawla M. Koro in female: A case report and a mini review. Eur J Psychiat. 2019;33(4):182-5.

Chapter 5

West Bengal Koro Epidemic 2010: A Tertiary Teaching Hospital Study

Sayanti Ghosh, Saswati Nath, Arabinda Brahma, Arabinda N Chowdhury

INTRODUCTION

Koro is a culture-bound syndrome endemic to Southeast Asian countries. Authors have extensively researched several Koro epidemics over the last several decades. It was initially recognized as a culture-bound syndrome in the 8th edition of Kraepelin's Textbook of Psychiatry in 1909. It described clinical pictures later labeled as culture-bound syndromes, namely *latah*, *Koro*, and *amok*.[1] Interestingly, the sociocultural changes and advancements in general knowledge have influenced symptomatology, modes of spread, information sharing, and help-seeking behavior patterns in all these epidemics. Comorbid psychiatric diagnoses have also been studied and researched in detail in these epidemics depending on prevailing standardized diagnostic systems for mental disorders. That Koro has been included in "Other Specified Obsessive-compulsive and Related Disorder" in the latest Diagnostic and Statistical Manual of Mental Disorders, Fifth Edition (DSM-5) manual of the American Psychiatric Association[2] reflects this view. Similar conceptual shifts have been proposed in other culture-bound syndromes (CBS).

The fifth Koro epidemic in India occurred in 2010 and probably started in the Northeastern Indian states. The epidemic's epicenter was Assam,[3] then Mumbai, and then transmitted by migrant laborers to West Bengal. On October 26th, 2010, Mid-Day, a news daily in Mumbai reported: "Mass panic at labor camp in Goregaon as 25 men suffer from "retracting" genitalia.[4] The Aarey milk colony is situated in Goregaon East, Mumbai, and houses several labor camps, where people came to work from different parts of India. At least 25 workers (all male) reported similar symptoms. Most of the victims were from West Bengal and Orissa states. These incidents created an air of panic in the camp. The news also received high publicity in other media and blogs in Mumbai,[5] in Assam,[6] and West Bengal.[7] It is worth noting that there was a mass-scale Koro affliction reported from Assam immediately preceding this incident in Mumbai. It is also noted that the media are overreporting, thus helping spread the illness. Duarah[8] reported how this epidemic speeded inside rural Assam and how people from all walks of life adhered to the folk preventing practices: "Quite, unfortunately, the local media hype regarding this syndrome has created an uncalled for situation that has put every educated individual to shame. On tour around the bustling capital city, ... one will bump into all sections of people with lime smeared on the ear lobe to shield oneself from the "dangerous disease." From the well-dressed men and women to the salesman in a sleek mall and the daily wage laborers, everyone is sporting lime spots on their ears, and the more paranoid ones are immersing themselves in water holes." October is the month of the Great festival of Durga Puja for Hindus and Ramadan for Muslims. Usually, the laborers get leave from work and visit their native homes. Few of these affected persons in Aarey Colony were indeed from West Bengal, and they returned to their homes during the festival leave.

THE EPIDEMIC SCENARIO

From the first week of November 2010, several districts of West Bengal were affected, mostly Darjeeling (Siliguri) and West Dinajpur.[9] At least 4,000 people were affected in those districts.[10.] The present report regarding is based on patients from Kolkata and adjoining districts who attended RG Kar Medical College, Kolkata, West Bengal.[11] The study was carried out from November 2010 to January 2011. A total of 60 cases had attended the emergency and other outdoor departments of RG Kar Medical College (a general teaching hospital), Kolkata, during this period. It was later referred to the psychiatry department for detailed assessment and management. Five cases were not Koro; hence, they were not included in this study of 55 patients. This study which included the demographic details, salient clinical features, beliefs regarding the illness, and different folk therapeutic measures adopted by the affected and nonaffected persons, was done after interviewing patients and accompanying family members and neighbors. Written consent from each patient was obtained to publish their data, maintaining anonymity. Diagnostic assessments were done following ICD 10 criteria.[12]

SOCIODEMOGRAPHIC FEATURES

Of the 55 cases, 52 were males, and 3 female patients were reported **(Table 1)**. All the female cases reported vaginal symptoms. The district of North 24 Parganas reported the maximum number of subjects (30 males) in the age range of 9–42 years. Muslim cases were predominant (25) compared to Hindus (10), and married (20) cases were more. Regarding the districts of South 24 Parganas, there were 15 males and 2 reported females in the age range of 16– 35 years, of whom 14 were Hindus compared to 3 Muslims. 13 persons were married. Kolkata reported 5 males and 1 female case in the age range of 23–35 years. All the cases were Hindus, and 4 were married. The district of Howrah had 2 male cases, 21 years of age, both Hindus and married. Hence, case distribution was highest in North 24 Parganas (54.54%), followed by

TABLE 1: Demographic pattern of the Koro cases (n = 55).

Area (% of cases)	*Age range (years)*	*Gender*		*Marital status*		*Religion*	
		Male	*Female*	*Single*	*Married*	*Hinduism*	*Islam*
North 24 Parganas (54.5)	9–42	30	0	10	20	5	25
South 24 Parganas (30.9)	16–35	15	2	4	13	14	3
Howrah (3.6)	21	2	0	0	2	2	0
Kolkata (10.9)	23–35	5	1	2	4	6	0
Total		52	3	16	39	27	28
Total%		94.5	5.5	29.1	70.9	41.1	50.9

South 24 Parganas (30.90%), Kolkata (10.90%), and Howrah (3.63%). 75% of cases were from an urban area in and around Kolkata, and 25% had a rural background. Most of the patients were illiterate or had only primary education. Only one male patient was a graduate. Except for two males who were students, most patients were either unskilled or semiskilled laborers. Females were all housewives. 95% of patients used tobacco (either smoked bidi or cigarette or oral tobacco—*Khaini*). Harmful use of alcohol (F10.1) was found in 21.15% of cases, of which 27.3% of persons fulfilled the ICD criteria for Alcohol Dependence (F10.24). Regular cannabis use was found in 3.84% of cases, though occasional use of alcohol and cannabis was reported by 30.76% of patients.

CLINICAL PRESENTATION

All male patients presented with acute penile shrinkage and retraction and pain and pulling sensation in genital region. A "Flu-like" syndrome with fever (described as "Disco fever"), tremor, headache, burning sensation all over body with increased temperature over the lower part of the body below the waist, sweating and dryness of throat, was reported by 80% of the cases. Since most patients' standard form of self-medication was submersion in cold water up to the neck level for long hours; some patients felt that the fever and associated symptoms could have been a result of such therapy. The acute penile pull was described as sudden retraction with pain in the lower abdomen that lasted for 10–15 minutes with resultant shortening of the penis (in 7.7%, shortening /reduction of the scrotum also). 95% of cases reported one attack, but 5% had several attacks (2–3) on the same day. One male patient also reported a shrinking feeling of both arms, legs, and ears (as if there is a pull from inside) along with penile symptoms. Associated fear of impending death was reported in 43.6% of cases. The remaining cases feared the "dissolution" of their male organ. One patient was fearful of dying due to the severe respiratory distress and palpitation rather than his penile retraction. Other complaints, among all patients, in order of frequency were difficulties in micturition (74.5%), heat emanating from the head and body (67.3%), generalized body weakness (54.5%), breathlessness (47.3%), vertigo (20%), and pain in the genital area and lower abdomen (7.7%). Many patients reported more than one symptom. Among the male patients' complaints of frequent loss of semen through urine (Dhat syndrome) were found in eight cases (15.38%). Erectile dysfunction (11.5%) and masturbatory guilt with intense anxiety (regarding future sexual life) were also reported in 5.8% of cases.

A 9-year-old male child was brought by his parents to the hospital with complaints of shrinkage of the penis and pain abdomen. His anxious mother confirmed the shrinkage. The child watched a Hindi action movie on television when he suddenly felt his penis was shrinking. On questioning, he revealed that he had heard discussions in the neighborhood about a recent illness of penile shrinkage a few days ago. However, the two female cases did not have such associated sexual anxiety; their concern was more focused on disfiguring their body and fear of some severe future health malady. Two female patients had symptoms of retraction of nipples. One case also reported an associated "peculiar sensation" in the vagina and vaginal discharge.

On MSE, 80% of patients had moderate-to-severe anxiety, mean HAM-A score 22.70 ± 3.52[13] regarding the illness, especially its outcome. One male patient presented with extreme agitation with symptoms of acute stress reaction (F43.0), fearing some fatal bodily ailment and imminent death. Hypochondriacal preoccupation with genital symptoms was seen in 56.4% of cases and associated moderate-to-severe depression, with a mean HAM-D score of 21.42 ± 2.46 (Hamilton, 1960). One male patient (with comorbid Dhat syndrome) had intense suicidal ideation. Definite features of body dysmorphic disorder (F45.2) regarding penile size and disfigurement were seen in 5.8% of male patients.

Regarding past psychiatric history and premorbid personality pattern, perception of excessive emission of semen via urine (Dhat syndrome) before the attack of Koro was the most common feature reported (15.38%). Of these cases, six were Hindu, two were Muslim, age was 21 ± 3.7 years, and all were single. Among these Koro cases with preexisting Dhat syndrome, three cases met the criteria for diagnosis of depression (one with severe depression without psychotic symptom (F32.2), two with Moderate Depressive episode with somatic syndrome (F32.11); one with Generalized Anxiety Disorder (F41.1) and two with Mixed Anxiety and Depressive Disorder (F41.2). Two cases had Hypochondrical Disorder (F45.2). One had Body Dysmorphic disorder F45.2 (firm conviction and deep concern about physical appearance, mainly small size of penis and scrotum, bordering onto the delusional belief of having a small penis). The last two cases had a history of multiple health consultations, both modern and traditional. Even though all Dhat syndrome cases had acute anxiety with the perception of penile pull, none had a fear of impending death. 34.54% of patients reported excessive masturbation and associated guilt. Three patients (5.54 %) had an anxious-avoidant personality, F60.6 (described as "mentally weak") and two cases (3.63 %) had obsessive-compulsive personality traits (F60.5). Four cases were referred from other departments: Three from dermatology (two received treatment for gonorrheal infection and had a perception of penile shrinkage, and the other had herpes simplex infection (HSV2) with symptoms of feverish feeling, tingling sensation in the penis with a perception of intermittent retraction of the penis, and pain on passing urine). One was from the medicine department (with Dhat syndrome and extreme fear of "penis-illness" infection from the current Koro epidemic). None of these patients had typical Koro symptoms such as sudden onset, penile pull from inside, acute anxiety, and fear of impending death. The case with HSV2 infection may be categorized as intermittent Koro-like symptoms. One 7-year-old male child was brought by his mother with the complaint of penile retraction. The boy had no complaint, but the mother was firmly convinced that since that morning, her son's penis gradually retracted and became "too small to grasp." There are some similar cases reported from her locality, she said.

MANAGEMENT

Most of the patients were treated with SSRI (selective serotonin reuptake inhibitor) antidepressants (Fluoxetine 60 mg or Citalopram 60 mg daily) and benzodiazepine (Clonazepam 500 µg twice/thrice or Alprazolam 0.25/0.50 mg twice or thrice daily). Supportive psychotherapy was initially provided to all patients. Two cases (severe depression and hypochondriasis) were offered a more structured form of psychotherapy. Family therapy was done. 18 cases attended follow-up (up to 12 weeks), and all of them reported doing well with complete remission of Koro symptoms.

MODE OF SPREAD OF KORO IN BENGAL AND EXPLANATORY MODEL

All the patients had prior information about this illness (Disco fever) mostly from neighbor's and some through newspapers. In one of the male patients, the illness started after receiving a phone call from a friend who worked in Mumbai and who first informed him that such an illness was occurring at his workplace. Though he received the information with disbelief, after 2 hours, he felt his genitals shrinking. Another male subject went to help his friend who had a Koro attack and while pouring water on his head, he developed Koro symptoms. The mode of referral to this hospital was as follows: 43.64% self-referral, 36.36% by "Quack doctors" (unregistered medical practitioners) and 20% by "Primary Care Physicians. 42.3% attributed their penile retraction and associated bodily symptoms to "bodily weaknesses." They also related this "weakness" with "body heat" as its consequence. 27.27% patients reported "Viral infection" as a probable causative factor. They used the term "Disco fever" to designate Koro symptoms. They believed that touching any person suffering from Koro would spread the disease. This belief created a panic atmosphere in that locality to such an extent that unaffected persons remained home-bound and did not even go out to work till the attack in the vicinity subsided. It is interesting to note that this area evidenced large-scale epidemics of Bird-flu (avian influenza from H5N1 virus) twice (2008 and early part of 2010). The concept of "viral infection/fever" most probably has a connection with these social experiences. One patient who vaguely associated his symptoms with AIDS, but could not explain it in more detail, admitted to having had extramarital affairs and sexual intercourse with prostitutes, increasing his fear of illness. 21.15% of cases believed the causative factor is excessive loss of semen, either by habitual masturbation or by sexual intercourse or due to weak Dhat (semen). Two patients reported a prior suspicion and deep concern that their penis was smaller than average, which they thought was a precursor condition for developing this illness. Anxiety regarding future marital life was present in both cases. One male patient felt that supernatural powers were responsible for such ailments, which indicated that "the world was coming to an end soon by 2012." He describes himself as an unfortunate target of this "evil power."

HELP-SEEKING BEHAVIOR AND FOLK TREATMENT MODALITIES

Some interesting observations are noteworthy. 74.54% of the patients initially consulted faith-healers, quacks, and local religious heads such as Priests or Moulavis, 25.45% consulted primary care physicians. Besides this, prophylactic folk measures were also taken by unaffected persons living in the same locality where the disease occurred.

The most common therapy (Water Therapy) adopted by 95% of patients, was to submerge the body up to neck level in water usually in local ponds **(Fig. 1)**, holding the penis and pulling it for approximately 5 minutes to 6 hours. Later, cold water was poured or ice was placed on the head by family members. Besides this, "cooling drinks" such as sugar water, medicinal water (prescribed by local faith healers or obtained from places of worship) was taken to combat the excessive heat believed to accumulate in the body due to the disease.

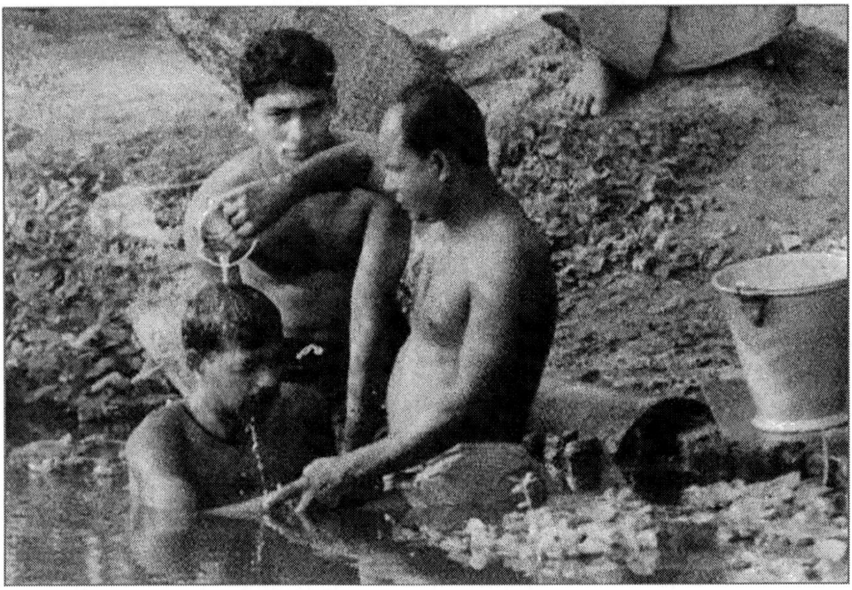

Fig. 1: Water therapy of a Koro patient in a pond, Kolkata.[14]

Herbal amulets, Armlets, amulets, and talisman containing medicinal herbs were also prescribed by Hindu priests and Muslim Moulavis for both, as therapeutic and prophylactic measure. It is reported that in Barasat town, 25 km from Kolkata city, many people were affected by genital shrinkage illness.[14,15] A wave of mass-hysteria was observed, where people rushed to purchase chanted amulets to prevent the disease. Ginger and root of Arum (*Arum triphyllum,* locally known as 'Mankachu') was taken together, tied up in a piece of cloth to be worn around the waist, by a red thread. Crushed seeds of bottle-gourd (*Lagenaria siceraria,* locally known as Lau) to be worn within an armlet was also advised. Manasa (Sij plant, belonging to the cactus family of *Euphorbia* genus), and Basil (*Ocimum basilicum,* locally called Tulsi) leaves were taken together and tied up in a string at mid-arm position. Muslim patients were mostly prescribed the Manasa leaves whereas Hindus priests preferred Tulsi. Tulsi is regarded as a holy plant by Hindu religious tradition and is worshipped by Hindus at large. All these herbs and vegetables were sold at high prices locally at that time! Lime (Calcium hydroxide) paste smearing on the forehead, throat and earlobes was also a popular preventive measure adopted by many patients and persons **(Fig. 2)**.

In some regions of the South 24 Parganas districts of West Bengal, from where most of the Muslim patients came, holy papers containing lines from the holy Koran were distributed by a local photocopy shop. A local Moulavi gave the initial writing to the shop owner. This created such an impact that some patients living in other areas rushed and procured the paper at high costs after hearing from friends over the telephone about this therapy. This piece

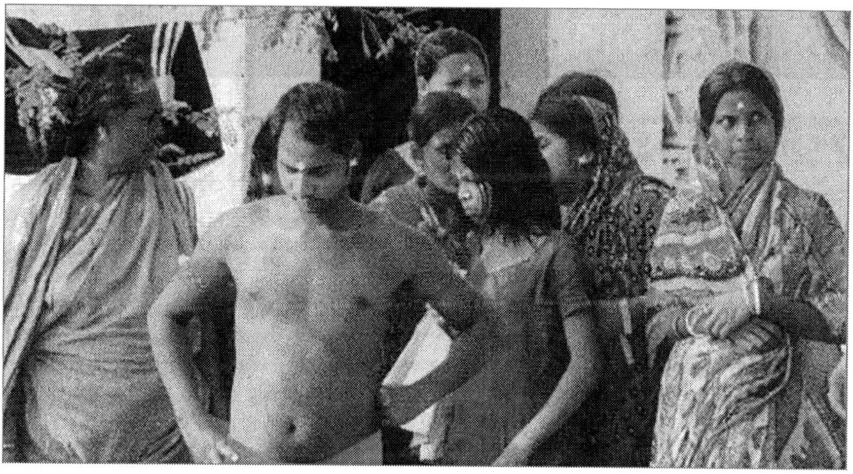

Fig. 2: Smearing of lime paste on forehead and ear lobules among the nonaffected persons in Kolkata.[15]

of paper was meant to be inserted into the armlets and worn all the time to prevent genital symptoms. The idea behind this therapy was the belief that people who had developed the symptoms had sinful thoughts in their minds, but keeping these holy lines would redeem them from their wicked thoughts. Similar incidents were also reported from Barasat town[14] where one Gunin (folk healer) wrote a chant (*Mantra*) on a paper and advised to copy it and keep it within an amulet to wear and keep one copy at home to protect family members. There were long queues in front of different Xerox (Copier) shops in Barasat town to procure a copy of this chanted paper. The typical cost of a document was Rs.1, but at that time, these chanted paper copies were sold at Rs. 20–30. Another prophylactic measure adopted by some patients was to massage the penile shaft with herbal massage oil (a herbal preparation called "German oil," sold as an aphrodisiac over-the-counter). The preparation was sold in large numbers with an escalating cost.

DISCUSSION

This Koro outbreak added some new clinical dimensions to our understanding of the psychiatric epidemic. Information gathered from this epidemic may help combat a future one.

The Migration Route of Psychic Infectivity of Koro

It is evident here that the first epidemic focus was Guwahati, Assam, from where the epidemic spread to Mumbai (air distance of 2,746 km) and then to West Bengal (1,662 km from Mumbai). This interstate spread occurred through migrant laborers. In recent times, because of the easy transport, people have rapid movement to distant places, and so is the psychic infectivity.

It is similar to an organic infection epidemic, e.g., the transcontinental spread of Severe Acute Respiratory Syndrome—from China-Vietnam-Singapore-Taiwan-Canada, the spread of COVID-19 pandemic from initial focus in Wuhan, China. This is a new dimension of Ecopsychiatry[16] where rapid transit and information systems (media, television, fax, cell phone, etc.) influence the quick spread of the psychiatric epidemic (news) over a wide geographical area.[17]

Reporting of Koro from Muslim Subjects

Muslim persons and Maulavis in advocating religious treatment for Koro is a new finding. In previous Koro epidemics from India, no Muslim patients were reported. The present epidemic-time coincided with Ramadan fasting in the Muslim community, and interestingly, a recent study said, "Ramadan fasting triggering koro-like symptoms during acute alcohol withdrawal: a case report from Oman."[18] This area needs further research.

Sexual Psychopathology

AIDS phobia,[19] sexual guilt,[20] and sexual preoccupation[21] of hypochondriacal concern[22,23] and generalized anxiety disorder[24] or Panic disorder[25] are pretty common comorbid psychopathology in Koro patients, and the same is evidenced among the current epidemic cases. Hypochondriacal concern about penile morphology or function is known to cause Koro vulnerability.[26] One case here had excessive guilt because of his long-continued extramarital sexual involvement and was found to be quite apprehensive that some sexual deformity may result from his behavior. The most familiar precipitating factor 23.5% reported among 162 Koro patients of the North Bengal epidemic was "extramarital intercourse."[27] Genital pain often accompanied a Koro attack.[28]

Koro and Comorbidity Factors

Empirical relation of any culture-bound syndromes (CBS) with a designated psychiatric disorder is essential.[29] The CBS often coexists with other psychiatric disorders, as many psychiatric disorders do with each other. Delineation of comorbidity factors will help in clinical decision-making and shed light on the phenomenology of the CBSs. Koro has offered a unique opportunity to study comorbidity in CBS. Over the years, Koro has been reported from diverse cultures and ethnicities with varieties of comorbid pathology, both mental and physical.[30] Dhat syndrome, a CBS reported from the Indian subcontinent, is based on the conviction that semen mixes with urine and is excreted through urination. It has a strong cultural belief that the loss of semen is harmful because it depletes the body of physical and mental energy.[31] Dhat syndrome often has a complicated psychosexual loading with multiple comorbidities.[32] In eight cases of Dhat syndrome with Koro here, different psychiatric comorbidities were found, which guides the clinical decision to treat these symptoms in addition to Koro complaints. These findings also help to develop insight into the psychodynamic psychopathology about sexual neurosis in the cultural context. In a recently reported case of Koro and Dhat syndrome with comorbid OCD in a young Muslim male,[33] the authors have discussed how initial Dhat and Koro symptoms camouflaged the underlying OCD symptoms in the patient. His mother brought the child for alleged Koro symptom, an example of Munchausen by proxy. By fabricating symptoms (nonexisting), the mother tried to convince the medical providers that her child was sick. In a psychoanalytical way, she displaced her sexual anxiety onto the child. Similar cases have been reported from the 1982 Indian epidemic[34] and the 1967 Singapore epidemic (mother came with a 4-month-old baby).[35] A very similar epidemic scenario is reported from coastal Vietnam, where some mothers observed that the penis and testes of their children had shrunk after swimming. This had created a social panic in several coastal communities. Some mothers tried to pull out the penis and testes manually or even with hooks, which resulted in severe penile injury in some boys.[36] Health professionals should have insight about Munchausen or Factitious disorder by proxy[37] while dealing with alleged Koro in children, especially during epidemic times.

Koro and Koro-like Symptoms

Careful delineation of classic symptoms of Koro is crucial to differentiate it from Koro-like symptoms (KLS)[38,39] or states.[40] Since Koro involves sexual organs, many individuals with varied psychopathology (and accompanied emotionality ranging from depression-anxiety-hypochondriasis to body dysmorphic perception, etc.) may present as if they are suffering during the epidemic wave from Koro. "Koro-like symptoms" are an accepted diagnostic category since Berrios and Morley[41] first described it in 1984. In KLS, symptoms are less dramatic and usually do not have a vital cultural context, and are generally seen in association with other neuropsychiatric disorders.[42] Association of KLS with varieties of psychiatric and nonpsychiatric disorders has been reported, e.g., with recurrent depressive,[43] mood-disorder,[44] generalized anxiety disorder and panic,[45] schizophrenia,[46,47] intellectual disability with fixated pedophilia,[48] voyeurism,[49] HIV infection,[50] genital pain[51] and prostatic enlargement.[52] Clinicians should be cautious about this differential diagnosis because the correct cultural formulation is essential to understand the CBS in its cultural context.[53,54] The other point of clinical interest is the difference between the delusional belief of penile retraction in Koro[55] and the perception of the small penis.[56] Common clinical mistakes are to merge both. Delusion of retracting (and thus small) penis may be either manifestation of body dysmorphic disorder[57] or penile dysmorphophobia, as in Koro,[58,59] and a "Small penis syndrome"[60,61] and often present with varieties of urogenital pathology[62] hypochondriasis and even in an otherwise normal person.[63] These are static penile perceptions over a long period of time, but in Koro, the penile retraction and consequent shortening is a sudden, acute dynamic perception with manifest acute anxiety, and the course of illness is short. The prominence of cultural context is absent in the former while present strongly in the latter.

Koro Perception

One of the several attempts to classify CBS is "taxon categories" (set of similar syndromes which share common or related symptoms.[64] Koro was placed under the "genital retraction taxon" where retraction is the key criterion. It was thus proposed to replace the term Koro with Genital Retraction Syndrome.[65] A "Koro-like" symptom affecting the tongue was reported from Malaysia,[66] suggesting that retraction taxon can involve other organs (and may not always be culture-bound). Complementary to this concept, we propose "Koro perception," where retraction from the inner pull within the body (of any organ) is the prime clinical presentation. In addition to penile symptoms, one case in this study complained of "Koro perception"—a shrinking feeling of arms, legs, and ears. This is a new finding.

Body Heat Explanatory Model

42.3% cases of this epidemic implicated "body heat" generated from the "body weaknesses" as the cause of their penile retraction. Excessive "body heat" was predominantly implicated by the patients (54.5%) as the cause of penile shrinkage in the 1982 Koro epidemic also.[67] In this epidemic, almost all the victims complained of body heat before the Koro attack. Body cooling, the prevailing folk therapy, was thus advocated by Priests, Gunins, and Maulavies and was well accepted by all, including the nonaffected family members of the victims and the general public. In fact, because of this excessive water submersion for hours, many Koro patients became seriously ill with respiratory distress. Similar ill effects and health hazards of folk therapy were also noted in the previous Koro epidemic in West Bengal.[68] The heat-cold concept in Koro is a standard social cognition and is also reported from Mumbai and Assam cases as well.

Folk Rituals

Folk therapeutics is a crucial component of any CBS. In addition to water cooling by water submersion **(Fig. 1)** or ice bath, one other ritual utilized was the advanced technology of copier machines. Both Koro and non-Koro subjects, in massive numbers, procured a copy of the chanted paper and a page containing lines from the holy Koran. This is a new finding of social responsibility to prevent the Koro infectivity. Interestingly, in the 1984–85 Koro epidemic in Guangdong, China, folk therapy consisted of feeding red pepper jam, black pepper, or ginger juice.[69] Social excitement with panic and anxiety in the neighborhood is a decisive environmental risk factor for any psychiatric epidemic.[70,71] Community's perception of infectivity of Koro is a dynamic force[72,73] that speeds the epidemic observed here in mass panic reaction and adopting folk preventive measures in massive numbers. Many avoided going out or were absent from work. Previous social experience with the viral epidemic (Bird flu) added further uncertainty and anxiety in the population. The price of bottle gourd in the local vegetable markets reached an astonishing level (from the usual cost of 4–6 to ₹ 40–45), and people from all categories of life put the lime-paste spots on the ear lobule and forehead **(Fig. 2)**. This practice was also observed in Assam and during the previous Koro epidemic in West Bengal.[74] This mass reactivity highlighted Koro's social anxiety, which has further fueled its spread in the neighborhood. The role of local health agencies timely intervention by health advocacy is an important measure to check the spread of any epidemic, be it medical or psychiatric. In this regard, the role of the medical community is crucial.[75] Unfortunately, the extreme dilemma and poor response from local health administration was noted in the present epidemic. This might be one of the reasons which have not only prolonged the epidemic wave but pushed people to adhere to folk explanation and therapy.

Role of Media

Media is a compassionate and powerful pathway by which epidemic news percolates through society.[76] Assam Tribune made a cautious statement on this issue, and in West Bengal too, during the first week of the epidemic, almost all the news daily of Kolkata, Television channels covered this epidemic with very ambiguous and sensational headlines for at least 4–5 consecutive days. This helped spread the news of this "strange and mysterious disease" in a broader public circle rapidly. The epidemic waves stayed for about 8 weeks.

CONCLUSION

Epidemics of Koro have followed the above-reported epidemic from Bengal in 2010. In 2014, it was reported from Assam[77] and again in West Bengal in 2017.[78] Previously at least five Koro epidemics occurred in India, and the states of West Bengal and Assam were affected repeatedly. Therefore, the population of these states has Koro vulnerability of epidemic proportion. The health administration and professionals should learn from these Koro episodes and equip themselves adequately for preventive strategies so that in the future, they can act proactively to restrict the epidemic spread of Koro and also to provide appropriate treatment to the affected population at the hour of need. This would also prevent the chronicity of the problem.[79,80] Mental health professionals should transmit the knowledge of Koro illness and pathology to other nonpsychiatric colleagues to enhance their clinical perception and precision in diagnosis[81] and treatment.[82] Mental health professionals should play a leading role in the education of the local health agencies in management principles and support media and others to enhance their limited or faulty knowledge about the subject of Koro.

Rapid cultural mingling in the modern world owing to enhanced communication and information technology is emerging as a key factor in modifying symptomatology of various culture-bound syndromes, and Koro is no exception. The cultural elements should be respected and addressed when diagnosing and managing the condition. Further, multiple media faculties should be more amenable to health advocacy and aid in the education of the public to mitigate mass fear and anxiety and enhance the spread of rational information.

REFERENCES

1. Jilek WG. Psychiatric Disorders: Culture-Specific. In: Neil J. Smelser, Paul B. Baltes (Eds). International Encyclopedia of the Social Behavioral Sciences Pergamon. 2001. pp. 12272-7.
2. American Psychiatric Association. Diagnostic and statistical manual of mental disorders (5th ed.). Arlington, VA: APA; 2013.
3. Roy D, Hazarika S, Bhattacharya A, Das S, Nath K, Saddichha S. Koro: Culture bound or mass hysteria? Aus NZ J Psychiat. 2011;45:683.
4. Ranga K. The curious cases of shrinking genitalia: Mass panic at labour camp in Goregaon as twenty five men suffer from 'retracting' genitalia. Mid-Day, 26 Oct,2010. Available at: http://www.mid-day.com/news/2010/oct/261010-labour-camp-Goregaon-Aarey-Colony- Koro-mumbai.htm
5. Wellsphere. (2010). Koro epidemic strikes Indian labour camp, 2 November, 2010.[online] Available from http://www.wellsphere.com/mental-health-article/koro-epidemic-strikes-indian-labour-camp/1267762. [Last accessed April, 2023].
6. Assam Tribune. (2010). It's a cultural syndrome, say doctors, 30 November, 2010. [online] Available from http://www.assamtribune.com/scripts/detailsnew.asp?id =sep 3010/city06. [Last accessed April, 2023].
7. The Statesman. (2010). Symptomatic stupidity, 27 November, 2010. [online] Available from http://www.thestatesman.net/index.php?id=350062&option =com_content&catid=39. [Last accessed April, 2023].
8. Duarah K. (2010). Ignorance causes panic among certain people. Assam Tribune, 30 September, 2010. [online] Available from http://www.assamtribune.com/scripts/detailsnew.asp?id=sep3010/city05. [Last accessed April, 2023].
9. Bera NK. North Bengal Medical College. Personal communication, 22 January, 2011.
10. Chakraborty R. District Hospital, West Dinajpur. Personal communication, 22 January, 2010.
11. Ghosh S, Nath S, Brahma A, Chowdhury A. Fifth Koro epidemic in India: A review report. Worl Cul Psychiat Res Rev. 2013;8(1):8-20.
12. ICD-10 Classification of mental and behavioural disorders: Clinical descriptions and diagnostic guidelines. Geneva: WHO; 1991.

13. Hamilton M. The assessment of anxiety states by rating. Br J Med Psychol. 1959;32:50-5.
14. Bartaman P. Lucrative business of amulets and talisman for the unknown disease. Kolkata edition, 13 October, 2010; pp. 1.
15. Bartaman P. The state is struggling with unusual 'illness' but health department is still unalert. Kolkata edition, 12 October, 2010; pp. 6.
16. Chowdhury AN, Jadav S. Ecopsychiatry: Culture, mental health and ecology with special reference to India. In: Chavan BS, Gupta N, Arun P, Sidana AK, Jadav S (Eds). Comprehensive Textbook on Community Psychiatry in India. New Delhi: Jaypee Brothers Medical Publishers (P) Ltd; 2012. pp. 521-41.
17. Colizza V. (2009). People interact. They travel. And diseases might travel with them. [online] Available from http://www.airneth.nl/index.php/columns/people-interact-they-travel-and-diseases-might- travel-with- them.html. [Last accessed April, 2023].
18. Al-Sinawi H, Al-Adawi S, Al-Guenedi A. Ramadan fasting triggering koro-like symptoms during acute alcohol withdrawal: A case report from Oman. Transcul Psychiat. 2008;45:695-704.
19. Chand SP. Koro associated with phobia for AIDS. Int J Psychiat in Med. 1998;28:353-6.
20. Chowdhury AN. Sex guilt cognition in the genesis of Koro. Arch Ind Psychiat. 1996;3:52-9.
21. Chowdhury AN. Psychopatho-sexuality in Koro patients. J Ind Acad Appl Psychol. 1992;5:71-83.
22. Chowdhury AN. Neuroticism, extraversion and sex-guilt cognition in the genesis of Koro. J Ind Psychoanal Soc. 1989;43:57-64.
23. Chowdhury AN. Clinical analysis of 101 Koro cases. Ind J Soc Psychiat. 1992;7:67-70.
24. Chowdhury AN. Trait anxiety profile of Koro patients. Ind J Psychiat. 1990;32:330-3.
25. Chowdhury AN. Koro: A state of sexual panic or altered physiology? Sexual Marital Therapy. 1996;11:165-71.
26. Rosenthal S, Rosenthal PA. Koro in an adolescent: Hypochondriasis as a stress response. Adoles Psychiat. 1982;10:523-31.
27. Chowdhury AN. Biomedical potential for symptom choice in Koro. Int J Soc Psychiat. 1989;35:329-32.
28. Wilson S, Agin C. Genital pain associated with genital retraction: A case of koro syndrome. J Pain Symp Manag. 1997;13:176-8.
29. Guarnacca PJ, Rogler LH. Research on culture-bound syndromes: New directions. Amer J Psychiat. 1999;156:1322-7.
30. Chowdhury AN. Definition and classification of Koro. Cul Med Psychiat. 1996;20:41-65.
31. Aktar S. Four culture bound psychiatric syndromes in India. Int J Soc Psychiat. 1988;34:70-4.
32. Bhatia MS, Choudhary S, Shome S. Dhat syndrome. Is it a syndrome of Dhat only? J Ment Health Hum Behav. 1997;2:17-22.
33. Ghosh S, Chowdhury AN. A case of two culture-bound syndromes (Koro and Dhat syndrome) coexisting with obsessive-compulsive disorder. Ind J Psychiat. 2020;62(2):221-2.

34. Nandi DN, Banerjee GA. Psychoanalytical study of Koro. J Ind Psychoanal Soc. 1986;40:94-104.
35. Mun CT. Epidemic Koro in Singapore. Brit Med J. 1968;1:640-1.
36. Kar N. Cultural variations in sexual practices. In: Kar N, Kar GC (Eds). Comprehensive Textbook of Sexual Medicine. New Delhi: Jaypee Brothers Medical Publishers; 2005.
37. Ostfield BM, Feldman MD. Factitious disorder by proxy: Awareness among mental health practitioners. Gen Hosp Psychiat. 1996;18:113-6.
38. Garlipp P. Koro—a culture-bound phenomenon. Intercultural psychiatric implications. Germ J Psychiat. 2008;11:21-8.
39. Chowdhury AN. Cultural Koro and Koro-like symptom (KLS). Germ J Psychiat. 2008;11:81-2.
40. Mukherjee T. Koro-like states. Brit J Psychiat. 1987;150:881.
41. Berrios GE, Morley SJ. Koro-like symptom in a non-Chinese subject. Brit J Psychiat. 1984;145:331-4.
42. Freudenmann RW, Schonfeldt-Lecuona C. The syndrome of genital retraction from a transcultural psychiatric point of view. Chinese suo yang, Indonesian koro and non-Asian forms (koro-like symptoms). Der Nervenarzt. 2005;76:569-80.
43. Freudenmann RW, Schonfeldt-Lecuona C. Koro-like symptoms in a recurrent depressive disorder. Nervenartz. 2005;76(7):885-7.
44. Damodaran SS, Nizamie SH. Incomplete Koro. A forerunner for mood disorder: Two case reports. Ind J Psychiat. 2005;35:60-2.
45. Al-Hmoud N. Koro-like syndrome in a Jordanian male. East Mediter Health J. 1999;5:611-3.
46. Maslowski J. Koro-like syndrome in Maltese subject on the basis of chronic schizophrenia. Bull Inst Maritime Trop Medin Gdynia. 1988;39:108-10.
47. Ntouros E, Ntoumanis A, Bozikas VP, Donias S, Giouzepas I, Garyfalos G. Koro-like symptoms in two Greek men. Brit Med J Case Reps. 2010;1:1.
48. Faccini L. The incredible case of the shrinking penis: A Koro-like syndrome in a person with intellectual disability. Sexual Disab. 2009;27:173-8.
49. Witztum E, Bersudsky Y, Mayodovnik H, Kotler M. Koro-like syndrome in a Bedouin man. Psychopathol. 1998;31:174-7.
50. Heyman I, Fahy TA. Koro-like symptoms in a man infected with the human immunodeficiency virus. Brit J Psychiat. 1992;160:119-21.
51. Caballero JM, Avila A, Cardona X, Sastre F, Maho P, Bello J. Genital pain without urogenital pathology: The Koro-like syndrome. J Urol. 2000;163:243.
52. Naim M. Penile retraction in non psychiatric patients. Brit Med Journal Case Rep. 2010;22:4.
53. Chowdhury AN. Hundred years of Koro: The history of a culture-bound syndrome. Int J Soc Psychiat. 1998;44:181-8.
54. Yang H, Tranulis C, Freudenreich O. Keeping culture-bound syndromes in cultural context: The case of Koro. Int J Cul Ment Health. 2009;2:86-91.
55. Ungvari GS, Mullen RS. Koro: The delusion of penile retraction. Urol. 1994;43:883-5.
56. Chowdhury AN. Variations in the perception of penis. J Sexual Health. 1993;3:156-60.
57. Phillips KA. Body dysmorphic disorder: Recognizing and treatment of imagined ugliness. World Psychiat. 2004;3:12-7.

58. Chowdhury AN. Penile perception of Koro patients. Acta Psychiatrica Scand. 1989;80:183-6.
59. Chowdhury AN. Dysmorphic penis image perception: The root of Koro vulnerability. A longitudinal study. Acta Psychiatrica Scand. 1989;80:518-20.
60. Murtagh J. The small penis syndrome. Aus Fam Physician. 1989;18:218-20.
61. Wylie KR, Eardley I. Penile size and the 'the small penis syndrome'. Brit J Urol Int. 2007;99:1449-55.
62. Shamloul R. Treatment of men complaining of short penis. Urol. 1995;65:1183-5.
63. Lee PA, Reiter EO. Genital size: A common adolescent male concern. Adoles Med. 2002;13:171-80.
64. Simons RC, Hughes CC (Eds). The culture-bound syndromes: Folk illnesses of psychiatric and anthropological interest. Dordrecht: D. Reidel Publishing Company; 1985.
65. Edwards JW. Indigenous Koro, a genital retraction syndrome of insular Southeast Asia: A critical review. Cul Med Psychiat. 1984;8:1-24.
66. Chin CN, S'ng KH. "Koro". Like syndrome affecting the tongue. A case report. Med J Malaysia. 1995;50:175-7.
67. Chowdhury AN. Ethnomedical concept of heat and cold in Koro: Study from Indian patients. Worl Cul Psychiat Res Rev. 2008;3:146-58.
68. Chowdhury AN. Medico-cultural cognition of Koro epidemic: An ethnographic study. J Ind Anthropol Soc. 1991;26:155-70.
69. Tseng WS, Mo KM, Hsu J, Li LS, Ou LW, Chen GQ, et al. A sociocultural study of Koro epidemics in a Guangdong, China. Am J Psychiat. 1988;145:1538-43.
70. Chowdhury AN. Psychic infectivity: The role of positive illness cognition in psychiatric epidemic. J Person Clin Stud. 1992;8:125-8.
71. Cheng ST. Epidemic genital retraction syndrome: Environmental and personal risk factors in southern China. J Psychol Hum Sexuality. 1997;9:57-70.
72. Chowdhury AN. Koro social response (urban): A longitudinal study of North Bengal Koro epidemic. Ind J of Psychiat. 1992;34:46-52.
73. Tseng WS, Mo KM, Li LS, Chen GQ, Qu LW, Zheng HB. Koro epidemic in Guangdong, China. A questionnaire survey. J NervMent Dis. 1992;180:117-23.
74. Chowdhury AN, Pal P, Chatterjee A, Roy Das M, Chowdhury BB. Analysis of North Bengal Koro epidemic with three years follow up. Ind J Psychiat. 1988;30:60-72.
75. Chowdhury AN. Role of medical cognition in psychiatric outbreaks: Study from North Bengal Koro epidemic. Ind J Behav Sc. 1991;1:64-7.
76. Small GW, Borus JF. The influence of newspaper reports on outbreaks of mass hysteria. Psychiatric Quart. 1987;58:269-78.
77. Kumar R, Phookun HR, Datta A. Epidemic of Koro in North East India: an observational cross-sectional study. Asian J Psychiat. 2014;12:113-7.
78. Dan A, Mondal T, Chakraborty K, Chaudhuri A, Biswas A. Clinical course and treatment outcome of Koro: A follow up study from a Koro epidemic reported from West Bengal, India. Asian J Psychiat. 2017;26:14-20.
79. Chowdhury AN, Brahma A. Chronic Koro. East J Psychiat. 2004;8:57-9.
80. Kar N. Chronic koro-like symptoms. Two case reports. BMC Psychiatry. 2005b;5:34.
81. Chowdhury AN. Diagnostic nosology of Koro. J Personal Clin Stud. 1990;6:207-9.
82. Chowdhury AN. Koro and the Indian Psychiatrists. Ind J Soc Psychiat. 1995;11:78-80.

ABSTRACTS OF PUBLISHED STUDIES OF 2010 KORO EPIDEMIC IN WEST BENGAL

1. Chakraborty S, Sanyal D: An Outbreak of Koro among 19 Workers in a Jute Mill in South Bengal

*Industrial Psychiatry Journal. 2011;20(1):*58-60

This is a valuable paper so far as the Koro demography in an epidemic setting is concerned. The authors provided many vital details of 19 jute mill workers, all male, from southern West Bengal. No timeline of the epidemic is reported. They also provide details of two case reports. Essential points the authors provided are: (1) 84.2% were single. (2) 63.2% did not complete their secondary education. (3) 12.5% had premorbid substance abuse. (4) 12.5% had a premorbid psychotic illness. (5) 15.8% admitted homosexual activity. (6) 12.5% had commercial sex worker exposure. (7) Majority of the cases believed that the disease was caused by overindulgence to masturbatory practices or nocturnal emission. (8) In 57.9% of the case, the primary health-seeking behavior was water immersion. (9) 5.26% of cases attempted mechanical penile traction resulting in abrasive injury on the glans penis. (10) None of the cases did meet any Axis I diagnosis of DSM IV. (11) All cases believed that the disease occurred due to increased heat accumulated within the body that needed to be cooled down. (12) 26.3% of cases said, "mobile phone as the initial information tool."

2. Sinha M: Resurgence of Koro: Perception of Mankind

*Asian Journal of Psychiatry. 2011;4(2):*153-4.

This is a descriptive account of the 2010 Koro epidemic in West Bengal, India. The author provided a firsthand account of the clinical symptoms, the demography of the affected persons, the epidemic spread, and the community's preventive measures. Koro was known as "Disco" in the city. A significant female (breast symptoms only) population was also affected. Some presented with a tingling sensation all over the body associated with the penis retraction, few complained of heat emanating from the body with a rise of body temperature. The age range was from 7 to 70 years. In rural areas, this illness news provoked some overvalued ideas bordering to a shared delusion. Folk treatment of water pouring and wearing of amulets contains charmed seeds of bottle gourd was widely prevalent. In some communities:

"They have perceived it as a miraculous phenomenon created by "Allah" or "The Almighty" which has occurred due to some wrongdoings or misgivings in their daily life. To prevent further recurrences, the village leaders urged the folks to pray and read the holy "Koran" (p.153).

Chapter 6

Mumbai Koro Epidemic of 2010

Arabinda N Chowdhury

There is no published study on the Mumbai Koro epidemic, except a few media reports. There was a mini-Koro epidemic (at least 25 men were affected) among the migrant construction workers in a camp at Aarey Colony in Goregaon (E), which is a locality in the Mumbai Suburban district **(Fig. 1)**.[1]

On October 26th, 2010, the Mid-Day, a news daily in Mumbai reported: "Mass panic at labor camp in Goregaon as 25 men suffer from 'retracting' genitalia."[2] The Aarey milk colony is situated in Goregaon East, Mumbai, and houses several labor camps, where people come to work from different parts of India. Mr Rai, one of the victims who came from Orissa, said: "On Sunday night, I experienced extreme heat emanating from my body. My genitalia was retracting, and I was really worried. Later, on my friends' advice, I jumped into a tub of iced water and sat there for 3–4 hours." He also said, "We all are from Orissa, Bengal, and Kolkata, but I have noticed that men from Orissa and Bengal are suffering the most." Another victim, who came from Assam, said, "I am shivering because of the cold and the heat that is emanating from my body. But I will sit in the water only. My relatives in Assam guided me on the disease and now I am feeling better." At least 25 other workers (all male)

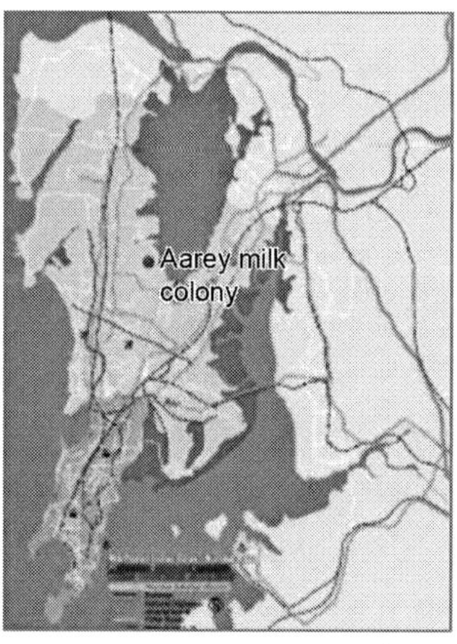

Fig. 1: Aarey milk colony.[1]

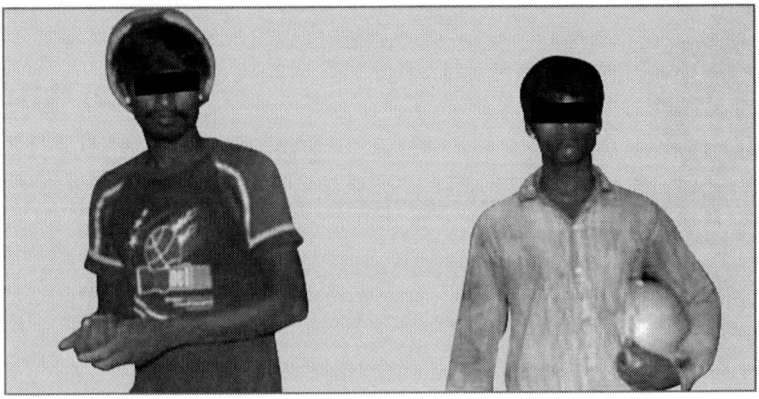

Fig. 2: Media Report in Mumbai on 26.10.10.
Source: https://archive.mid-day.com/news/2010/oct/261010-labour-camp-Goregaon-Aarey- Colony-Koro-mumbai.htm.

reported similar symptoms, with most victims coming from West Bengal and Orissa states. These incidents created an air of panic in the camp. The news also received high publicity in other media and blogs in Mumbai (Wellsphere, 2010; Now Public Staff, 2010) and also in Assam (Assam Tribune)[3,4] and West Bengal (The Statesman).[5] Though no details were found about the index case at Aarey Colony, it is worth noting that there was a mass scale Koro affliction reported from the labor colony. Interesting to note that the Aarey colony news was instantly communicated by the victims over mobile phones to their relatives in West Bengal and Assam, which also precipitated a Koro epidemic in both states.[6,7] The role of mobile phones in the instant transmission of epidemic news is a research area in the cause and spread of psychiatric epidemics in this technological age. One case of a sporadic Koro with Dhat syndrome was reported from Mumbai in 2012.[8]

The following are the media reports from Mumbai. Interestingly, one may note the lime paste marking on the ear lobules of both the migrant workers **(Fig. 2)**.

Mid-day

2010-10-26
Mumbai

GENITALS SHRINK AT CONSTRUCTION SITE

The Curious Case of Shrinking Genitalia

By: Ketan Ranga, Date: 2010-10-26, Place: Mumbai

Mass panic at labor camp in Goregaon as 25 men suffer from "retracting" genitalia.[2]

Several laborers living in a workcamp near the Aarey Colony in Goregaon have been spending sleepless nights since Saturday after they found that the size of their genitals have been gradually reducing and getting inside the lower abdomen **(Fig. 3)**. The panicked sat in a bathtub and family members poured water on them to cure them.

The relatives of the afflicted told Mid-Day that the workers have been suffering from Koro since Saturday. Govind Rai, a recent victim of Koro, said, "On Sunday night, I experienced extreme heat emanating from my body.

My genitalia were retracting and I was really worried. Later, on my friends' advice, I jumped into a tub of iced water and sat there for 3–4 hours."

Rai added that the treatment worked and he was cured of the deadly disease by yesterday evening. Further investigations revealed that at least 25 people were suffering from the same ailment.

"We all are from Orissa, Bengal, Kolkata, but I have noticed that men from Orissa and Bengal are suffering the most," said Rai.

The construction site manager said, "We called the doctor last night but he, too, was unaware of the reason for the ailment."

One of the victims of Koro said, "I am shivering because of the cold and the heat that is emanating from my body. But I will sit in the water only. I am unaware why I am suffering from this disorder. My relatives in Assam guided me on the disease and now I am feeling better."

Police officials from Aarey Colony came to the labor camp around 1 AM and started questioning the laborers. They also took down the statements of the victims and other camp workers.

Inspector Girish Ahvankar said, "We will record the statement of the victims. However, this is not a police case."

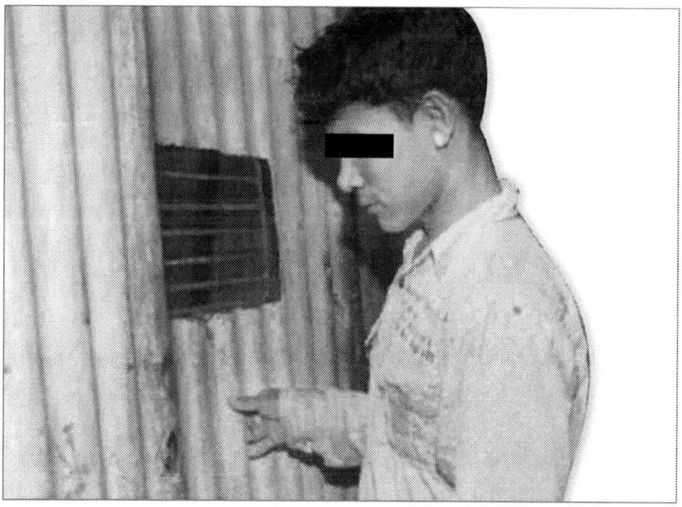

Fig. 3: An aggrieved laborer enters the site for treatment.

Initial enquiry ruled out infection to be the cause of the epidemic, as no chemicals or detergents were present at the site.

A representative from the PR agency that looks after the publicity of the builder for whom the laborers work, said, "We were not aware that the workers were suffering from such an ailment.

A doctor was sent and we will look into the matter." ....

MEDIA REPORT IN MUMBAI ON 2.11.10

Providentia

A Biased Look at Psychology in the World

November 02, 2010

Koro epidemic strikes Indian labor camp: Workers at a labor camp in the Aarey Milk Colony near Mumbai, India have recently begun complaining that their genitals are shrinking and retreating into their bodies. One victim, Govind Rai reported feeling "extreme heat emanating from my body. My genitalia were retracting and I was really worried. Later, on my friends' advice, I jumped into a tub of iced water and sat there for 3–4 hours." The treatment was apparently successful and Rai had a complete cessation of all symptoms. At least 25 other workers (all males) reported similar symptoms with most victims coming from the Bengal and Orissa areas of India. While a medical doctor was called in on the case, no cause for the outbreak could be determined and medical treatment provided little relief. The possible role of chemical or infectious agents at the work site has also been ruled out. In many cases, victims sought advice from relatives who advised them to use iced water based on old folk remedies. A police investigation has been carried out although the matter is not seen as suspicious.

While outbreaks of KORO (a culture-specific syndrome involving belief that the genitals are shrinking and retreating into the body) are most common in China and other parts of south-east Asia, sporadic cases have also been reported in other countries such as Thailand, India, and even western nations such as Canada. Typically involving Chinese immigrants, possible cultural diffusion have led to cases involving non-Chinese victims as well. Shrinking penis epidemics have also been reported in African nations and outbreaks of workplace-related mass hysteria remain well-documented in clinical and historical literature.

Source: https://drvitelli.typepad.com/providentia/2010/11/koro-epidemic-strikes-indian-labour-camp.html

REFERENCES

1. Ujjal K. (2019). Mumbai oxygen supply cutting down. September 1, 2019,Infotonline. [online] Available from https://infotonline.com/mumbai-oxygen-supply-cutting-down/. [Last accessed March, 2023].

2. Ranga K. (2010). The curious cases of shrinking genitalia: Mass panic at labour camp in Goregaon as twenty five men suffer from 'retracting' genitalia. Mid-Day, 26. October, 2010. [online] Available from http://www.mid-day.com/news/2010/oct/261010-labour-camp-Goregaon-Aarey-Colony-Koro- mumbai.htm. [Last accessed March, 2023].
3. The Assam Tribune. (2010). It's a cultural syndrome, say doctors. 30 September, 2010. [online] Available from http://www.assamtribune.com/scripts/detailsnew.asp?id=sep3010/city06. [Last accessed March, 2023].
4. Duarah K. (2010). Ignorance causing panic among certain people. 30 September 2010. The Assam Tribune. [online] Available from http://www assamtribune.com/ scripts/detailsnew.asp?id =sep3010/city05. [Last accessed March, 2023].
5. The Statesman. (2010). KMC move to treat Koro patients. 10 November 2010. [online] Available from http://www. thestatesman.net/index.php?option=com_content&view=article&id=348109&catid=73. [Last accessed March, 2023].
6. Roy D, Hazarika S, Bhattacharya A, Das S, Nath K, Saddichha S. Koro: Culture bound or mass hysteria? Aust & NZ J Psychiatry. 2011;45(8):683.
7. Ghosh S, Nath S, Brahma A, Chowdhury AN. Fifth Koro epidemic in India: A review report. World Cult Psychiat Res Rev. 2013;8(1):8-20.
8. Kalra GS, Bansod A, Shah NB. A case report of dhat and koro: A double jeopardy. ASEAN J Psychiat. 2012;13(1):91-5.

Chapter 7

Assam

INTRODUCTION

Assam[1] is situated in Northeastern India, south of the eastern Himalayas range along the Brahmaputra and Barak River valleys **(Fig. 1)**. Assam covers an area of 78,438 km^2 (30,285 sq mi) with 41 administrative districts. Geographically, it has both national and international borders. The state is bordered by Bhutan and Arunachal Pradesh to the north; Nagaland and Manipur to the east; Meghalaya, Tripura, Mizoram, and Bangladesh to the south; and West Bengal to the west via the Siliguri Corridor, a 22 km-wide strip of land that connects the state to the rest of India.

As per the 2011 census, the total population of Assam was 31,169,272. Religious division was: 61.47% Hindus, 34.22% were Muslims, and 3.7% Christians. The literacy rate was 73.18% (male: 78.81% and female: 67.27%). Assamese is the official and most commonly spoken language, followed by Bengali. Assam is one of the highest tea-producing areas globally, contributing

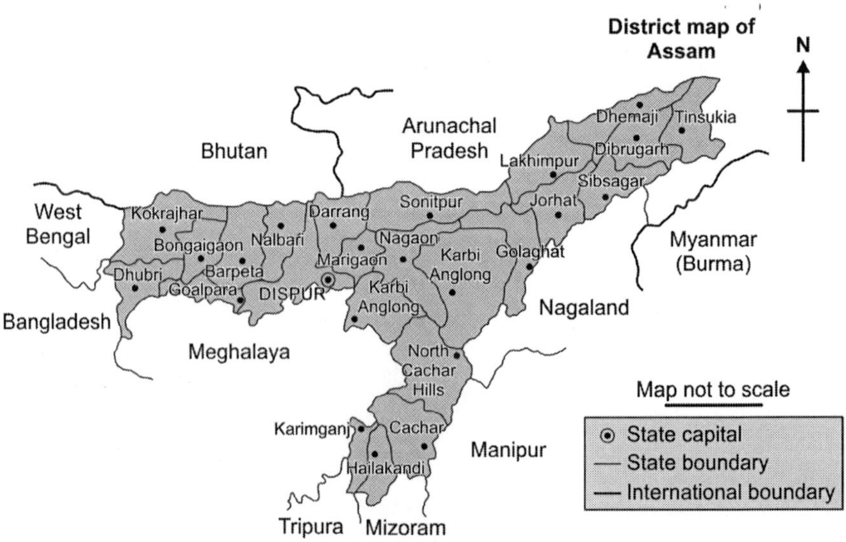

Fig. 1: Map of Assam.
Source: https://www.researchgate.net/figure/District-map-of-Assam_fig1_242209612.

80% of India's export and 55% of the country's total tea production. The state has a unique biodiversity with a huge river system, mountain range, and home for diverse animals, wildlife including world-famous National Parks. Assam has an extended historical past and is associated with many mythological histories and traditions. Guwahati is one of the fastest-growing cosmopolitan cities in India. It is situated on the south bank of the Brahmaputra. The state capital Dispur is situated in Guwahati. It is well connected by roads, railways, and an international airport. It is called the "Gateway to Northeast India."[2] Guwahati derives its name from the Assamese word "Guva" derived from the Sanskrit word *Guvaka*, meaning areca nut and its plant, and "Hati" representing rows, the rows of areca nut trees.[3]

REFERENCES

1. Assam. [online] Available from https://en.wikipedia.org/wiki/Assam. [Last accessed March, 2023].
2. Guwahati a gateway to the exotic North East. (2011). [online] Available from https://mumbaimirror.indiatimes.com/mumbai/other/Guwahati-a-gateway-to-the-exotic-North- East/articleshow/16183684.cms. [Last accessed March, 2023].
3. Sharma MM. Inscriptions of Ancient Assam. Assam: Department of Publication, Gauhati University; 1978; p. 137.

COMMENTARY ON 1982 ASSAM KORO EPIDEMIC

Hemendraram Phookun

It was the morning of June 1982; we sat at Psychiatry OPD, Gauhati Medical College Hospital, attending to patients. Outside the OPD, there was a hue and cry, and a young boy of around 16 years was brought (somewhat physically lifted) by four attendants, one of them firmly holding his penis. They put the boy on the examination table but did not let go of the grip on his penis. They frantically shouted, "Sir! Please save him, his penis is retreating inside his abdomen, and he will die." I proceeded to examine the boy. After that, with a lot of patience and assurances, I convinced the patient and the attendants that it would not retreat inside and succeeded in letting go of the firm grip of the patient's father from his penis. The attendants were relieved to see that the penis did not retreat. After about an hour, we disposed of the case with some anxiolytic prescribed for 2–3 days. At that moment, I failed to make a diagnosis but vaguely remembered reading somewhere in the *Comprehensive Textbook of Psychiatry (CTP)*, a similar description of some cases. After coming back from duty, I consulted the CTP and finally found the definition of a condition called "Koro." I was quite surprised as this has been a culture-bound syndrome in only some southeast Asian countries and Chinese populations. How did it come to Assam that intrigued me? Since then, from June to September 1982, we came across many such cases, so I took it up as a project to let the world know that Koro has also been reported from Assam.

The findings of the study is depicted as follows:

As described in a textbook of psychiatry, Koro is "an acute anxiety reaction characterized by the patient's desperate fear that his penis is shrinking and will disappear into his abdomen, and he may die. Almost invariably, the affected person secures a strong hold of his penis by tying a ribbon around it or clamping it into a wooden box. Females correspondingly may experience the feeling of shrinkage of their breast and labia."[1]

As early as 1834, Pao described this condition as a severe state of emergency requiring immediate treatment, failing which death might ensure.[2] Yap,[3] in his series of 19 cases of Koro collected over 15 years stressed a number of points, i.e., affected persons having poor education, possessing immature, dependent personalities, and lacking confidence in his masculinity are more likely to be involved. He emphasized the need to recognize it as a class of "a typical culture-bound psychogenic psychosis," to which Koro belongs.

So far, Koro was confined to the South Chinese population of lower Yangtze valley and amongst the Chinese population in Southeast Asia, especially Malaysia and Indochina.[3-5] Sporadic cases have been reported to occur in Canadians,[6,7] in an American schizophrenic,[8] in Sudanese[9] and in Indian population.[10,11] Koro occurring in epidemic form in Singapore in 1967 reported by Ngui,[12] who said a series of 228 cases confirming the predominance of the disease in the Chinese population and also the presence of the personal and cultural concept of Koro in that culture as important predetermining factors in the development of this disease.

In the early eighties, the State Health of Assam faced a unique situation as dozens of SOS messages kept pouring in from doctors working in rural, subdivisional and district hospitals and petitions from public leaders. One wireless message from a subdivisional office in the later part of June 1982 came, stating "Shrinkage of testicles of males and nipples of females affected eight villages since mid-June. No definite disease could be established. No death reported, no relapse reported. Please send expert." A team of experts consisting of senior physicians and neurologists, and neurosurgeons visited the affected area of Assam. They opined that there is no disease, only a fear psychosis based on rumor related to the first case of Koro. He was a 16-year-old Assamese Hindu schoolboy from North Kamrup who was bought for a consultation to the Department of Psychiatry, Gauhati Medical College and Hospital. He was a panic-stricken adolescent boy who was seen firmly grasping his penis by his hand. Since then, we have encountered many cases of Koro, often coming in batches to our outpatient department as well as in private clinics.

This disease started with a tingling sensation over the legs, so in Assamese, we named it as Jinjinia bemar; *Jinjinia* means tingling, and *bemar* means disease. After diagnosing this epidemic as an epidemic of Koro, a team was immediately formed that decided to undertake the following steps to combat the outbreak.

- A unique history sheet was improvised to have a uniform case record
- Arrangements were made for the on-the-spot study of the area affected by the epidemic.
- A uniform plan of treatment and management were envisaged.
- Mass education and consultation with the State Government Health Secretariat press notes were released through various mass media.
- Contacts were established with all practitioners of the affected area.

We had a total of 83 cases which we examined either in the psychiatry outpatient department or in private clinics and also in on-the-spot study tours of the affected areas. Using a semistructured interview schedule, all cases were interviewed independently, at least by two of our psychiatrists. Cases were managed using both psychological and pharmacological methods of treatment. Reviews were made as and when necessary. A detailed history was taken from the accompanying persons regarding predisposing and precipitating factors.

Four districts of lower Assam were under the grip of the epidemic from the later part of June 1982 to the middle of September 1982. The symptomatology of the condition in any of these particular areas lasted for 3–5 days. No new cases were reported after 11 September 1982. This coincided with massive public awareness and health education measures through print and visual media in the first week of September. For interior places, microphones were used for general education and awareness.

Four districts of Assam, viz., Goalpara, Kamrup, Darrang, and Nagaon were mainly affected out of 10 districts of Assam at that time. The epidemic spread from west to east. Considering the degree of panic generated among the population, the number of cases seen by us was relatively small. The reason probably is that the condition's nature was such that most of the patients got cured without any medical help.

Interestingly, the epidemic appeared to jump from one village to a distant village leaving many villages in between miraculously "escaped" from its grip, despite their proximity to the affected areas.

As far as sex distribution is concerned, 64 out of 83 cases (77.1%) were males, and 23.9% were females. Analysis of age variation ranged from $1^{1/2}$ to 40 years. This youngest one and 1/2-year-old Hindu male child was undoubtedly the victim of his mother's anxiety. Another 4-year-old Christian boy actually complained of penile shrinkage in his colloquial terms. 43 out of 83 cases (55.4%) belonged to the age group of 20–29 years. There were 29 cases in the age group of 10–19 years. No single case was recorded above the age of 40 years. 49 out of 83 cases (59%) were unmarried, whereas 33 (41%) cases were married. One case was a widow. 69 out of 83 cases (83.1%) were Hindus, 13 (17.3%) were Muslims, and one Christian. 51 (61.4%) belonged to the Assamese community, 20 (24.1%) were Bengalis, and one Rajasthani.

It was found that 22 (26.5%) out of 83 were skilled workers, and 22 out of 83 were unskilled workers; of which 19 cases were students of various standards, 12 were homemakers, 6 were semiskilled workers, and two were minor children.

Socioeconomic status showed that 48 (61.3%) out of 75 belonged to the middle-income class and 22 (26.5%) belonged to the lower economic class. In 8 cases, socioeconomic status was not recorded.

In our data, 37 out of 83 (44.6%) were educated up to higher secondary level, 8 were graduates, one was an engineering student, law-cum-chartered accountant student, and radiographer. Hence, education provided no immunity to the misconception circulating around human reproductive biology.

The data found that 53 out of 73 (74%) attacks started at home, 20 while they were engaged in outdoor activities and in educational institutes. In 10 cases, there were no records of the place of occurrence.

As regards the time of occurrence 58 out of 73 cases (79.4%) showed the first manifestation during the hour 6 PM to 6 AM, with a full record between 7 PM to 1 AM, while they were either studying or sleeping. In 15 cases, attacks occurred during the day. In 10 cases, the time of occurrence were not recorded. These tally with Ngui's (1969)[12] findings that Koro attacks are more prone to develop at night when a person gets more time for introspection, sexual fantasies, sexual stimulations, and sexual acts.

Regarding the presence of a history of hearsay or witnessing a Koro attack: In 60 (72.3%) out of 83, there was a definite history of hearsay, discussion, or witnessing a Koro case. Most cases admitted apprehension or preoccupation with fear of contracting this so-called dreadful and killer disease.

The attack's duration lasted from 5 minutes to 5 hours with an average of 25 minutes. Symptoms found in Koro cases were classified under three subgroups:

1. *Genital symptoms:* Shrinkage and the inward pull of penis in males and shrinkage and the inward pull of breast and labia in females.
2. *Anxiety symptoms:* Fear, apprehension, palpitation, sweating, sinking feeling, air hunger, extreme retrosternal pain, excessive thirst, restlessness, and sense of impending death.
3. *The disturbed state of consciousness:* Tingling sensation starting from the toes creeping upward leading to dizziness and fainting attack, which may vary from a semiconscious state with bizarre movements or with total dissociation of variable duration.

Nine out of 19 female cases (47.3%) suffered from genital symptoms in the form of shrinkage or pull of breast and labia. 12 out of 19 cases (69.1%) reported retrosternal pain and other anxiety symptoms leading to dissociation of varying degrees and duration. In almost all cases, anxiety symptoms manifested first. 33 out of 47 (70.1%) male cases came with shrinkage and invert pull of the penis. Three of them tied their penis with rubber bands and ribbons. Complete dissociation was not seen in male cases. Almost all male cases came wearing a dhoti, lungi, or gamosa (towel) for easy accessibility to the genitals as and when required to be grabbed by them. Only 10 out of 83 cases (12.04%) had a history of relapse within 30 days of initial illness. They had relapses of one to five times, and every time came for reconsultation. Most of the cases relapsed with anxiety symptoms only. Only two out of 10 cases came with relapse of genital symptoms.

The treatment procedures which were adopted mainly were supportive psychotherapy and reassurance. Only cases with moderate-to-severe symptoms were given mild doses of antianxiety medicines, and occasionally antidepressants were indicated.

REFERENCES

1. Freedman AM, Kaplan JH, Saddock DJ Koro. Comprehensive Textbook of Psychiatry, 2nd edition. Baltimore: Williams and Wilkins; 1976; pp. 1127-731.
2. Gwee AL. Koro a cultural disease. Singapore Med J. 1963; 4:119.
3. Yap PM. Koro a culture bound depersonalization syndrome. Brit J Psychiat. 1965;111:43.

4. Kiev A. Trans cultural psychiatry. New York: The Free Press, and London: Collier-Macmillan Limited; 1972. pp. 4,79.
5. Rin H. Koro: A consideration of Chinese concepts of illness and case illustrations. Trans Psychiatric Res. 1965;15:23-5.
6. Dow TW, Silver E. A drug induced koro syndrome. J Florida Med Assoc. 1973;60:32.
7. Lapierre YD. Koro in a France Canadian. Can Psychiat Assoc J. 1972;17:333-4.
8. Edward JG. The koro pattern of depersonalization in an American schizophrenic patient. Med J Psychiat. 1970;126(8):1171-3.
9. Baasher TA. The influence of culture on psychiatric manifestation. Trans. Psychiat Res Rev. 1963;15:51-2.
10. Shukla JD, Mishra DN. Koro-like syndrome. Ind J Psychiat. 1981;23:96-7.
11. Chakravarty PK. Koro a peculiar anxiety neurosis (a case report) Ind J Psychiat. 1982;24:192-3.
12. Ngui PW. The koro epidemic in Singapore. Aus NJ J Psychiat. 1969;3:263-6.

ABSTRACTS OF PUBLISHED STUDIES OF 1982 AND 2010 ASSAM KORO EPIDEMICS

1. PS Sachdev, A Shukla: Epidemic Koro Syndrome in India
Lancet, 1982, II, 1161.

It is a brief report of the 1982 Koro epidemic of Assam. The authors reported a cohort of 60 Koro cases from a village near Guwahati (Assam) from 600 households, with a detailed analysis of 30 patients (17 males and 13 females). The majority of cases were from the age group of 20–40 years, and about two thirds of them were married and were mainly from the lower economic class. The disease was locally termed "*Jhinjhinia bimari*", meaning a tingling illness or condition as the onset symptom was a tingling sensation in the legs. The authors report different social modes of treatment, viz., cold water pouring, lime juice drinking, and holding of the shrinking penis.

2. D Dutta: Koro Epidemic in Assam
British Journal of Psychiatry, 1983, 143, 309-310.

It is a brief report on the Koro epidemic of lower Assam, India, reported in response to three epidemic psychoses reported by Harrington (BJP 1982, 141: 98-99). She mentioned some interesting observations on the Assam Koro epidemic (June 1982). The local name of the disorder was 'Jinjina Bemar' (tingling illness). She mentioned the role of a local rumour to precipitate the epidemic—"a lethal disease had struck the people bringing instant death or making the person impotent." She mentioned different indigenous strategies to combat the disease as "pouring copious cold water, drinking gallons of lemon water, smearing of chalk paste or lime paste over the ear lobules and also over the private parts." Both sexes were affected. The intensity of the epidemic faded away in the middle of September this year.

3. D Dutta, HR Phookan, PD Das: The Koro Epidemic in Lower Assam
Indian Journal of Psychiatry, 1982, 24, 370-374.

This is a report of the Koro epidemic of Assam, which took place from June to September 1982. Four districts (Goalpara, Kamrup, Darrang, and Nagaon) out of ten were affected mostly by this epidemic **(Fig. 1)**.

This is a comprehensive report of the first Koro epidemic on Indian soil and provides detailed features of both the individual and the outbreak from Indian culture and Assamese ethnicity. The authors describe 83 cases, 64 males and 19 females. The main findings are grouped under the following headings.

Demographic Characteristics

The age range was 4–40 years, where most cases (55.4%) were between 20 and 29 years. Marital status: 59% of the patients were single and 41%

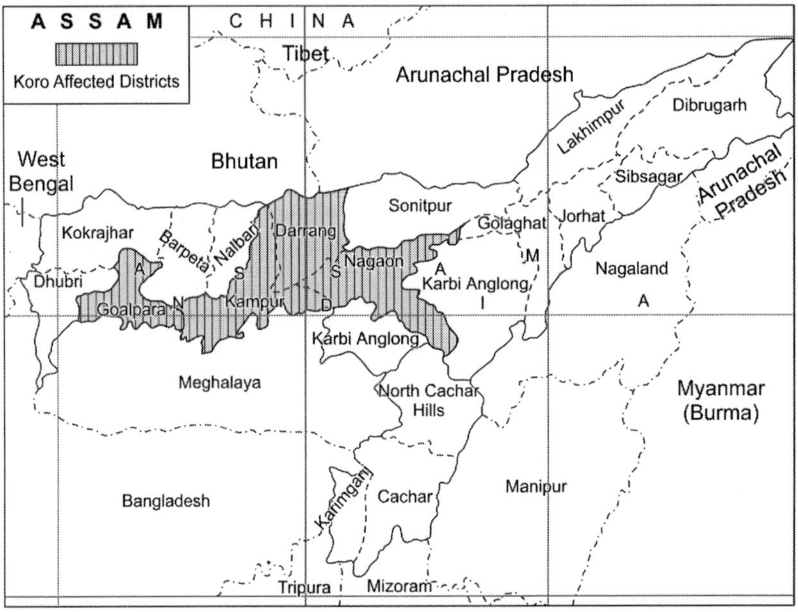

Fig. 1: Koro-affected districts.

married. Religion: 83.1% were Hindus, 15.7% Muslims, and 1.2% Christians. Ethnicity—61.4% were Assamese (Hindu, Muslim, and Tribal), 24% were Bengalese, and 1.2% were Rajasthanis. Education: 3.6% were students of some professional courses (Engineering, Law, and Chartered Accountancy), 9.6% were graduates, 44.6% were educated up to secondary level, and 19.3% were illiterate.

Occupation: 43% had no work, including two minors and 12 homemakers, 33.8% were workers, and 23.8% were students. Socioeconomic status: 61% from middle economic classes, 27% lower economic class, and 6% were from the upper level.

Clinical Characteristics

- *Time and place of attack:* 74% started indoors while 24% were outdoors. In 10 cases, there was no record. 79.4% of attacks occurred between 6 PM and 6 AM, with a maximum record between 7 AM and 1 PM.
- *Presence of hearsay history or witnessing a Koro patient:* 72.3% of the cases had definite exposure to gossip, discussion, or seeing a Koro case on the day of their attack or within the previous 2–3 days. Most of the subjects showed great apprehension about the infective nature of the illness.
- *Duration of attack:* Koro attacks lasted from 5 minutes to 5 hours, with an average duration of 25 minutes.
- *Symptoms:*
  - *Genital:* Shrinkage and the inward pull of the penis in males and shrinkage or inward pull of the breast in females were the main

presenting features. Out of the 19 females, only nine (47.3%) had Koro breast symptoms, and no one had genital complaints. The remaining female cases showed varieties of anxiety symptoms. 33 males (70.1%) had shrinkage and the inward pull of the penis.

- *Anxiety symptoms:* Different psychosomatic expressions of anxiety were present. These are fear, apprehension, palpitation, sweating, sinking feeling, air hunger, extreme retrosternal pain, excessive thirst, restlessness, and a sense of impending death.
- *Disturbed consciousness:* A tingling sensation started from the toes with upward radiation in some cases. It was followed by a dizziness and fainting spell, which varied from a semiconscious state with abnormal movements to total dissociation of variable duration.
- *Relapse:* 12% of cases had a history of relapse within 30 days of the first attack.

The author failed to trace any significant contribution in the cases of overt sexual perversions or overindulgence. The illness earned a local Assamese name—"Jhin-Jhinia" in the community. Mass education initiatives by media and administration were instrumental in mitigating the epidemic's spread beyond 11 September 1982.

4. R Kumar, HR Phookun, A Datta: Koro: A Culture Bound Syndrome: An Anxiety Disorder

Indian Journal of Psychiatry, 2013, 55 (Suppl.1): S131-S132 (Poster 18.17).

A study report of 20 Koro patients attended the hospital in the background of an ongoing epidemic in Assam, India. Most of the patients were young single males of lower socioeconomic strata. The three most prominent symptoms were: (1) Tingling sensation originated from the thigh and spread to the abdomen or other body parts; (2) shortening of the penis; (3) Severe degrees of anxiety with increased worrying about genitalia, restlessness, increased sweating, and fear of death. This episode was of very severe intensity and short lived. The authors commented that this presentation is well befitting with an acute anxiety state, and most of them responded positively with psychoeducation and benzodiazepine. They were very eager to be treated immediately.

5. R Kumar, HR Phookun, A Datta: Epidemic of Koro in North East India: An Observational Cross-Sectional Study

Asian Journal of Psychiatry, 2014, 12: 113-117.

This is a 2010 Koro epidemic report from India. It is a very comprehensive and detailed reporting of Koro epidemic (70 cases, including two females), as observed in the Gauhati city, Assam.

The description of Koro demography is essential:

A percentage of 61.4% lied within the age group of 21–30 years and 70% were single. 68.5% presented at the hospital casualty department. 64.2% were from Hindu religion, 34.3% were of Islamic faith, and 1.4% was Sikh. 62.8% were from lower socioeconomic status. 71.4% had education above high school. The authors provided a detailed clinical description as follows:

- 82.8% of cases had prior knowledge of Koro.
- 30% witnesses Koro attacks in the community.
- 85.7% of attacks occurred at home.
- 72.8% of attacks were at night.

A host of anxiety symptoms accompanied the Koro attack: Tingling sensation (90%); restlessness (85.7%), sweating (75.7%), and palpitation (70%). The attack itself was comprised of: (1) feeling of retraction or shortening of the penis; (2) tingling sensation originated from the thigh and radiating to the body; and (3) severe anxiety about genitalia and fear of death. Two female patients complained about the shortening and retraction of nipple and female genitals inward with fear of death. The local name was "Jhinjhinia Bemar," and people believed that "bad air" or "bad spirit" was the cause of the illness.

Patients were successfully treated with pharmacotherapy, psychotherapy, and mass education program. The photograph of traditional treatment (victim carried in a giant water bucket) is unique and enriched the presentation. The presentation is very standard and touched all the relevant issues of clinical significance. One crucial point is that the authors excluded some cases (numbers not mentioned) who have coexisting "schizophrenia, delusional disorder, other psychosis, or some significant medical or surgical genital's illness." Information on these patients may offer precious insight into the clinical diversity of secondary Koro cases. This is a fair reporting of the 2010 Assam Koro epidemic.

Chapter

8

Koro Epidemics in Tripura

INTRODUCTION

Tripura[1] is a landlocked state in Northeastern India. It is the third-smallest state in India **(Fig. 1)**. It covers an area of 10,491.69 km^2 (4,050.86 sq mi) and is bordered by Bangladesh to the north, south, and west, and the Indian states of Assam and Mizoram to the east. In 2011, the state had 3,671,032 residents, with 1,871,867 males and 1,799,165 females, constituting 0.3% of India's population. As of 2012, the state had eight districts, 23 subdivisions, and 58 development blocks. Agartala is the capital of Tripura and is the most populous city. The state has a long history of monarchy-ruling dynasties.

According to the 2001 census of India, Bengalis represented almost 70% of Tripura's population while the Tripuri population amounted to 30%. In the

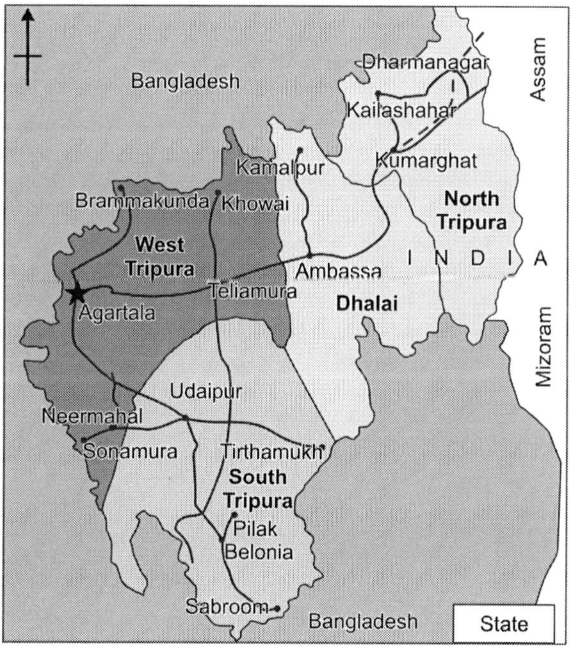

Fig. 1: Map of Tripura.
Source: https://www.traveldealsfinder.com/tripura-maps.html.

2011 census, Hinduism was a significant religion—83.40% of the population. Muslims made up 8.60% of the people, Christians 4.35%, and Buddhists 3.41%.

The state's official languages are Bengali, English, and Kokborok (Tripuri). Bengali is the most widely spoken language, while Kokborok is the most prominent language among the Tripuri people. According to the 2011 census, Tripura is one of the most literate states in India, with a literacy rate of 87.75%.

Agartala, the state capital is located on the banks of the Haora River, near the Bangladesh border [about 90 km (55 mi) east of Bangladesh's capital Dhaka]. Agartala is India's third international internet gateway after Mumbai and Chennai.[2] As of the 2011 Indian Census, Agartala had a total population of 400,004 (200,132 males and 199,872 females). One domestic airport is located 12 km northwest of Agartala, and it is the second busiest airport in northeast India after Guwahati. There are direct flights to Kolkata, Imphal, Delhi, Shillong, Guwahati, Bangalore, Chennai, Ahmedabad, and Mumbai. Only one major road, the National Highway (NH8), connects Tripura to the rest of India. National Highways (NH) connect Agartala to Assam and the rest of India by road, also known as the lifeline of Tripura. The highways (NH44, NH 44A) connect Agartala with other capitals of North-Eastern states: Silchar (317 km), Guwahati (599 km), Shillong (499 km), Dharmanagar (200 km), and Aizawl (443 km). Tripura has an 856 km (532 mi) long international border with Bangladesh. A bus service connects it to Dhaka (150 km). Railway connection with Assam from the north side of the state. From 2016 trains run from Agartala to Kolkata and Delhi.

REFERENCES

1. Tripura. [online] Available from https://en.wikipedia.org/wiki/Tripura. [Last accessed March, 2023].
2. Times of India. (2016). Agartala becomes India's third int'l internet gateway. 25 March 2016. [online] Available from https://timesofindia.indiatimes.com/city/agartala/Agartala-becomes-Indias-third-intl-internet-gateway/articleshow/51544682.cms. [Last accessed March, 2023].

KORO EPIDEMICS: A RECURRING TREND IN TRIPURA

Dipayan Sarkar, BK Bhowmic, JM Ghosh, Sakal Kumar Gupta

PREAMBLE

Koro is a culture-bound psychogenic disorder in which individuals firmly believe that their sex organs are retracting and will disappear, despite the lack of any actual shrinkage or retraction of their genitals. In males, it involves mainly the penis and often the scrotum, and in females, it consists of the vagina or breasts.[1] Tripura, a Northeastern state in India, evidenced four distinct episodes of Koro epidemic in different parts of the state in 1998, 2005, 2008, and 2015. It involved both males and females. The symptoms were subsided by early intervention from the Government of Tripura and a team from the Indian Psychiatric Society. No death was recorded.

INTRODUCTION

Koro is a culture-bond psychogenic disorder. It is also known as "shrinking penis syndrome" or "genital retraction syndrome" throughout the globe. The word Koro is derived from Malay term, which means head of the turtle refers to how it looks when they retract their heads into the shells.[2] Koro is classified as an "Other specified Obsessive-Compulsive and Related Disorders" (ORCD) in the Diagnostic and Statistical Manual of Mental Disorders 5 edition (DSM 5). In DSM-IV, it was incorporated in "Culture-bound Syndromes."

It has been described as primary in sporadic or epidemic context when it appears only with genital retraction symptoms with fear of death or sexual disability. It is associated with some comorbid mental, neurological, or urological diseases in secondary Koro. Koro is often present without a clear history of psychosis or psychiatric conditions. Some studies have demonstrated a clear link between psychosis and other psychiatric disorders. Koro has also been observed in patients with schizophrenia, depression, obsessive compulsive disorder (OCD), body dysmorphic, somatization disorder, depersonalization, sexual disorders not otherwise specified, conversion reaction, poor intellectual functioning, and voyeuristic tendencies.[3-6]

SOCIOCULTURAL SCENARIO

Tripura is a Northeastern state of India with around 37 lakh population. It is encompassed by Bangladesh almost on all three sides with a narrow strip through Assam and Mizoram states. It is terrain hills covered with dense forests and valleys. Its economic progression is hindered due to geographical isolation from the rest of the country. Surprisingly, the literacy rate of Tripura in 2011 was 87.75%, higher than the national average of 74.04 % and third best among all the states. The climatic condition is generally hot and humid. The main occupation of people is cultivation, tea, and rubber plantation. The primary inhabitant of the state is Bengali (60–70 %), a Tribal community (30%), and a minority group comprising Buddhists, Muslims, and Christians mainly. The people living in valleys are mostly mixed populations. They share some of their social values and rituals. Peoples' lives of all sections are influenced by ancient beliefs of God, ghosts, etc. In crises, especially in hill and rural areas, a small fraction still rushes to a faith healer and seeks help for remedies. However, a rapid change toward scientific upgradation was observed in the last decade.

EPIDEMICS IN TRIPURA

Recordable first episode of koro occurred in 1998 in Agartala town and was restricted to about a 20 km radius around Agartala, capital of Tripura. Hundreds of young males and females were affected with complaints of the retracted penis in the abdomen and retraction of breasts in the chest cavity in females. As per verbal eyewitness of that episodes, the victim visited faith healers who tied up a red or yellow ribbon around the right wrist of males and the left wrist of females, with chanting mantras in their dialects and sprinkled water on the victim's head and body. All of them were from the Tribal community. No deaths were reported.

Most of the people believed that the disease occurred because of the evil eyes of ghosts and would stopped automatically when the ghost moved away from the particular area to elsewhere.

The second episode occurred in 2005 July, in Taibandal area under the then West district (presently comes under Sipahijala district). Information collected from the practicing doctors of that time posted in Melaghar Subdivisional hospital and a nearby hospital reveals that around 30 patients came to OPD with similar symptoms in 1 week. The episode finished with the timely intervention of administration and medical officers working there. The administrative staff talked to patients and warned local quacks to stay away from them.

The third episode occurred in 2008 August, in Dhalai district of Tripura. The episode is restricted to two small adjacent villages Laljhuri and Shahilpara about 8 km from Ambassa town. They were mostly of a mixed population of Tribal and Bengali community with average education of 5–6 years of schooling. Eight individuals were affected within a span of 12 days in a chain reaction. No apparent precipitating factors were noticed. A team of psychiatrists from the government and a team from Indian Psychiatric Society, Tripura State Branch, moved to the affected area immediately, did IEC (Information, Education, and Communication) activity, and tried to treat the symptoms. The index case was 40 years married male of Mog community (a section of the Tribal community). Before the onset, a rumour spread among the inhabitants of two villages that a peculiar and severe type of disease that spreads through harmful elements of air of ghosts involving the penis started in nearby villages about 5 km away from the village. On hearing this, the people of the two villages became alert, searched and stopped going out of their village. Some of the young men shouted at night, saying "ayere ayere" meaning coming (of the cursed illness). The inhabitants were already anxious, and it aggravated the situation. The episode primarily began after the sunset, and all the victims felt shivering for 2–3 minutes, followed by a tingling sensation in the penis and mild lower abdominal pain. Thinking this as fatal, they tried to pull their penis to resist its ingoing and simultaneously shouted for help, while others became anxious and tensed. Nearby people rushed to the victim's spot, out of curiosity and sympathy; *Ojha* and *Tantric* were called for remedial measures, but that provided no improvement in the situations. During the attack, they were anxious, and restless; perspiration with hurried respiration, palpitation, and tremor and became preoccupied with impending death. All were in a panic state. Each episode lasted 2–4 minutes with an average of three to five times during 4–5 days.

The fourth episode occurred in 2015, March-July, in Shantirbazar area in the South district. Many cases were recorded in the Karbook subdivision.[7] Three villages were affected, and at least 20 patients had similar classical symptoms of genital retraction, and all were males. A team headed by a psychiatrist soon rushed to the spot and did counseling to restore their cognition which was difficult due to poor education and their spiritual beliefs. Local administration was strict to faith healers and local spiritual Gurus. Their condition came into control in 20 days with very few residual anxiety symptoms.

IMPORTANCE OF PROMPT INTERVENTION

The experience showed that most of the affected people turned to local healthcare providers for their treatment. There is a wide network of different types of healers in the community such as Gunin, Priest, Ojha, Tantrik, and faith healers. Virtually, they provide the first line of clinical contact for the vast majority of the village-living population. Unfortunately, these people's ignorance and low literacy rate were exploited by these so-called treatment providers and strengthened the illness's false beliefs among the affected and nonaffected people. They prescribed different types of magicoreligious rituals and incurred some costs as well. Both because they believed in magicoreligious phenomena and distance and unfamiliarity with the modern allopathic treatment hospital, the major section of affected persons preferred local healing rituals. It is also evident that prompt intervention by the team of doctors from the local health centers yielded good results. The use of different psychotherapeutic processes with IEC materials was quite helpful to cure the Koro-affected subjects and help to ameliorate community fear and anxiety, and thereby mitigate the spread of the epidemic in the locality. In all the four epidemics mentioned above, the active intervention by the local health team helped to contain the epidemic spread within a few weeks, and the affectivity rate was controlled.

CONCLUSION

It is interesting to note that Tripura had four Koro epidemics. So, it is a serious research issue why there is a recurring trend of Koro epidemics in this land-locked state of India. It is also of concern that two neighboring states, viz., Assam and West Bengal also have a history of repeated Koro epidemics. Tripura has easy access with frequent land and air communication with these two states. The recent upgraded technology of mobile phone connection may be a crucial factor in easy transmissibility of epidemic news between the states.[8] This may be a risk factor for these recurrent Koro epidemics in Tripura.

REFERENCES

1. Chowdhury AN. Definition and classification of Koro. Cult Med Psychiat. 1996;20:41-65.
2. Chowdhury AN. Koro: Clinical and historical developments of the culturally defined genital retraction disorder. Switzerland: Palgrave Macmillian, Springer Nature; 2021.
3. Yap, PM. Koro-a culture-bound depersonalization syndrome. Brit J Psychiat. 1965;111(470):43-50.
4. Cohen S, Tennenbaum, Teitelbaum SY, Durst AR. The koro (genital retraction) syndrome and its association with infertility: A case report. J Urology. 1995;153(2):427-28.
5. Silva L, Rapso-Lima C, Soares C, Cerqueira JJ, Morgado P. Koro syndrome in an obsessive compulsive disorder. European Psychiat. 2016;33:(Suppl S618).
6. Rin H. A study of the aetiology of Koro in respect to the Chinese concept of illness. Int J Soc Psychiat. 1965;11:7-13.
7. Debbarma S, Das SK, Kumar A, Debbarma D, Das A, Reang T. Koro epidemic: A descriptive study. J Evolution of Medical Dental Sc. 2016;5(76):5634-8.
8. Ghosh S, Nath S, Brahma A, Chowdhury, AN. Fifth Koro epidemic in India: A review report. World Cul Psychiat Res Rev. 2013;8(1):8-20.

PUBLISHED REPORTS OF KORO EPIDEMICS IN TRIPURA

Two study reports on the Tripura Koro epidemic are available. It seems that there are at least four Koro epidemics occurred in the state, viz., in 1998, 2008, 2010, and 2015.

1. AK Nath, BK Bhowmic, JM Ghosh: A Sociocultural Study of 'Koro' Epidemic in Certain Villages of Tripura

*Brochure of Conference of Indian Psychiatric Society, East Zone, 2011:*29-30.

This short reporting of Koro is from two villages of Kamalpur district of Tripura, at the background of a Koro epidemic in the adjacent villages. They reported eight male Koro cases that happened within 12 days. Five cases belonged to tribal ethnicity, and three were from the Bengali community. The two adjacent small villages were Laijury north and west and Sashipal para, about 8 km away from this spot. Three of the victims were married, and five were single. The age range was from 12 to 38 years. Five victims were students, and three were cultivators. Each episode lasted 2–4 minutes, with an average of three to five times in 4–5 days. After the sunset, most of the attacks began with shivering for 2–3 minutes and then a tingling sensation in the penis and inward pull with heightened anxiety and fear of death. Local faith healers like Tantrik and Ojha were consulted and provided traditional treatment.

From the description, it appears that all of them had recurrent Koro attacks within a specified time of 4–5 days. The authors also mentioned, "The people of the state still vividly remember the episode of Koro in 1998 when hundreds of young males and females were affected restricted to about 20 km radius around Agartala, Capital of Tripura."

2. S Debbarma, SK Das, A Kumar, D Debbarma, A Das T. Reang: Koro Epidemic: A Descriptive Study

*Journal of Evolution of Medical & Dental Sciences, 2016, 5 (76):*5634- 5638.

This is a relatively comprehensive report of the March to July 2015 Koro epidemic of Tripura. The authors reported detailed psychosocial demography of 57 cases (49 males and 8 females) from the Karbook (Gomti district) subdivision. The epidemic was also documented from other areas such as Shantir Bazar, Belonia (South district) subdivision, and villages of the Bishalgarh subdivision under Sepahijala district.

The salient findings of Koro demography are as follows: 1. Age group-50.9% in 17–30 years; 2. 78.6% married; 3. 50% with primary education; 4. 78.6% Hindu, 21.4% Buddhist and 5. 49.1% Day-laborer and 35.1% unemployed

Reported Symptoms

Shrinking of the penis was the predominant clinical presentation among the 49 male cases and retraction of the breast (no vaginal symptom) among the 8 female cases; all had a fear of impending death. Besides, 20% of cases complained of "feeling cold, and 45% of reduced sexual function." Traditional folk treatment preferred treatment seeking from Ojhas, Tantric, local quacks, and priests. The predominant beliefs were that the illness was due to black magic, witchcraft, or spells of "mantra." Very few cases turned to the hospital. Many victims offered "poojas" and religious worship rituals for a cure. The hospital patients responded well with small doses of benzodiazepine (clonazepam 0.5 mg/alprazolam 0.25 mg twice or thrice daily). The vast majority of the affected villages believed that the disease might infect them if closer to the affected person. So avoidance behavior and restricted movement of persons in the community were advised. People also used traditional prophylactic measures to prevent affliction—herbal amulets or chanted paper containing "mantras" from the priest inserted in their armlets were used by many and was of high demand in the community. One important incident was reported that some people in the neighborhood were charged with allegations that they were causing this malady by casting black magic, and they were physically attacked. The authors believe that these are due to some past familial ill-feelings and hostility in the community.

Chapter 9

Koro in South India

INTRODUCTION

South India[1] is a region consisting of the southern part of India, which encompasses five States (Andhra Pradesh, Karnataka, Kerala, Tamil Nadu, Telangana), and the Union Territories (UT) of Lakshadweep and Puducherry. South India comprises 19.31% of India's area (635,780 km^2 or 245,480 sq mi) and 20% of India's population. South India is bounded by the Bay of Bengal in the east, the Arabian Sea in the west, and the Indian Ocean in the south.

The region's geography is diverse, with two mountain ranges—the Western and Eastern Ghats. Many major river systems traverse the entire area. The majority of the people in South India speak at least one of the four major Dravidian languages: Telugu, Tamil, Kannada, and Malayalam. Some states and UTs also recognize a minority language: Urdu in Telangana and French in Puducherry. English is also used by central and state governments for official communications and is used on all public signboards.

Kerala[2] state is on the Malabar Coast of India and spread over 38,863 km^2 (15,005 sq mi), with 33 million inhabitants (2011 Census). Kerala is the 13th largest Indian state by population. The state of Karnataka borders it to the north and northeast, the state of Tamil Nadu to the east and south, and the Lakshadweep Sea to the west. It has 14 districts, with the capital at Thiruvananthapuram. Other major cities are Kozhikode, Kochi, Kollam, and Thrissur. Malayalam is the most widely spoken language and is the state's official language. Agriculture, fisheries, industries including information technology are the main livelihood measures in the state. The state has well-knit roads, railways, and waterways with four international airports. Kochi has a metro rail system also. Hinduism is Kerala's most widely professed faith, with significant Muslim and Christian minorities. As of 2015, Kerala has a Human Development Index of 0.770, which is in the "high" category, ranking it first in the country.[3] According to the 2011 census, Kerala has a 93.9% literacy. The 2020 data showed 96.2% literacy in Kerala and emerged as the most literate state in the country.[4]

KORO

Koro is not so prevalent in South Indian states as in Northeast India. Since 2020, three sporadic Koro cases have been reported from South India. The first one was from Puducherry (in 2014),[5] the second one was from Thrissur, Kerala (in 2018)[6] and the third was from Bengaluru (in 2018).[7] Interestingly, there are two reports on the Koro epidemic from South India: one from Kochi, Kerala in (2010)[8] and the other from Bengaluru in (2020).[9] Dr K Promodu has kindly provided a full report on the Kochi epidemic, and the Bengaluru study by Banerjee et al. (2020) is abstracted.

Interestingly, both the Koro epidemics affected the migrant worker population in their camps. In both instances, the victims had a kinship link with the Northeastern Indian states (West Bengal, Assam, and Odisha). Mobile phone messages played a vital role in both epidemics.

REFERENCES

1. South India. [online] Available from https://en.wikipedia.org/wiki/South_IndiaSouth. [Last accessed March, 2023].
2. Kerala. [online] Available from https://en.wikipedia.org/wiki/Kerala. [Last accessed March, 2023].
3. Subnational HDI-Area Database. *Global Data Lab*. Institute for Management Research, Radboud University. [online] Available from https://globaldatalab.org/shdi/shdi/. [Last accessed March, 2023].
4. Firstpost. [online] Available from https://www.firstpost.com/india/at-96-2-kerala-tops-indias-literacy-rate-chart-again-andhra-pradesh-ranks-lowest-with-66-4-8796401.html. [Last accessed March, 2023].
5. Ramamourty PV, Menon V. Koro presenting as acute and transient psychosis: Implications for classification. Asian J Psychiat. 2014;10:116-7.
6. Megha AP, Antony JT, Beevi KS, Chakkalakkudy GG, Kuttichira PA. Case of sporadic Koro from Kerala. Ind J Soc Psychiat. 2018;34:90-1.
7. Garg K, Das N, Kumar CN. Koro in panic disorder: Beyond a culture bound phenomena. Asian J Psychiat. 2018; 31:73-4.
8. Promodu KK, Nair KR, Pushparajan S. Koro syndrome: Mass epidemic in Kerala, India. Ind J Clini Psychol. 2012;39:152-6.
9. Banerjee D, Sharma S, Antony S. Koro and migration: Observational study of an outbreak of Koro in a migrant population working in South India. J Psychosex Health. 2020;2(2): 174-8.

KORO SYNDROME: EPIDEMIC IN KERALA, INDIA

Kunjappan Promodu

INTRODUCTION

Koro is a culture-bound syndrome characterized by acute fear and anxiety that the external genital organ may retract into the body and even cause death. The affected male believes that his penis will recede into the abdomen or disappear, while the female believes that the vulva, labia, breasts, or nipples will retract into the body. Some affected patients assume that the culmination of this process leads to death. These beliefs are solid and irrational convictions but not delusions in their strict sense.

Koro had been reported in various countries like Hong Kong,[1] China,[2] Taiwan,[3] Singapore,[4] Thailand,[5] Philippines,[6] and Africa.[7] Koro had also been reported from various parts of India like Assam,[8,9] West Bengal,[10-15] Tripura[16] Delhi[17] and Kerala.[18] The term Koro originated from the Malaysian word "kora" meaning "the head of the turtle."[19] Koro is prevalent in southwest Asia and predominantly among the Chinese.[2] In Cantonese, this is called "Suk-Yeong,"[1] meaning the shrinking of the penis.

It is usually accompanied by severe anxiety and often a panic state characterized by complaints of palpitations, sweating, precordial discomfort, trembling, and a firm belief or perception that his/her genitalia are retracting into the body and may disappear. Symptoms may last for 1/2 hour to 1 or 2 days. Extremely anxious sufferers may perform indigenous methods. Some men have reportedly tied the penis to an external object, and a few others used to hold it tight or pull the penis to prevent retracting inside. Male suffering from extreme anxiety can experience loss of erection, reduction in the length and girth of their penis. This is a part of the physiological response to the accompanying anxiety-provoking cognitive state. Vasoconstriction is usually caused by severe anxiety and even by cold temperatures. So, it is pretty natural for a male suffering from Koro to feel receding of his penis into the body as it might have already shrunk due to the state of anxiety. Associated symptoms may include perception of alteration of penile shape, loss of erection or muscle tone, shortening of the penis, and paresthesia of genital organs. A female with Koro syndrome would experience her breasts and nipples receding into the body. Some women may even grab their breasts or keep pulling out their nipples. The associated anxiety itself will cause a momentary pulling up of the scrotal sac and shrinkage of the penis in men and shrinkage of nipples, areola, and breast in women, which may further worsen the anxiety thus form a vicious cycle for worsening the symptoms. Due to severe distress, fear, and anxiety, patient may attempt self-harm. Personality factors, family environment, social milieu, literacy level, cultural beliefs, psychosexual conflicts (sexual inadequacy, lack of erectile confidence, misconceptions), and guilt associated with masturbation may play a pivotal role in the etiology of Koro.

KORO: A CULTURE-BOUND SYNDROME

Koro is known as a culture-bound syndrome. Sociocultural factors influence the symptoms of all psychiatric disorders. The cross-cultural difference is evident in almost all anxiety-related disorders. The initial medical reporting of Koro came from the writings of Dutch physicians in the 20th century.[20,21]

Kerala and the Background of the Epidemic

Kerala **(Fig. 1)**, popularly known as "God's own county," is a southern state of India, famous for its scenic beauty and culture, lying between the Arabian Sea and the Western Ghats. The Arabian Sea flanks Kerala on the west, Karnataka on the north and northeast, and Tamil Nadu on the east. Kerala has a population of 35.8 million as per the 2021 estimate, with a rich history of art and cultural heritage, known for its foreign trade for the last several years. It has the highest literacy rate and has unique achievements in education, healthcare, gender equality, social justice, law, and order.

Kerala's high literacy rate, technical education, and professional competence paved the way for many Keralites to migrate to other countries worldwide, especially to the middle east.

This led to the shortage of laborers in Kerala to perform skilled, semiskilled, and manual work. Since the 1990s, hiring large laborers from other Indian states has become common. In the late 90s and early 2020s, lakhs of people from Assam, Odisha, Bihar, and West Bengal were either brought or migrated to Kerala to carry out the above work. They were provided with group accommodation in lodges or temporary shelters with bare minimum facilities near their workplaces. Usually, they visit home for a few days, once a year, especially during the festivals. Agents or mediators supplied migrant laborers during the early migration days to different sites and workplaces as required. Some laborers worked in the same place or with the same job providers for several months to years. Other groups of more educated people and/or those capable of seeking or engaging in their jobs or businesses. Many such workers have brought families together and live in independent houses.

Location of the Epidemic

Ernakulam is one of the 14 districts located in the central part of Kerala, with a population of 3.46 million as per the 2021 estimate. Ernakulam, the commercial capital of Kerala, is also known as Kochi, and people often use these terms interchangeably. Kochi is one of the fast-developing metropolitan cities with massive construction work underway. Kakkanad is the center of Ernakulam with the district administration and almost all government offices

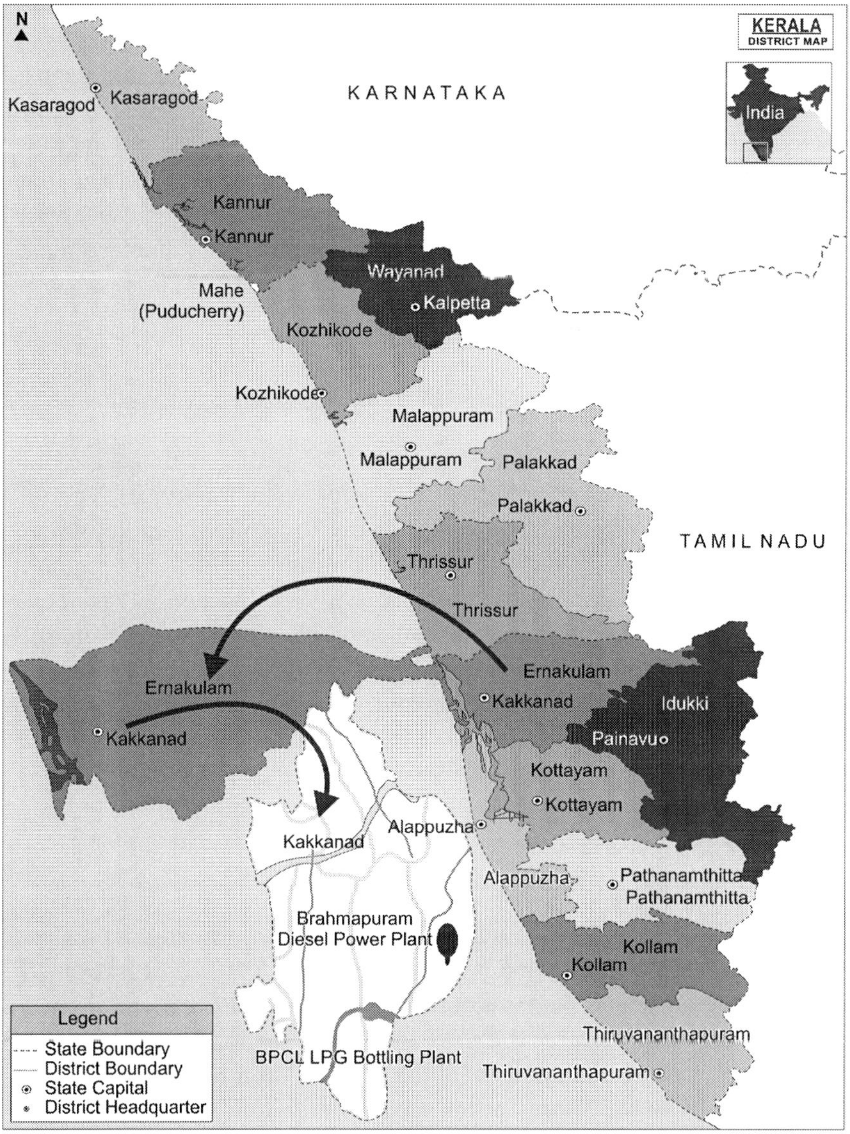

Fig. 1: Map of Kerala.

and other establishments. Tens of thousands of laborers have been working in the construction sites and living in the adjacent labor camps in Kakkanad. Men living in this environment were affected by the Koro epidemic.

Outbreak of Koro

During August to September 2010, construction sites and other workplaces in Kochi experienced a shortage of workers. Suddenly, the rate of absenteeism hiked. Scarcity of workers was reported, and the inquiry for the above desertion revealed that several laborers from West Bengal suddenly fled to their home as they experienced severe anxiety accompanied by a feeling that the penis is receding into the body. After sharing the experience with friends, a few started experiencing similar symptoms. It gradually spread to the migrant workers hailing from West Bengal. The epidemic spread like wildfire within a month among the migrant workers from West Bengal. Though several men were reportedly affected by Koro, the exact number was unavailable as most had already left.

Method

The Sample and Period of Study

Though the affected population was in the 100s, actual statistics are not available as most fled or returned to their homes. The investigators could locate only 21 men, who had been suffering from symptoms, and four men had already recovered during this study. All of them belonged to migrant workers from West Bengal. The medical team could evaluate only 12 patients suffering from the Koro epidemic and four recovered from the symptoms, who expressed willingness to undergo a clinical interview and physical examination. Subjects were selected by purposive cluster sampling from 3 labor camps and were conducted on 12 victims suffering from the symptoms. The study period was from 1st to 16th September 2010.

Data Collection

A medical team under the leadership of the author, including a urologist, clinical psychologist, and male nurses, visited the affected location as well as the three labor camps on 1st and 2nd September, 2010. After 2 weeks on 15 and 16th September, follow-up was done to identify and study any additional patients suffering from the same illness. Before conducting the site visit and study, prior approval was taken from the Ethics Committee. Information was collected by survey, observation, clinical interview, the case study of the victims, eyewitnesses, friends, roommates, coworkers, camp leaders, managers, adjacent shop keepers, and the local inhabitants. The medical examination was conducted for the victims. The team could identify 19 victims suffering from the epidemic at the time of the study. Only 12 gave consent to undergo a clinical interview and physical examinations out of them. During the follow-up, four recovered patients were identified and cooperated for the investigation. After the joint and separate clinical interview of the victims by the medical team, the urologist conducted the relevant medical evaluation focused on examining external genitals. Living conditions at the labor camps were also evaluated.

Epidemic Scenario

In August 2010, sudden mass absenteeism was reported at the work sites. Many workers were in a panic state, fearing the penis retracting into the body. For relief, they engaged in group worship, offerings, and poojas (religious rituals). It became a significant labor problem within a few days, and the construction work at a few sites came to a standstill due to the mass absenteeism. Many affected workers returned to their hometowns due to panic and fear of transmission. Television channels and daily newspapers reported the news. More people, including the local inhabitants, became panicky due to the fear of unknown diseases and their transmission. Reportedly the symptoms started with a sudden feeling of the penis shrinking and receding into the body. Affected persons experienced a panic state characterized by extreme fear, apprehension, palpitation, sweating, and tremors. It was also reported that friends helped a few victims by holding the penis to prevent it from retracting inside. In some other instances, plenty of water was poured on the head of the victims. On average, within 1/2–1 hour, most affected persons became normal; though, for a few, symptoms such as anxiety and fear persisted up to 2 days. They took rest for 1 or 2 days in their room by confining to bed or engaged in worship. Several victims returned to their hometown on the next day itself.

Clinical Interview of the Victims

The medical team examined 12 affected victims, and four patients recovered from Koro state during the visit. All of the victims selected for the study underwent general physical checkups with a specific focus on genital examination by the urologist. Clinical psychologists conducted a clinical interview, including case history recording and mental status examination.

Findings and Observations

The patient's age range was 18–48 years with a mean age of 27.3 years and education from illiteracy to 10th class with a mean of 6 years of schooling. All of them hailed from remote villages of West Bengal and belonged to lower socioeconomic strata. None of them reported a family history of mental disorders or suicide. Clinical examination did not reveal any medical abnormality. Examination of the external genitals of all victims was normal. The prominent symptoms observed were severe fear of receding the penis into the body, preoccupation with the thoughts of retraction of the penis, palpitation, feeling of apprehension, sweating, tremors of limbs, giddiness, and extreme tiredness, and a feeling of "going to die" in a few. Some of them expressed feelings of sadness and fear of death due to the retraction of the penis. Most of them were observed to be engaged in prayers and religious rituals to get rid of the symptoms or confined to bed. The main corrective measures adopted by the victims were bed rest, pouring cold water into the genital area, and holding or pulling out the penis to prevent it from receding into the body.

During the clinical interview, one of the patients revealed that he belonged to Hoogly District of West Bengal and a similar disease was prevalent in his village a few months ago. The person who complained of Koro symptoms first in the camp also belonged to his village. Others could not believe it when they complained of the symptoms and mocked the victim. To their surprise, more natives of West Bengal reported similar symptoms. Later on, others also got affected gradually. Within 2 weeks, it spread to others in the three labor camps. The majority of them reportedly fled to their home at the onset of the symptoms. Hence, the medical team could not identify the exact number of the affected cases. One person from Kerala was also affected and was admitted to the hospital. The medical examination could not detect any abnormalities. The patient reportedly recovered with the physician's reassurance after the physical examination. When the news spread in the local community, laborers from the index group were kept away by the local people.

Living Conditions at the Labor Camps

During the investigation, the living conditions at the labor camps were observed. Laborers lived in groups either in large rooms or the temporary shelters made of aluminum or fiber sheets and slept on temporary cots or on the floor using a mattress. Only minimum convenience facilities were available. Food was cooked by themselves with the help of a kerosene stove at the corner of the room. Purified potable water was not available. Drinking water was supplied in tanker lorries. Bathing and sanitary facilities were entirely inadequate. The level of occupational stress was extremely high. A few complained that they were not getting adequate wages. The whole scenario at the labor camp was very unsatisfactory.

DISCUSSION

The etiological factors, pathogenesis, and clinical manifestations in Koro are still not understood fully. There is a difference between primary and secondary Koro (sporadic or epidemic form).[22] Preoccupation with genital shrinking is the chief and presenting complaint in primary Koro,[13,22] In contrast, the secondary presentation is a part of other disorders such as anxiety disorder, schizophrenia, depression,[22,23] neurological diseases,[24,25] urological diseases, drug withdrawal, brain tumors, or epilepsy.[26,27] It is considered that genital retraction is intimately related to ethnocultural beliefs and the dramatic expression of acute anxiety and the fear of impending catastrophe or death.[12] The symptomatology of the epidemic that broke out in Kerala had a typical clinical picture of Koro syndrome reported elsewhere. Cognitive-behavioral and social learning models are better suited to explain the pathogenesis and symptomatology of the Koro epidemic in Kerala rather than by a psychoanalytic model.

The present study revealed that the index patients had the typical symptoms of Koro syndrome. In Kerala, it was first noticed among the laborers who migrated from the Hooghly district of West Bengal, who had previous knowledge of the same, as it had been prevalent in West Bengal. Almost all the affected men belonged to lower socioeconomic strata with low levels of education. It was reported earlier in other studies that most of the individuals affected by Koro in India had poor educational levels and belonged to lower socioeconomic strata.[25] The present study also found similar observations. Cultural attitudes, beliefs, news and rumors about Koro, and mass anxiety in the community are some critical risk factors for spreading the epidemic.[28,29] Gradually, the symptoms spread to other laborers in the camps. Illiteracy, low educational level, separation from family, severe occupational and economic stress, poor living conditions, and prior knowledge of the disorder are the major etiological factors in these cases. The literature already reported that stressful life events such as separation from family and loneliness in an unfamiliar environment preceded the onset of Koro syndrome.[22]

The victims, who remained in the camp, recovered spontaneously within a week. The medical examination of the victims and our team's group counseling helped relieve their anxiety and facilitated a speedy recovery. The spontaneous recovery and the quick response to the psychological intervention itself ruled out any organic cause behind this outbreak. After the news broke out, there was intervention from the local government authorities to improve the living conditions in the labor camps.

Patients afflicted with Koro syndrome were referred to urologists by primary care physicians. Some of them directly consulted urologists depending on their awareness and access. Therefore, understanding Koro syndrome among primary care physicians, urologists, clinical psychologists, and psychiatrists is of great value.

CONCLUSION

Signs and symptoms observed in patients affected by the Koro epidemic in Kerala were found to have symptomatology typical of that reported elsewhere. Etiology was purely psychogenic, and no organic factors could be identified. The majority of the patients belonged to lower socioeconomic classes with a low level of formal education. Previous knowledge of Koro syndrome combined with unhealthy premorbid personality traits, low socio-cultural-economic background, poor literacy rate, and stressful events led to the outbreak of this epidemic. Individuals with histrionic and anxious personality disorders or traits were more prone to such conditions. From a social and humanitarian perspective, it was an eye-opener to the poor living and working conditions prevailing in the labor camps, which needed closer supervision by the authorities to prevent future mishaps. Further research in this area will help to understand the gray areas. It will give insight into the issues related to the etiology, nosology, sociocultural and ethnic specificity, and the management of Koro syndrome.

REFERENCES

1. Yap PM. Koro—a culture-bond depersonalization syndrome. Brit J Psychiat. 1965;111:43-50.
2. Gelder M, Gath D, Mayou R. Oxford Textbook of Psychiatry, 2nd edition. Oxford: Oxford University Press; 1989. pp. 195-6.
3. Rin H. A study of the aetiology of koro in respect to the Chinese concept of illness. Int J Soc Psychiat. 1965;11:7-13.
4. Gwee AL. Koro—A cultural disease. Singapore Med J. 1963;4:119-22.
5. Jilek WG, Jilek-Aall L. A koro epidemic in Thailand. Transcult Psychiatr Res Rev. 1977;14:57-9.
6. Edwards JW. Indigenous koro, a genital retraction syndrome of insular south-east Asia. In: Simons RC, Hughes CC (Eds). The Culture Bound Syndromes. Dordrecht: Reidel; 1985. pp.169-91.
7. Ifabumuny OI, Rwegellera GGC. Koro in Nigerian male patient: A case report. African J Psychiat. 1979;5:103-5.
8. Dutta D, Phookan HR, Das PD. The koro epidemic in lower Assam. Ind J Psychiat. 1982;24:370-4.
9. Roy D, Hazarika S, Bhattacharya A, Das S, Nath K, Saddichha S. Koro: Culture bound or mass hysteria? Aus N Z J Psychiat. 2011;45:683.
10. Nandi DN, Banerji G, Saha H. Epidemic Koro in West Bengal, India. Int J Soc Psychiat. 1983;29:265-8.
11. Chowdhary AN. Medico-cultural cognition of Koro epidemic: An ethnographic study. J Ind Anthropol Soc. 1991;26:155-70.
12. Chowdhary AN. Clinical Analysis of 101 Koro cases. Ind J Psychiat. 1992;8:67-70.
13. Chowdhary AN. The definition and classification of Koro. Cul Med Psychiat. 1996;20:41-65.
14. Chowdhary AN. Ethnomedical concept of heat and cold in Koro: Study from Indian patients. World Cult Psychiatry Res Rev. 2008;3:146-58.
15. Sachdev PS. Koro epidemic in north-east India. Aust N Z J Psychiat. 1985;19: 433-8.
16. Chowdhury AN, Nath A, Chakraborthy J. An atypical hysteria epidemic in Tripura, India. Trancul Psychiatric Res Rev. 1993;30:143-51.
17. Bhatia MS. An analysis of 60 cases of culture bound syndromes. Ind J Medical Sc. 1999;53:140-52.
18. Promodu K, Nair KR, Pushparajan S. Koro syndrome: mass epidemic in Kerala, India. Ind J Clin Psychol. 2012;39:152-56.
19. AL-Hmoud N. Koro-like syndrome in a Jordanian male. East Mediter Health J. 1999;5:611-3.

20. Brero PCJ van. Naar Aanleiding van het Opstel Over 'Koro' van den Heer J. C. Blonk-in de Voring Aflevering van dit Tijdschrift. Geneeskunding Tijdschrrift voor Nederlandsch-Indie. 1896;36:48-54.
21. Mattelaer JJ, Jilek W. Koro—the psychological disappearance of the penis. J Sex Med. 2007;4:1509-15.
22. Ataly H. Two cases of koro syndrome. Turk Psikiyatri Derg. 2007;3:282-5.
23. Saji SD, Nizamie SH. Incomplete Koro—A forerunner for mood disorder: Two case reports. Ind J Psychiat. 1993;35:60-2.
24. Dzokoto VA, Adams G. Understanding the genital-shrinking epidemics in West Africa: koro, juju, or mass psychological illness? Cult Med Psychiat. 2005;29:53-78.
25. Kar N. Chronic koro like symptoms—two case reports. BMC Psychiat. 2005;5:34.
26. Bernstein RL, Gaw AC. Koro: proposed classification for DSM-IV. Am J Psychiat. 1990;12:1670-4.
27. Earleywine M. Cannabis induced koro in Americans. Addiction. 2001;96:1663-6.
28. Cheng ST. Epidemic genital retraction syndrome: Environmental and personal risk factors in Southern China. J Psychol Hum Sexuality. 1997;9:57-70.
29. Tseng WS, Mo KM, Hsu J, Li LS, Chen GQ, Jiang DW. A socio-cultural study of koro epidemics in Guangdong, China. Amer J Psychiat. 1988;145:1538-43.

ABSTRACT OF THE STUDY OF A MINI-KORO EPIDEMIC IN BENGALURU

Banerjee D, Sharma S, Antony S. Koro and Migration: Observational Study of an Outbreak of Koro in a Migrant Population Working in South India *Journal of Psychosexual Health, 2020:*2(2):174-8.

This is a very interesting study of a mini-Koro epidemic among migrant labor population, from Bangalore, South India. These migrant workers came from states of Eastern and central parts of India. It was a study of a cohort of 13 migrant workers (8 males and 5 females) from a population of 52, who attended the hospital within 2 weeks. The index case was a 29-year-old single mason who was having typical Koro symptoms. He believed that he had contracted this illness from a fellow worker who had this illness and with whom he shared a meal. There was no fear of imminent death, but fear of being infertile was there. To prevent this malady, he poured cold water on the penis several times a day. He disclosed that 5 of his fellow laborers also had the penis shrinking illness, but they kept secret out of fear, shame, and stigma. Subsequently, 12 more patients (7 males and 5 females) attended the hospital clinic with Koro symptoms. Males complained of penile and scrotal retraction, while females felt that their breasts and vagina were shortening and disappearing within the body. Females fear that they may be losing the ability to bear children or lose the capacity for breastfeeding. All the patients showed good recovery with treatment with fluoxetine 20 mg and clonazepam 0.5 mg. Ten patients were treated with a single 1-hour session of cognitive behavioral therapy (CBT). The authors provided a few important clinical details also. 84.6% had previous knowledge of Koro. They tried to classify the nature of genital shrinking belief: Delusional: 61.5%, Ideas: 23.1%, and Doubts: 15.4%. 76.9% had a fear of death. 69.2% belief the illness is contagious. The authors identified the stress of migration, social isolation, and stigmas are the environmental risk factors for this epidemic in a closed migrant colony.

Chapter 10

Culture-bound Syndromes: Pioneers of Koro Research

Arabinda N Chowdhury, Monali Chowdhury

INTRODUCTION

Professor Pow Ming Yap from Hong Kong first coined "culture-bound syndrome" (CBS) in the 1960s[1,2] to justify a compromise between Western psychiatric nosology and "atypical" mental presentations from the Asia-Pacific region. The late 19th century and early 20th century are marked by discovering three culture-specific syndromes, mainly reported from indigenous people of Malay, Indonesia, and Papua New Guinea. They are primarily the Amok, Latah, Koro, and another one was Tropical Neurasthenia written by the Dutch physicians from the then Nederlandsch-Indie (Indonesia).[3] The "Tropical neurasthenia" was a frequent diagnosis applied to Europeans only, who developed psychosomatic symptoms after posting in colonial outposts in the far East. In today's terms, this may be referred to as dysthymic disorder, minor depressive disorder, or cultural stress, and adjustment disorder.

For over a century, much debate was on CBS's psychiatric nosology, especially to fit it with the Western mental illness construct and disease categories. Some researchers viewed these cultural terms and nosologies of illnesses are the expression of academic colonization of indigenous distress of conditions or the medicalization of exotic deviances.[4,5] Marsella (1996)[6] provided a catalog of different confusing nosological terms used to define CBSs' in the mid-1990s. Gradually, a strong opinion was voiced by the work of many researchers for the need for inclusion of CBS's under the Western classificatory system.[7-9] They felt that all psychiatric disorders are culture-bound in a general sense, as no disease can escape local cultural encoding, shaping, presentation, and communicative style of distress experience.[10] These academic debates, logic, and counter logic led to the development of a new discipline, "Transcultural or Cross-cultural Psychiatry," which dedicatedly aimed to study the interface between culture and mental health globally.[11-13]

The culture-bound syndrome is a broad rubric that encompasses specific behavioral, affective, and cognitive manifestations seen in specific cultures.[14] Diagnostic and Statistical Manual of Mental Disorders, Fourth Edition

(DSM-IV)[15] first included CBS[16] in the American disease classification. It provided short clinical descriptions of 25 culture-bound syndromes, in the introduction to the Glossary of Culture-Bound Syndromes in appendix I of DSM-IV is as follows:

The term culture-bound syndrome denotes recurrent, locality-specific patterns of aberrant behavior and troubling experience that may or may not be linked to a particular DSM-IV diagnostic category. Many of these patterns are indigenously considered to be "illnesses," or at least afflictions, and most have local names.... culture-bound syndromes are generally limited to specific societies or culture areas and are localized, folk, diagnostic categories that frame coherent meanings for certain repetitive, patterned, and troubling sets of experiences and observations (p. 844).

In DSM-5 (2013),[17] the term culture-bound was replaced by the term "cultural concept of distress," but keeping the provision of CBS to be referred to as "folk illnesses" or "culture-specific disorders."[18]

The ICD-10[19] (Chapter V) of the World Health Organization (WHO), provided a framework for culture-specific disorders which should follow a set of features: (1) Categorization as a disease in the particular culture; (2) Widespread familiarity in the culture; (3) Complete lack of understanding or misunderstanding of the condition to people in other cultures; (4). There are no objectively demonstrable biochemical or tissue abnormalities; and (5) The condition is usually recognized and treated by the culture's folk medicine.

The American Psychiatry Association (APA) Dictionary of Psychology[20] defined Culture-bound Syndrome as follows:

"a pattern of mental illness and abnormal behavior that is unique to a specific ethnic or cultural population and does not conform to standard classifications of psychiatric disorders. Culture-bound syndromes include, among others, amok, amurakh, bangungut, hsieh-ping, imu, jumping of Frenchmen of Maine syndrome, koro, latah, mal de pelea, myriachit, piblokto, susto, voodoo death, and windigo psychosis, also called culture-specific syndrome."

Following is a brief note on three categories of CBS (Amok, Latah, and Koro) that initiated a protracted discussion on the inter-relation of culture and psychiatry, focusing on Koro.

AMOK

It is an acute condition of mental misbalance. The affected individual, usually a man, shows violent outbursts, moves around, and attempts to injure or kill others on his way. Martin[21] provides a detailed history of Amok: Captain Cook first reported his observations and recordings of amok in the Malay tribe members in 1770 during his around-the-world voyage. In Malay mythology, running amok was an involuntary behavior caused by the "hantu belian," or evil tiger spirit entering a person's body and compelling them to behave violently without conscious awareness.[21] Amok is etymologically related to the Malayan term "*meng-amuk,*" which means "to make a furious and desperate charge."[21] It was first reported from Malaysia and later said from other countries like Papua New Guinea,[22] Laos,[23] Philippines, Thailand, Indonesia, Polynesia (*cafard, cathard*), Puerto Rico (*mal de pelea*), and from the USA.[21,24,25] Even now, Indonesians use the term "gelap mata" (literally "darkened eyes") to refer to individuals with amok. "Gelap mata" or the Dark Eye, is also a common expression in Sumatra and Java to describe a curious and disturbing social incident.

Yap[1] described that amok behavior is preceded by a period of brooding. If the attacker survives the process, it leads to a state of exhaustion and collapse, and frequently the individual has amnesia for the event. This description points to a psychotic depression or dissociative disorder state. Carr[26] stated that *amok* is an expression of a common behavioral pathway after multiple precipitants (may or may not be related to any psychopathology). It represents a specific form and conceptualization linked to the social learning system and Malay beliefs. So, it is said that "Amok as a cultural prescription for violent behavior in response to a given set of conditions. It is not a disease but rather a behavioral sequence, perceived as illness, and; various etiological factors may precipitate that."[27]

LATAH

It is a combination of a complex of behaviors. It shows nonhabituating hyperstartling and other stereotypic behaviors such as coprolalia, echolalia, echopraxia, "forced obedience" (immediate obedience to commands), and hypersuggestibility. They were mainly reported from Malay or Indonesia.[28,29] Latah is originally a Malay term for a broad category of strange behaviors. Literally, it means "Tiklish," "Jumpy," or "Love-madness." Yap suggested that references to Latah in Malay literature date to the 14th century. In 1849, Logan was the first to write in English about Latah's behavior and described it as an uncontrollable startle reaction.[28]

Murphy[30] traced the history of Latah from European colonial times and tried to offer a psychiatric explanation of the disorder. In 1994, the Diagnostic and Statistical Manual of Mental Disorders or DSM-IV recognized Latah for the first time as a member of a new category of psychiatric illnesses known as culture-bound syndromes. Latah is a symbolic representation of marginality, and it is as appropriate to specific mythological and religious figures to the socially marginal people.[31] Latah provides a unique example of how neurophysiological, experiential, and cultural variables interact to produce a strongly marked clinical phenomenon.[32] Tanner and Chamberland,[33] from their extensive study of historical accounts of Latah in Indonesia, concluded that *latah* is a deviant social role and a unique Malayo-Indonesian idiom. Bakker and Tijssen[34] believe that from their study of three groups of startle syndromes, Latah is a "neuropsychiatric startle syndrome."

KORO

Dr JC Blonk is credited for the first publication on Koro in the Western medical press in 1895 from Dutch occupied Indonesia **(Fig. 1)**.[35] Still, a historical search showed that the symptoms of genital retraction (not by the name Koro) were first reported from Russia by A.A. Ivanov in 1885[36] and second was immediately after, written by TF Raven in 1886[37] from England published in Lancet. Blonk just used the term Koro first to address the clinical phenomenon of penile retraction. But it is also true that the number of Dutch physicians made a crucial clinical contribution of Koro pathology from their colony Nederlandsch Indie.

Dr PCJ van Brero, the second physician at the mental hospital in Buitenzorg (now Bogor city), West Java province, published two consecutive papers on Koro in 1896 and 1897.[38,39] He provided a detailed discussion and interpretation of the Koro case reported by Blonk.[35] He described Koro as "a strange compulsive idea." His two publications provided the first detailed clinical discussion on Koro. It is interesting to note that after 117 years, DSM-5[17] designated Koro as a form of OCD spectrum disorder ORCD ("Other specified Obsessive-Compulsive and Related Disorders"-300.3). **Figure 2** shows the first page of van Brero's 1986 publication in a Dutch Medical journal (Geneeskundig Tijdschrift voor Nederlandsch-Indie). In 1897, Dr AH Vorstman,[40] a medical officer in Palembang (Borneo), described two Koro case reports from Kalimantan of the Dutch Indies.

In the early part of the 19th century, two Dutch physicians again contributed significant knowledge on Koro from Dutch Indies. The first one was in 1935, Dr by JA Slot,[41] a government doctor in the South Celebes. He provided a detailed report on ethnomedical cognition of Koro etiology from the Macassaran area of Sulawesi **(Fig. 3)**. He designated Koro as the affliction of nerves (nerve-contracting disease). The second author was JGA Mulder,[42] who described Koro among the Sulawesi natives **(Fig. 4)**. He reported that the name Koro locally signifies "shriveling" meant by Macassars or Buginese people of South Celebes. He stressed the construct of the Chinese Yin-Yang principle as a strong primitive folk belief behind Koro among the Celebes people.

Dr PM van Wulfften Palthe **(Fig. 5A)**,[43-47] a Dutch physician, was the psychiatrist at the hospital for mental diseases at Bongor and Professor of Neurology and Psychiatry in the Medical Academy, is a well-known name in the area of early Koro research. His five papers (1934, 1935a, 1935b, 1936a,

KORO,

DOOR

J. C. BLONK,

Officier van Gezondheid 2e Klasse.

Onder dezen naam is bij de Boegineezen en Makassaren een ziektebeeld bekend, dat, naar ik meen, nog niet is beschreven. Ook is het mij niet mogen gelukken het voorkomen dier ziekte op Java, in de Padang'sche bovenlanden, en te Atjeh te constateeren.

Volgens lijders aan deze ziekte gevoelen zij op onregelmatige tijdstippen dat de penis neiging heeft zich in de buikholte terug te trekken. In de gevallen, waarin niet tijdig hulp wordt verstrekt, zoude dit ook werkelijk geschieden, en de patient dan tevens bezwijken. De lijders zijn daarvoor natuurlijk zeer bevreesd. Zoodra zij dan ook bemerken dat de eerste verschijnselen zich voordoen, nemen zij den penis in de hand om het terugtrekken te beletten. Soms echter kunnen zij dit zelf niet volhouden, en moet deze therapie door een ander worden overgenomen. Uren achtereen moet soms op die wijze de penis worden vastgehouden, terwijl in sommige gevallen een vrij sterke kracht moet worden aangewend.

Gedurende deze aanvallen worden de patiënten geplaagd door een hevig angstgevoel, terwijl zij, nadat de aanval geweken is, uiterst vermoeid en afgemat zijn.

Omtrent de aanleiding tot het optreden van een aanval kon ik niets te weten komen, ook niet op welkèn leeftijd gewoonlijk de eerste aanvallen zich voordoen.

Fig. 1: 1895 Publication of JC Blonk (first page).

1937) and a textbook chapter (1936b)[48] are the most valuable early Koro documents. These provide rich and elaborate information on the clinical, epidemic, and endemic aspects, the linguistic genesis of the term "Koro," and ethnomedical and cultural perspective of genital retraction syndrome **(Fig. 5B)**. Moreover, his multilingual publications like Dutch publication (1934); German psychoanalytic literature (1935b); French medical literature

Naar Aanleiding van het Opstel over „Koro" van den Heer J. C. Blonk in de vorige Aflevering van dit Tijdschrift.

DOOR

P. C. J. VAN BRERO,

2e Geneesheer aan het Krankzinnigengesticht te Buitenzorg.

De Heer BLONK beschreef in de laatste aflevering van dit tijdschrift een eigenaardig ziektebeeld, dat ik kortelijk hier memoreeren wil.

In het zuidelijk gedeelte van *Celebes* zag hij lijders, wier penis af en toe, zonder dat hem de aanleiding daartoe bekend was, neiging had zich in de buikholte terug te trekken, hetgeen, indien dit niet verhinderd werd, door dat of de lijders zelven of anderen de penis vasthielden, werkelijk gebeuren en dan den dood ten gevolge zou hebben. Deze aanvallen duurden soms uren, waren vergezeld van een hevigen angst, en werden door groote afgematheid gevolgd. De verschijnselen schenen bij menschen met een gestoord zenuwleven gevonden te worden, en werden door deze lieden uit een gevoel van schaamte verborgen gehouden. Omtrent herediteit, tijdstip van optreden was hem niets bekend; persoonlijk kon hij dergelijke aanvalleu niet te zien krijgen.

Deze interessante waarneming is belangrijk ten eerste als bijdrage tot de kennis der anthropologie van de bewoners in wier midden wij leven, en ten tweede als vermeerdering onzer kennis van die eigenaardige psychische stoornissen bekend

Fig. 2: 1896 Publication of PCJ van Brero (First Page).
Source: Adopted from Brero van PCJ. Naar Aanleiding van het Opstel Over 'Koro' van den Heer J. C. Blonk-in de Voring Aflevering van dit Tijdschrift. Geneeskunding Tijdschrrift voor Nederlandsch-Indie. 1896;36:48-54.

Koró in Zuid-Celebes [1] [2] [3],

DOOR

Dr. J. A. SLOT, *Gouvernements Arts.*

In the cage.
„What I say is, what I say!" I vociferate, as a Parrot in the great cage of the World, I hop screeching, „What I say is!" from perch to perch.
(L. P. SMITH, in „More Trivia").

In het midden van 1933 berichtte de Controleur van Gowa (Onderafdeeling van de Afdeeling Makassar) phonografisch, dat in een kleine kampong in zijn ressort de koró-ziekte was uitgebroken en verzocht mij ter plaatse een onderzoek naar den aard en de uitbreiding van deze ziekte in te stellen.

Alvorens mij in gezelschap van een Inlandsch hoofd op weg te begeven had ik gelegenheid door toedoen van Dr. H. DE ROOK kennis te nemen van een korte mededeeling, waarin de voornaamste verschijnselen van deze eigenaardige ziekte worden beschreven[4]).

Bij aankomst in de afgelegen, slechts te voet over sawahdijkjes bereikbare kampong deelde men ons mede, dat er inderdaad tegelijkertijd zes gevallen van koró waren voorgekomen, doch dat alle zieken hersteld waren en 3 hunner reeds weer op de sawah aan het werk waren gegaan. De overige drie bleken in hun woning aanwezig te zijn, zoodat het, dank zij de tegenwoordigheid van het Inlandsche hoofd, mogelijk was deze geheel volgens mijn wensch te ondervragen.

Het betrof in alle gevallen eenvoudige kampongbewoners, die op het land hun werk vonden en in geen enkel opzicht verplicht of gedwongen waren hun houding in en tegenover de westersche samenleving te bepalen. Een belangrijke, overigens voor de hand liggende reden tot het ontstaan eener neurose ontbrak derhalve.

De eerstondervraagde verstond nauwelijks Maleisch; hij was ongeveer 28 jaar oud, had een stevige, athletische lichaamsbouw en vertoonde geen grove somatische afwijkingen. Wat echter terstond opviel waren de vermoeide gelaatstrekken. Hij deed een omstandig verhaal van zijn ziekte, die hij vroeger ook reeds had gehad. De hoofdzaak bestond hierin, dat zijn membrum in volume afnam, hetgeen voor hem een aanleiding was om medebewoners te

[1]) Bij de redactie ontvangen 20 Febr. 1935. [2]) Aan de welwillende bemiddeling van de heeren NOEROEDDIN DAENG MAGASSING, medewerker van den taalkundige Dr. CENSE, en ACHMAD MARZOEKI DAENG MARALA, fiscaal griffier, beide te Makassar, dank ik voor het overgroote deel de gegevens, die aanleiding gaven tot de volgende bijdrage. [3]) Aanvullende opmerkingen bij het artikel van Prof. van WULFFTEN PALTHE: Koró, een eigenaardige angstneurose, Geneesk. Tijdschrift van Ned. Indië, 1934 No. 26. [4]) P. C. J. VAN BRERO. Die Nerven und Geisteskrankheiten in den Tropen, Mense's Handbuch der Tropenkrankheiten, 2e Auflage, 1914.

Fig. 3: 1935 Publication of Dr Slot.
Source: Adopted from Slot JA. Koro in Central Celebes. Geneeskundig Tijdschrift voor Nederlandsch-Indie. 1935;75:811-20.

Casuïstische Mededeelingen.

Over Koró [1]),

DOOR

J. G. A. MULDER, *Off. v. Gez. 1ste kl. Tjalang.*

In aansluiting aan het artikel in het Geneeskundig Tijdschrift van Nederlandsch-Indië van 25 December 1934 Aflevering 26 deel 74, handelende over een eigenaardige angstneurose genaamd „Koró", meen ik, gezien het vrij zeldzaam voorkomende ziektebeeld, een geval van Koró te moeten vermelden dat zich gedurende mijn praktijk te Bálikpapan voordeed. Ook deze patiënt was een welgestelde ontwikkelde Chinees.

Geboren in China, vestigde hij zich later in Singapore en vervolgens in Balikpapan, terwijl hij nog geregeld voor zaken China bezocht.

Patiënt was een neuroticus, zag elke klacht zoowel van zichzelf als van de overige familieleden zwaar in en had bij een van deze gelegenheden wel eens verteld van een Chinees in Singapore die gestorven zou zijn aan het naar binnen schieten van den penis. Niet bekend met het ziektebeeld werd door mij dan ook aan deze mededeeling niet veel waarde gehecht en geen verband gezocht met een latere klacht nl. over het uitblijven van erecties. Patiënt was voor de tweede keer getrouwd met een veel jongere vrouw. Ondanks nauwkeurig onderzoek werd door mij geen oorzaak voor deze klacht gevonden tot ik op een avond met den meesten spoed bij den Chinees aan huis ontboden werd. Patiënt lag te bed; groote angst was van het gelaat af te lezen en de geheele familie, om het bed gezeten, deelde in deze angst. Patiënt vertelde mij zeer opgewonden dat de penis naar binnen wilde schieten en hield dat lichaamsdeel dan ook stevig vast, terwijl ik hierbij weer het geval van Singapore te hooren kreeg. Patiënt had het zelf ook niet gezien, doch van hooren zeggen.

[1]) Bij de redactie ontvangen 8 Maart '35.

Gen. Tijdschr. Afl. 10 4

Fig. 4: 1935 Publication of Dr Mulder.
Source: Adopted from Mulder JGA. Over Koro. GeneesKundig Tijdschrift voor Nederlandsch-Indie. 1935;75:837-8.

(1936a) and Italian Journal of Psychiatric Anthropology (1937) and his work in a Dutch textbook of tropical medicine which was translated into English (1936b) opened the topic of Koro to British, German, and American academia. It is fascinating that local "Koro" from the Indonesian colonial landscape entered into a wider Western medical press and psychiatric academia.

Koro's cultural journey, defacto, started in 1951. It was *Professor PM Yap* of Hong Kong **(Fig. 6)**[1] whose relentless debate offers a psychiatric nosological standpoint of Koro as a culture-bound syndrome. Crozier[50] very rightly pointed out that "PM Yap's most significant intellectual achievement was his development of the concept of the culture-bound syndrome, which synthesized years of research into transcultural psychiatry, and situated this work within this field by drawing on an elaborated nosological schema that challenged some of the ethnocentric assumptions made by previous psychiatrists who had tried to understand mental illnesses that presented in non-western cultures." Chiu[51] acknowledged his contribution and honored him as "... A giant in psychiatry from Hong Kong."

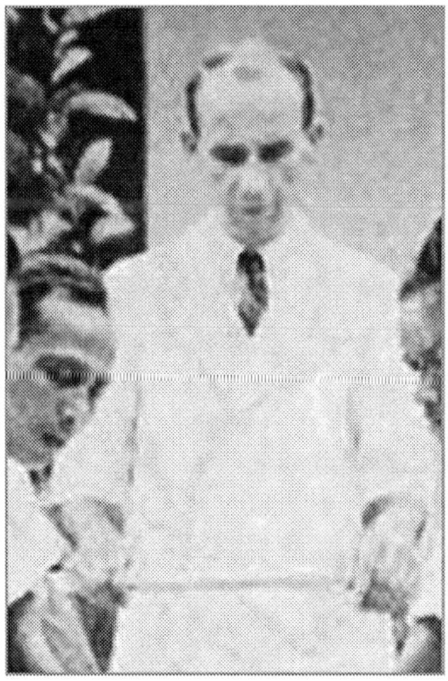

Fig. 5A: Professor PM van Wulfften Palthe in a shock-therapy setting (GTNI, 1937).
Source: Adopted from Indonesian Academy of Science[49] p. 282.

Prof Yap was born in 1921 in Malacca, Malaysia. He was a Fellow of the Royal College of Psychiatrists. He obtained his MB (Cambridge) in 1946, DPM (London) in 1948, MD (Cambridge) in 1957, and FRCP (Edinburgh) in 1963. He became a world authority on the phenomenology of culturally-related psychiatric syndromes such as koro, latah, and other conditions seen primarily in East Asia. He extensively researched these topics.

In 1948, Dr Yap took up residence in Hong Kong and was appointed Medical Officer in charge of Psychiatry. He was a Lecturer at the University of Hong Kong in 1952. He founded the Hong Kong Mental Health Association in 1961. He was the chief architect behind the mental health services in Hong Kong. He was active and instrumental in setting up psychiatry clinics in a general hospital, halfway houses with nongovernmental organizations, and passing the Mental Health Ordinance, 1950 (with the provision of voluntary admission), enacted in 1960. He has a very brilliant international academic career. From 1963, he was a member of the Expert Advisory Panel on Mental Health at the World Health Organization. From 1969 to 1971, he was an Associate Professor in charge of Transcultural Psychiatry at the Clarke Institute of the University of Toronto, Canada. He returned to Hong Kong in 1971 to become the first Professor of Psychiatry on the Island. In November 1971, while attending the Fifth World Congress of Psychiatry in Mexico, he passed away, and "with that, the world lost a brilliant man of science."[52]

Dr Hsien Rin from National Taiwan University Hospital, Taipei, strengthens the Chinese cultural dynamics in Koro. He blended psychoanalytical thoughts, especially the concept of psychosexual development (orality), symbolism, and castration fear, with traditional Chinese cultural construct of Koro. His three papers on Koro (1963, 1965, 1966)[53-55] strengthened the Chinese cultural background of Koro.

KORO.

Een eigenaardige angstneurose [1]),

DOOR

Prof. Dr. P. M. VAN WULFFTEN PALTHE.

In het Gen. Tijdschrift v. Ned. Indië van 1895 komt een artikel voor van den officier van Gezondheid J. C. BLONK getiteld.: „Koro". In anderhalve bladzijde beschrijft hij hierin een ziektebeeld, dat hem van hooren zeggen bekend is en dat bij Boegineezen en Makassaren zou voorkomen. Volgens de lijders aan deze ziekte gevoelen ze op onregelmatige tijdstippen, dat de penis neiging heeft zich in de buikholte terug te trekken. Als dan niet tijdig hulp wordt verschaft zou dit ook werkelijk gebeuren en de lijder dan tevens bezwijken. In hun vrees, dat dit geschieden zal, nemen zij de penis krachtig ter hand en laten zich, zoodra zij dit niet meer kunnen volhouden, hierbij door anderen bijstaan. Uren lang en met groote kracht wordt deze manoeuvre volgehouden. Het geheel gaat met groote angst gepaard en als na uren of dagen de aanval geweken is, voelen de patiënten zich afgemat en uiterst vermoeid.

BLONK meent, dat deze toestand zich op neurasthenischen bodem ontwikkelt en acht een verband met het geslachtsleven twijfelachtig.

Het geval, dat hem bij de beschrijving voor oogen stond, betrof een intelligente djaksa, die hem beloofd had te waarschuwen, wanneer er weer een aanval optrad, hetgeen echter niet geschiedde.

Hoewel dus slechts gegevens uit de tweede hand verstrekt werden, moeten wij toch dankbaar erkennen, dat BLONK de eerste geweest is, die op dit ziektebeeld de aandacht vestigde.

Dr. VORSTMAN geeft in 1897 een beschrijving van hetzelfde ziektebeeld, waargenomen in de Westelijke Afdeeling van Borneo. Hij neemt den naam Koro over, omdat een andere benaming daarvan ter plaatse niet bekend is. Zijn geval betrof een Inlandsche „grootheid", dien hij in bed aantrof omringd door gevolg en met een oud man aan het voeteneinde. VORSTMAN begreep eerst den aard van het lijden niet, maar werd door den hem begeleidenden Luitenant-Chinees ingelicht. Deze vertelde hem n.l., dat reeds gedurende acht dagen de penis van den patiënt neiging had vertoond naar binnen te schieten. De oude man aan het voeteneinde had hem vastgehouden en zou het leven van zijn meester gered hebben. Bij nadere informatie bij Inlandsche bestuursambtenaren kon hij omtrent dit ziektebeeld niets naders te weten komen. Slechts de toenmalige controleur van Nangoh - Pino kwam met het verhaal, dat hij in een kampong het lijk van een Inlander gezien had, die aan die ziekte

[1]) Bij de redactie ontvangen 24 September 1934.

Gen. Tijdschr. Afl. 26 2

Fig. 5B: 1934 Publication of Dr Palthe.
Source: Palthe, PM van W. Koro-Een Eigenaardige Angstneurose. Geneeskundig Tijdschrift voor Nederlandsch-Indie. 1934;74:1713-20.

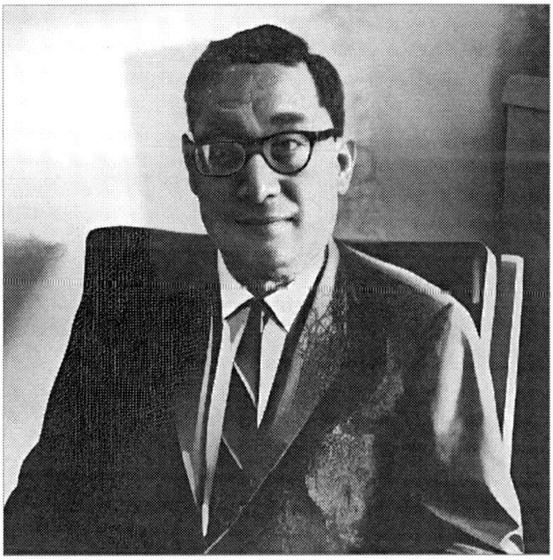

Fig. 6: Professor PM Yap (1921–1971).

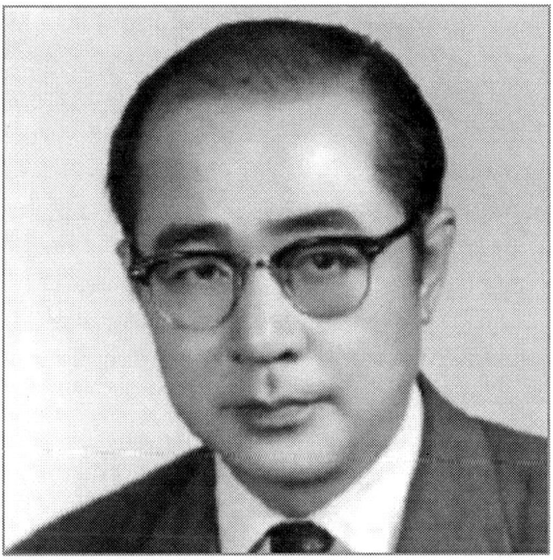

Fig. 7: Dr Gwee Ah Leng (1920–2006).

Dr Gwee Ah Leng, LMS Singapore (1949) MRCP (1954) MD (1964) FRCP (1967), was a very distinguished and respected physician in Singapore **(Fig. 7)**. He was the founding member of the Singapore Medical Journal. He was the Medical Unit head at Singapore General Hospital, from where he retired in 1971. In recognition of his continued interest and active involvement in medical education and public health service, the Government of Singapore awarded him the meritorious service medal in 1967. He was President of the Singapore Medical Association from 1972 to 1973. He was the founder of the

Academy of Medicine Singapore in 1957 and was elected master from 1961 to 1964. His contribution to the development of medical education in Singapore is immense.[56]

Dr Gwee introduced Koro solely as a "Chinese disease." He tried to explain Koro's psychodynamics in terms of Chinese cultures, including tracing the castration theme from Imperial Chinese history. His three publications on the Koro and Koro epidemic of Singapore (1963, 1968, 1970)[57-59] act as a bible to any Koro researchers in the field. Those papers are precious for their documentation of Chinese history, cultural explanation of Koro, and his clinical assessment for the disease. Koro researchers have extensively cited them since the 1970s. The second author communicated with him in the early part of 1984,[60] and he sent the reprints of all his articles and, in a very teacher-like way, advised to publish the research data as early as possible. We respect this great man whom all Koro researchers will be indebted to forever. *Dr PM Nugi,*[61] one of his colleagues, also contributed a detailed study of the Singapore Koro epidemic.

Dr Wen-Shing Tseng, a world-renowned Cultural Psychiatrist, provided two essential research papers on the Guandong Koro epidemic in South China. He was born in Taiwan in 1935, did his medical graduation from the National Taiwan University in 1961, and had additional training in psychiatry at the Massachusetts Mental Health Center of Harvard Medical School (1965–68). He taught psychiatry in Taipei from 1965–71 and then joined for 2 years as a research associate at the East-West Center in Honolulu in 1971. In 1972, he joined the University of the Hawaii School of Medicine's psychiatry faculty and became a professor in 2009. For many years, he was a principal ambassador for cultural psychiatry worldwide. He visited China in 1981 as a WHO fellow and later became a guest professor at the Institute of Mental Health at Peking University. He was chair of the Transcultural Psychiatry section of the World Psychiatric Association. He later was the founding President of the World Association of Cultural Psychiatry (WACP), when he organized several congresses worldwide, including the inaugural meeting of WACP in Beijing (2006) **(Fig. 8)**. His contribution to the academic discourse regarding Culture and Mental health is astounding. His life and work are always inspiring to any Koro researchers and cultural psychiatrist. He has authored or edited numerous books related to cultural psychiatry, such as *Handbook of Cultural Psychiatry, Clinician's Guide to Cultural Psychiatry, Cultural Competence in Clinical Psychiatry, Cultural Competency in Forensic Mental Health,* etc. His conceptual contribution to cultural psychiatry is original and opens up a healthy discourse of cultural psychiatry's clinical aspect in the multicultural world. His book "Handbook of Cultural Psychiatry" (2001)[62] is "regarded by international colleagues as the landmark book in the field of cultural psychiatry."[63]

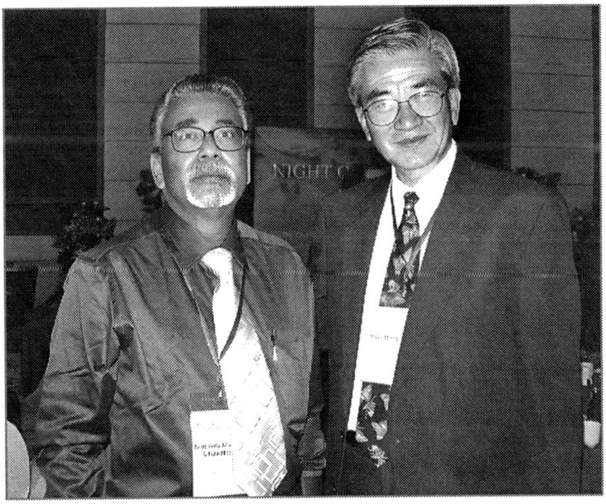

Fig. 8: First author with Professor W-S Tseng in Beijing WACP Conference, 2006.

The first author was privileged to get his support and encouragement in his research. In the 2008 WACP conference in Moscow, he expressed his desire to visit India's Sundarban region, where the first author worked on the World Bank's "self-harm prevention" research. The first author dedicated his research "Culture and stigma: Ethnographic case studies of tiger widows of Sundarban Delta, India"[64] to his sacred memory. His humanitarian advice to all cultural psychiatrists runs as follows: "It is time to move from merely studying the cultural aspects of psychopathology (fascinated by peculiar or exotic syndromes) to the provision of culturally competent care for all people of diverse cultures, in order to fulfill the contemporary mission of cultural psychiatry" (p. 571).[65]

Dr Wolfgang Jilek (Psychiatry, UBC)[66] (25.11.30-15.1.21), Clinical Professor Emeritus, Department of Psychiatry, University of British Colombia, Canada, was a great academic and social anthropologist. His six exploratory research studies (1982, 1977, 1985, 1986)[67-71] on Koro are precious to every Koro researcher. He and his wife Dr Louise Jilek-Aall, Clinical Professor Emerita, conducted several ethnopsychiatric field studies in East Africa, Haiti, South America, Thailand, Papua New Guinea, and Western Canada.

Four important publications related to Koro need to be mentioned here. The first one was by Edward (1984) who after an extensive research on Koro proposed a new term "Genital Retraction Syndrome" (GRS).[72] The second one was the book exclusively devoted to studying culture-bound syndromes with anthropological and social analysis by *Ronald C Simons* and *Charles C Hughes* (Eds).[73] Two other papers were on Koro by *Professor RH Prince* (Canada).[74,75] All these publications are examples of scholarly masterwork in cultural psychiatry and are of high value to all students of transcultural psychiatry.

In the Indian context, *Professor Dipali Dutta,*[76] Head, Department of Psychiatry, Guwahati Medical College, and later Director of Medical Education, Government of Assam, and *Dr PS Sachdev*[77] reported a detailed research study of the 1982 Koro epidemic of Assam. *Professor Ajita Chakraborty*[78-80] **(Fig. 9)** and *Professor DN Nandi*[81,82] **(Fig. 10)** from West Bengal reported a series of research studies on the 1982 Koro epidemic of West Bengal state, India. Professor Nandi explained the Koro phenomena in terms of psychoanalytical construct, viz., castration anxiety. Professor Chakraborty suggested a hypothesis linking Koro with internal displacement as well as loss of agricultural land and threats to cultural identity among the indigenous farming population of North Bengal.[83] The first author was

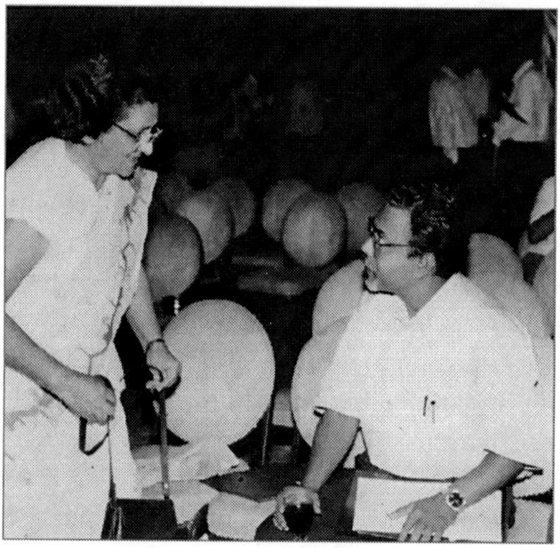

Fig. 9: The first author with Professor Ajita Charaborty in an International Workshop on 'Mental Health Service in Primary Care Level', Feb., 2005 at Institute of Psychiatry.

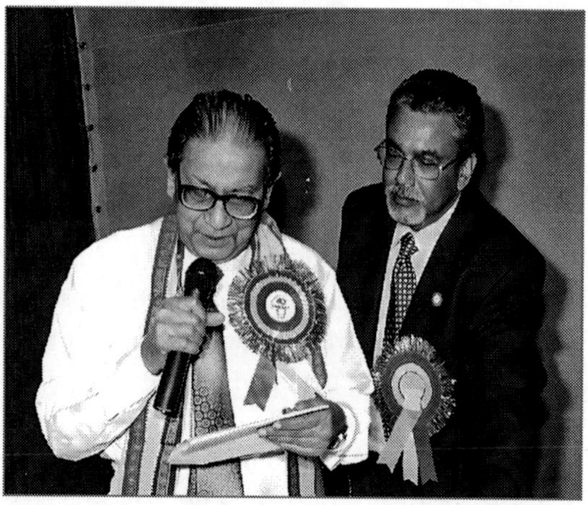

Fig. 10: First author with Professor DN Nandi at a National Conference on Suicide Prevention, Kolkata, 2005.

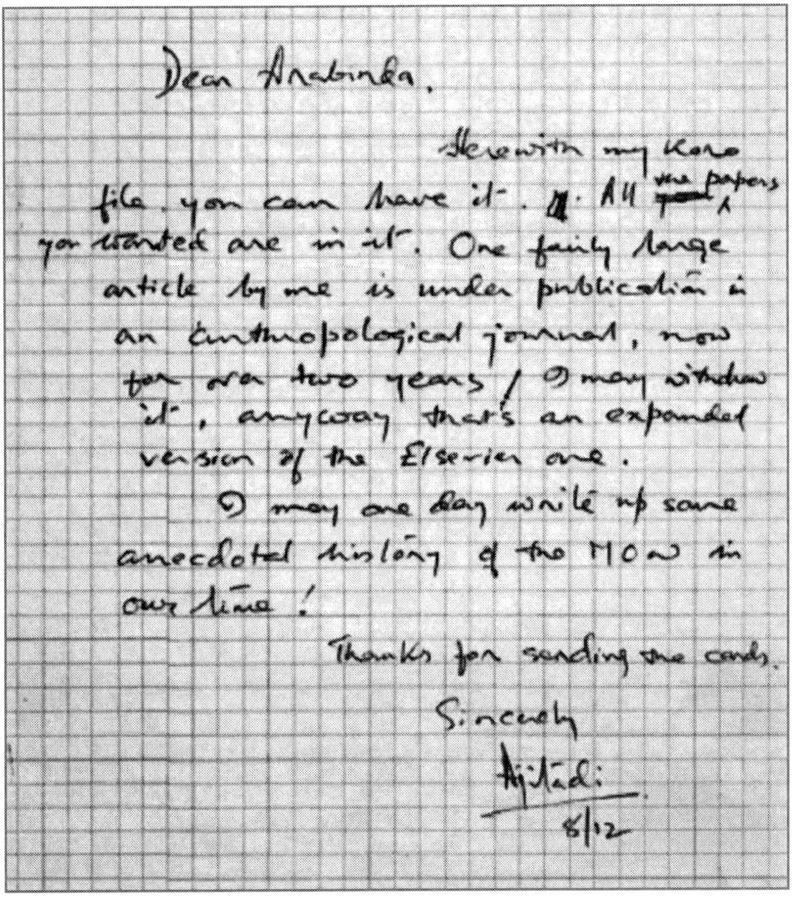

Dear Arabinda,

Herewith my Koro file, you can have it. All the papers you wanted are in it. One fairly large article by me is under publication in an anthropological journal, now for over two years / I may withdraw it, anyway that's an expanded version of the Elsevier one.

I may one day write up some anecdotal history of the MOW in our time!

Thanks for sending the cards.

Sincerely

Ajita

8/12

Fig. 11: Letter of Professor Ajita Chakraborty in December 1987.

privileged to receive Professor Chakraborty's support and encouragement in his Koro research. In fact she gave her personal Koro file to the first author for use **(Fig. 11)**.

Other authors such as Dr Amitav Dan,[84] Dr Sayanti Ghosh,[85] Chakraborty and Sanyal[86] [(2011 from West Bengal, Debbarma et al. (Tripura)],[87] and Dr K Promodu[88] from Kerala, Banerjee et al.,[89] from Bengaluru, reported valuable research studies on Koro epidemic from their respective states. Some of their studies are also included in this book. The first author did a series of studies on the 1982 North Bengal Koro epidemic and recently published a book on Koro, the first of its kind in the world of Koro literature.[90] All these Indian studies made a valuable contribution to the deep understanding of Koro psychopathology.

REFERENCES

1. Yap PM. Mental disorders peculiar to certain culture: a survey of comparative psychiatry. J Mental Sc. 1951;97:313-27.

2. Yap PM. The culture-bound reactive syndrome: In: Caudill W, Lin TY (Eds). Mental Health Research in Asia and the Pacific. Honolulu: East-West Centre Press; 1969. pp. 33-53.
3. Bartelsman M, Eckhardt PP. Mental illness in the former Dutch Indies-four psychiatric syndromes: Amok, latah, koro and neurasthenia. Ned Tijdschr Geneeskd. 2007;151(51):2845-51.
4. Bartholomew RE. Disease, disorder or deception? Latah as habit in a Malay extended family. J Nerv Ment Dise. 1994;182:331-8.
5. Bartholomew RE. The medicalization of exotic deviance: A sociological perspective on epidemic koro. Transcul Psychiat. 1998;35(1):5-38.
6. Marsella AJ. Culture-bound syndromes. In: Corsini R, Auerbach A (Eds). Concise encyclopedia of psychology, 2nd edition. New York: Wiley; 1996. pp. 223-4.
7. Prince RH, Tcheng-Laroche F. Culture-bound Syndromes and International Disease Classification. Cul Med Psychiat. 1987;11:3-19.
8. Kirmayer LJ. The place of culture in psychiatric nosology: Taijin Kyofusho and DSM-IIIR. J Nerv Ment Dis. 1991;179:19-28.
9. Levine RE, Gaw AC. Culture-bound syndromes. Psychiatric Clin North Amer. 1995;18(3):523-36.
10. Littlewood R. DSM-IV and culture: is the classification internationally valid? Psychiatric Bull. 1992;16:257-61.
11. Teodoro T, Afonso P. Culture-bound syndromes and cultural concepts of distress in psychiatry. Revista Portugugesa de Psiquiatria. 2020;6(3):118-30.
12. American Psychiatry Association Resource Document. (2013). Manual. Resource Document on Cultural Psychiatry as a Specific Field of Study Relevant to the Assessment and Care of All Patients. [online] Available from https://www.psychiatry.org/psychiatrists/search-directories-databases/library-and-archive/resource-documents. [Last accessed April, 2023].
13. Tseng W-T, Streltzer J (Eds). Introduction: culture and psychiatry, in Cultural Competence in Clinical Psychiatry. Washington, DC: American Psychiatric Publishing; 2004. pp. 1-20.
14. Pal Y, Balhara S. Culture-bound syndrome: Has it found its right niche? Ind J Psychological Med. 2011;33(2):210-5.
15. American Psychiatric Association. Diagnostic Criteria From DSM-IV. American Psychiatric Press Inc.; Washington, DC 1994.
16. Guarnaccia PJ, Rogler LH. Research on culture-bound syndromes: New directions. Am J Psychiat. 1999;156:1322-7.
17. Diagnostic and Statistical Manual of Mental Disorder, 5th edition. Arlington, USA: American Psychiatric Association; 2013.
18. Bonnie NK, Weaver LJ. Culture-bound syndromes, idioms of distress, and cultural concepts of distress: New directions for an old concept in psychological anthropology. Transcul Psychiat. 2019;56(4):589-98.
19. ICD-10 Classification of Mental and Behavioural Disorders. Clinical description and diagnostic guidelines. World Health Organization, Geneva: Delhi: Oxford University Press; 1992.
20. APA Dictionary of Psychology. [online] Available from https://dictionary.apa.org/culture-bound-syndrome. [Last accessed April, 2023].
21. Martin MLS. Running Amok: A modern perspective on a culture-bound syndrome. Prim Care Companion J Clin Psychiatry. 1999;1(3):66-70.

22. Burton-Bradley BG. The amok syndrome in Papua and New Guinea. Medical J Aust. 1968;1(7):252-6.
23. Kon Y. Amok. Brit J Psychiat. 1994;165(5):685-9.
24. Tseng WS. Culture-related specific psychiatric syndromes. In: Gelder MJ, Andreasen NC, Lopez-Ibor Jr JJ, Geddes JR (Eds). New Oxford Textbook of Psychiatry. New York: Oxford University Press; 2009. pp. 979-85.
25. Imai H, Ogawa Y, Okumiya K, Matsubayashi K. Amok: a mirror of time and people. A historical review of literature. Hist Psychiat. 2019;30:38-57.
26. Carr JE. Ethno-behaviorism and the culture-bound syndromes: The case of *amok*. Cult Med Psychiat. 1978;2:269-93.
27. Tan EK, Carr JE. Psychiatric sequelae of amok. Cul Med Psychiat. 1977;1(1):59-67.
28. Bakker MJ, Tijssen MAJ. Latah. In: Kompoliti K, Metman LV (Eds). Encyclopedia of movement disorders. USA: Elsevier; 2010. pp. 120-2.
29. Winzeler R. Latah in South-East Asia: The history and ethnography of a culture-bound syndrome. Cambridge University Press; 1995.
30. Murphy HBM. History and the Evolution of Syndromes: The Striking Case of Latah and Amok. In: Hammer M, Salzinger K, Sutton S (Eds). Psychopathology: Contributions from the Social, Behavioral, and Biological Sciences. New York: Wiley; 1972.
31. Kenny MG. Latah: the symbolism of a putative mental disorder. Cult Med Psychiat. 1978;2(3):209-31.
32. Simons RC. The resolution of the Latah paradox. J Nerv Ment Dis.1980;168(4): 195-206.
33. Tanner CM, Chamberland J. Latah in Jakarta, Indonesia. Mov Disord. 2001;16(3):526-9.
34. Bakker MJ, Dijk, JG, Pramono, A, Sutarni, S, Tijssen, MAJ. Latah: an Indonesian startle syndrome. Mov Disorder. 2013;28(3):370-9.
35. Blonk JC. Koro. Geneeskunding Tijaschrift voor Nederlandsch-Indie. 1895;35:5623.
36. Ivanov AA. Vetjagivanie Polov Chlena (Retraction of Sex Organ). Vrach. 1885;423.
37. Raven TF. Retraction of the penis. Lancet. 1886; August 7, 250.
38. Brero van PCJ. Naar Aanleiding van het Opstel Over 'Koro' van den Heer J. C. Blonk-in de Voring Aflevering van dit Tijdschrift. Geneeskunding Tijdschrrift voor Nederlandsch-Indie. 1896;36:48-54.
39. Brero van PCJ. Koro, eine Eiggentuemliche Zwangsv-Orstellung. Allegemeine Zeitschrift fur Psychiatric und Psychischgerichtliche Medicin. 1897;53:569-73.
40. Vorstman AH. 'Koro' in de Westerafdeeling van Borneo. Geneeskundig Tijdschrift voor Nederlandsch-Indie. 1897;37:499-505.
41. Slot JA. Koro in Central Celebes. Geneeskundig Tijdschrift voor Nederlandsch-Indie. 1935;75:811-20.
42. Mulder JGA. Over Koro. GeneesKundig Tijdschrift voor Nederlandsch-Indie. 1935;75:837-8.
43. Palthe van PMW. Koro-Een Eigenaardige Angstneurose. Geneeskundig Tijdschrift voor Nederlandsch-Indie. 1934;74:1713-20.
44. Palthe van PMW. Koro-Eine Merkwurdige Angsthysterie. Internationale Zeitschrift fur Psychoanalyse. 1935a;21:249-57.
45. Palthe van PMW. Anauvulling op Het Artikel "Koro", een Eigenaardige Angstneurose. Geneeskundig Tijdschrift voor Nederlandsch-Indie. 1935b;75:836-7.

46. Palthe van PMW. "Koro". Une Maladie Imaginaire et Une Phobie Orientale. La Presse Medicale. 1936a;44(67):1331-2.
47. Palthe van PMW. Psychiatry and Neurology in the Tropics. In: de Langen CD, Lichtenstein A (Eds). A Clinical Textbook of Tropical Medicine. Batavia: G. Kolff and Company; 1936b. pp. 525-47.
48. Palthe van PMW. It Significanto Forense del 'Koro'. Archivio Di Anthropological Criminale. Psychiatry Medicina Legale. 1937;57:173-82.
49. Bergen van L, Hesselink L, Verhave JP (Eds). The medical journals of the Dutch Indies. A platform for medical research. Jakarta: Indonesian Academy of Sciences; 2017.
50. Crozier I. Making up koro: Multiplicity, psychiatry, culture, and penis-shrinking anxieties. J Hist of Med Allied Sc. 2012;67(1):36-70.
51. Chiu HFK. Professor Pow-Meng Yap: A giant in Psychiatry from Hong Kong. Asia-Pacific Psychiat. 2012;4:84-6.
52. Margetts EL. Pow Meng Yap (1921-1971). Can Psychiatric Asso J. 1972;17(3):253-4.
53. Rin H. Koro: A consideration on Chinese concepts of illness and case illustrations. Transcul Psychiatric Res Rev. 1963;15:23-30.
54. Rin H. A study of the aetiology of Koro in respect to the Chinese concept of illness. Int J Social Psychiat. 1965;11:7-13.
55. Rin H. Two forms of vital deficiency syndrome among Chinese male mental patients. Transcul Psychiatric Res Rev. 1966;3:19-21.
56. Loh RCK. Dr. Gwee Ah Leng, July 17, 1920–March 31, 2006. A tribute to our first editor. Singapore Med J. 2006;47(5):447-9.
57. Gwee AL. Koro—A Cultural Disease. Singapore Med J. 1963;4:119-22.
58. Gwee AL. Koro—Its origin and nature as a disease entity. Singapore Med J. 1968;9:3-6.
59. Koro Study Team (Chairman: AL Gwee). The Koro epidemic in Singapore. Singapore Med J. 1969;10:234-42.
60. Gwee AL. Personal Communication to second author, 1984.
61. Ngui PW. The Koro epidemic in Singapore. Aust NZ J Psychiat. 1969;3:263-6.
62. Tseng WS. Handbook of Cultural Psychiatry. San Diego, CA: Academic Press; 2001.
63. World Psychiatric Association-Transcultural Psychiatry Section. (2013). In memoriam Wen-Shing Tseng. [online] Available from https://www.wpa-tps.org/about-wpa-tps/in-memoriam/wen-shing-tseng/. [Last accessed April, 2023].
64. Chowdhury AN, Mondal R, Biswas MK, Brahma A. Culture and stigma: Ethnographic case studies of tiger-widows of Sundarban Delta, India. World Cull Psychiat Res Rev. 2014:9(3):99-22.
65. Tseng WS. From peculiar psychiatric disorders through culture-bound syndromes to culture-related specific syndromes. Transcul Psychiat. 2006;43(4):554-76.
66. In Memoriam: Dr. Wolfgang Jilek, Clinical Professor Emeritus. [online] Available from https://psychiatry.ubc.ca/2021/02/19/in-memoriam-dr-wolfgang-jilek-clinical-professor-emeritus/.
67. Jilek W, Jilek-Aall L. A Koro epidemic in Thailand. Transcul Psychiatric Res Rev. 1977a;14:57-9.
68. Jilek W, Jilek-Aall L. Mass Hysteria with Koro Symptom in Thailand. Schweizer Archieve Neurologic Neurochirurgie und Psychiatrie. 1977b;120: 257-9.

69. Jilek WG. Culture: "Pathoplastic" or "Pathogenic"? A key question of comparative psychiatry. Curare. 1982;5:57-68.
70. Jilek W, Jilek-Aall L. The metamorphosis of "Culture-bound" syndromes. Soc Sc Med. 1985;21:205-20.
71. Jilek WG. Epidemic of "Genital Shrinking" (Koro): Historical review and report of a recent outbreak in South China. Curare. 1986;9:269-82.
72. Edwards JW. Indigenous Koro: A genital retraction syndrome of insular South East Asia: A critical review. Cul Med Psychiat; 1984;8:1-24.
73. Simons RC, Hughes CC (Eds). The Culture-bound Syndromes: Folk Illnesses of Psychiatric and Anthropological Interests. Dordrecht, Netherlands: Dordrecht Reidel Publishing Company; 1985.
74. Prince RH. Koro and the fox sprit on Hainan Island (China). Transcul Psychiatric Res Rev. 1992a;29:119-32.
75. Prince RH. A symposium on the vulnerable male: Cultural variations on the castration theme. Transcul Psychiatric Res Rev. 1982b;29:87-90.
76. Dutta D, Phookun HR, Das PD. The Koro epidemic in Lower Assam. Ind J Psychiat. 1982;24:370-4.
77. Sachdev PS, Shukla A. Epidemic Koro syndrome in India. Lancet. 1982:1161.
78. Chakrabarty A, Das S, Mukherjee A. Koro makes an epidemic appearance in India. Transcul Newsletter III. 1982;3-4 December.
79. Chakraborty A. An epidemic of Koro in West Bengal (India). Ind J Psychiat. 1983;25:138-9.
80. Chakrabarty A, Bag DC. Genesis of the Koro epidemic in West Bengal and Assam: Implication of Turtle Cults. Human Sc. 1989;38:142-9.
81. Nandi DN, Banerjee G, Saha H, Boral GC. Epidemic Koro in West Bengal, India. Intl J Soc Psychiat. 1983;29(4):265-8.
82. Nandi DN, Banerjee G, Bera S, Nandi S. Mode of spread of epidemic Koro in a village of West Bengal. Ind J Psychiat. 1984;26331-4.
83. Bhattacharya D, Bhattacharya R. Professor Ajita Chakraborty MB, DPM, FRCP (Ed.) FRCPsych. Formerly Director of Postgraduate Medical and Research Institute, Professor and Head of the Department of Neurology and Psychiatry, Calcutta, India. Brit J Psych Bull. 2016;40(2):109.
84. Dan A, Mondal T, Chakraborty K, Chaudhuri A, Biswas A. Clinical profile and outcome of Koro: A follow up study from a Koro epidemic in West Bengal, India. Ind J Psychiat. 2016;58(Suppl 1):571.
85. Ghosh S, Nath S, Brahma A, Chowdhury AN. Fifth Koro epidemic in India: A review report. World Cul Psychiat Res Rev. 2013;8(1):8-20.
86. Chakraborty S, Sanyal D. An outbreak of Koro among 19 workers in a jute mill in South Bengal. Industrial Psychiat J. 2011;20(1):58-60.
87. Debbarma S, Das SK, Kumar A, Debbarma D, Das A, Reang T. Koro epidemic: A descriptive study. J Evolution of Medical & Dental Sc. 2016;5(76):5634-8.
88. Promodu K, Nair KR, Pushparajan S. Koro syndrome: Mass epidemic in Kerala, India. Ind J Clin Psychol. 2012;39:152-6.
89. Banerjee D, Sharma S, Antony S. Koro and migration: Observational study of an outbreak of Koro in a migrant population working in South India. J Psychosexual Health, 2020;2(2):174-8.
90. Chowdhury AN. Koro: Clinical and historical developments of the culturally defined Genital Retraction Disorder. Palgrave Macmillan, Switzerland: Springer Nature; 2021.

Index

Page numbers followed by *f* refer to figure, *fc* refer to flowchart, and *t* refer to table.

A

B

C

Q

R

S

T

U

V

W